Health Informatics: an overview

Edited by

Evelyn J S Hovenga RN PhD AFCHSE
Senior Lecturer, Section Head, Health Informatics and Management,
Faculty of Health Sciences, Central Queensland University, Rockhampton

Michael R Kidd MBBS MD DipRACOG DCCH FRACGP
Professor, Department of General Practice, University of Sydney

Branko Cesnik MBBS MD
Associate Professor and Director of Medical Informatics,
Faculty of Medicine, Monash University

Foreword by

Ian Graham MBBS MHP FRCMA AFCHSE
Director, Centre for Health Informatics and Deputy Director
of Medical Services, Austin and Repatriation Medical Centre Chair, HISA

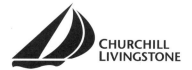

CHURCHILL
LIVINGSTONE

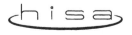

Health Informatics
Society Australia Inc.

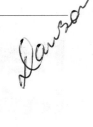

CHURCHILL LIVINGSTONE
An imprint of Pearson Professional

Pearson Professional (Australia) Pty Ltd
Kings Gardens
95 Coventry Street
South Melbourne 3205 Australia

Copyright © Pearson Professional (Australia) Pty Ltd 1996
First published 1996

National Library of Australia Cataloguing-in-Publication Data

Health informatics: an overview.

ISBN 0443 05430 4.

1. Medical informatics. 2. Medical informatics - Australia.
I. Hovenga, E. J. S. (Evelyn J. S.) 1945-. II. Kidd, Michael 1959-.
III. Cesnik, Branko, 1956-.

025.0661

The
publisher's
policy is to use
paper manufactured
from sustainable forests

Cover designed by Jan Schmoeger, Designpoint
Produced by Churchill Livingstone in Melbourne
Printed in Singapore

iv

Foreword

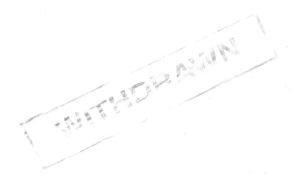

Data, information and knowledge are the essence of modern health care. Every hour of every day in the homes of patients or clients, in consulting rooms, clinics, practices, hospitals and health services, information is collected, processed, stored, retrieved and exchanged. Health informatics concerns itself with all these activities and with the optimal use of health related information in support of clinical decision making, problem solving and the assurance of excellence in healthcare.

Health informatics faces special challenges in a health care system that must span a country the size and diversity of Australia. Modern information and communication technologies offer the opportunity to link healthcare providers with their patients and clients, with colleagues, researchers and educators, regionally, nationally and even internationally. Their success will depend on the coordination, promotion and development of the field of health informatics. To this end, the Health Informatics Society of Australia (HISA) was formed in 1993.

HISA brings together a range of health professionals, information specialists, information technology vendors, academic and research staff, all with a common interest in the field of health informatics. It also provides the opportunity to assemble a body of knowledge about health informatics and its application in Australia. *Health Informatics: an overview* provides a comprehensive review of that body of knowledge.

Health Informatics: an overview surveys health informatics from a historical and global perspective and relates it to the practice of health care in Australia. It reviews the basic concepts of informatics and the application of the technologies and methodologies of the information sciences in health care. The use of health informatics and its implications for clinical practice, health care management, research and education are explored by health informatics practitioners from throughout Australia.

I commend *Health Informatics: an overview* to anyone with a personal, professional or academic interest in the field of health informatics. It provides a foundation of knowledge upon which the future of health informatics will be built, enhancing the quality, accessibility and cost effectiveness of health care in Australia and beyond.

Ian Graham

Preface

This text was compiled primarily for health professionals who now require knowledge about how computing, communications technologies and information science may be used to enhance their practice. It aims to provide an overview of the health informatics discipline. The contents reflect what we consider are the basics for continuing education purposes and for inclusion into any curriculum which prepares the student for practice in any of the health professional disciplines. It is suitable for use as a basic text in both undergraduate and post graduate curricula. Each chapter can be expanded upon as required.

This text is not all inclusive or exhaustive; most of the chapters could be expanded individually into a book on its own. The field of health informatics is extensive. For example at the Eighth World Congress on Medical Informatics held in Vancouver in 1995, over 400 papers were presented and classified into any one of 48 different topics. They covered a range of applications from a vast array of health professionals working in diverse health care disciplines. Areas ranged from clinical, management, administrative, to policy and research, and they were based in both community and institutional settings.

The text has deliberately avoided a focus on any one of the health professions. This is because of the trend towards integrated systems and the use of a 'professional' or 'clinician workstation' to reflect the use of patient focused systems in place of discipline specific or departmental systems. This is in line with current Australian health policy which promotes patient focused organisational structures.

The book is divided into five sections: an overview of the discipline, basic informatics concepts, the application of health informatics in clinical practice, management, and research. We first present the history of computing in health and outline some of the basic principles underlying this emerging health discipline, including the need to balance the technology with our underlying commitment to patient care. We then discuss the basic concepts which need to be grasped about computing and explain how these apply to the health professions. The following three sections demonstrate how these new technologies can assist in your daily work, in clinical practice, management, education and research.

Contributors

Rita Axford RN PhD FRCNA
Professor, Director Centre for Graduate Studies in Clinical Nursing
Subfaculty of Nursing, Monash University, Melbourne

Erica Bostock RN BA ML
Lecturer in Nursing, Faculty of Health Sciences
Australian Catholic University, Mackillop Campus, Sydney

J Michael Brittain BA MA(Hons) PhD
Professor of Information Management
School of Communication and Information Studies
University of South Australia, Adelaide

Branko Celler PhD
Associate Professor, Biomedical Systems Laboratory
School of Electrical Engineering
University of New South Wales, Sydney

Branko Cesnik MBBS MD
Associate Professor and Director of Medical Informatics
Faculty of Medicine
Monash University, Melbourne

Moya Conrick RN DipAppSci (NEd) BNurs MC LinEd
Lecturer, School of Nursing, Griffith University, Nathan Campus
 Queensland

Jeff Cooke MSc Mathematics CSOption MIEEE
Senior Lecturer in Information Systems, Faculty of Business
Central Queensland University, Rockhampton

Gary F Egan PhD
Centre for Positron Emission Tomography
Austin Hospital, Melbourne

Peter Feeney RN
Client Support Consultant, Polyoptimum Inc., Sydney

Joanne Foster RN DipAppSc BN
Lecturer, Queensland University of Technology, Kelvin Grove Campus, Brisbane

Shirley Gregor BSc GrDipComp MAppSc
Senior Lecturer in Information Systems, Faculty of Business
Central Queensland University, Rockhampton

Gary Grunwald PhD
Lecturer, Department of Statistics, University of Melbourne, Melbourne

Lynn M Hall MBBS MFamMed
General Practitioner, Melbourne

Terry J Hannan FRACP
Consultant Physician, Health Informatics Consultant, Sydney

Jennifer L Hardy RN Bsc MHPEd
Lecturer in Nursing, Faculty of Health Sciences, Australian Catholic University
Mackillop Campus, Sydney

Mark Harris MBBS DRACOG FRACGP MD
Professor of General Practice, University of New South Wales, Sydney

Evelyn J S Hovenga RN PhD AFCHSE
Senior Lecturer, Section Head, Health Informatics and Management
Faculty of Health Sciences, Central Queensland University, Rockhampton

Rob Hyndman PhD
Lecturer, Department of Statistics, University of Melbourne, Melbourne

Graham Ivers BBus GradDipMgt MInfSys FCPA
Senior Lecturer in Information Systems, Faculty of Business
Central Queensland University, Rockhampton Qld

Rohan Jayasuriya MBBS MPH MD(Comm Med)
Senior Lecturer, Department of Public Health and Nutrition
University of Wollongong, Wollongong

Michael Richard Kidd MBBS MD Dip RACOG DCCH FRACGP
Professor, Department of General Practice, University of Sydney

Teng Liaw MBBS DipObst GrDipPHC FRACGP
Senior Lecturer, Department of Public Health and Community Medicine
University of Melbourne, Melbourne

Trevor Lord MBBS FRACGP
General Practitioner, Rockingham, WA

Jo Luck BSc GradDipCmtg, GradDipAppComp MACS PCP MInftech(QUT)
Lecturer in Information Systems, Faculty of Business
Central Queensland University, Rockhampton

Geraldine Mackenzie LLM
Solicitor, Senior Lecturer, Faculty of Law, Queensland University of Technology
Brisbane

Bill McGuiness RN DipT(Nursing) BEd(Nursing) MNS
Lecturer in Nursing, Centre for Nursing Therapies and Practice, School of
Nursing, Faculty of Health Sciences, La Trobe University, Melbourne

Rory R McNeill BBSc BCol MBA McG
Lecturer in Information Systems, Faculty of Business
Central Queensland University, Rockhampton

Wendy McPhee
Deputy Director of Medical Informatics, Faculty of Community Medicine
Monash University, Melbourne

Debra O'Connor BA BS(Melb)
Committee Member Victorian Consumer Health Voice (Previously Association of
District Health Councils) and General Committee of Consumer Health Forum
(National peak body)

Malcolm Pradhan MBBS PhD Candidate
Section on Medical Informatics, Stanford University California
1991–92 Project Manager, 1992 Consultant, Medical Computing
Faculty of Medicine, University of Adelaide, Adelaide

David Ranson BMedSci BM BS LLB MRCPath FRCPA DMJ(Path)
Assistant Director, Victorian Institute for Forensic Pathology, and Honorary
Clinical Associate Professor, Department of Forensic Medicine,
Monash University, Melbourne

Gurpal K Sandhu RN RM BA BScN MScN GDipDrHlthSc
Senior Lecturer, Post Graduate Studies Co-ordinator, School of Health Sciences
Monash University, Gippsland Campus, Churchill, Victoria

Christopher Silagy MBBS PhD FRACGP FAFPHM
Professor and Head, Department of General Practice, School of Medicine
Flinders University, Adelaide

Gray Southon Msc PhD MComm
Consultant in Health Management Research and Analysis, Sydney

Don C Walker MBBS
Medical Practitioner, Research Associate
Faculty of Medicine, University of Adelaide, Adelaide

Gregory K Whymark Bsc Msc PhD MACS PCP MASOR MACM MTIMS
Associate Professor and Section Head Information Systems
Faculty of Business, Central Queensland University, Rockhampton

Contents

1

Introduction

1

Introduction

Health informatics in Australia

EVELYN J S HOVENGA, MICHAEL R KIDD

Health Informatics is defined as 'an evolving scientific discipline that deals with the collection, storage, retrieval, communication and optimal use of health related data, information and knowledge.'The discipline utilises the methods and technologies of the information sciences for the purposes of problem solving, decision making and assuring highest quality health care in all basic and applied areas of the biomedical sciences' (Graham 1994).

Now the new 'professional' workstations support both independent discipline specific tasks and interdependent interactions with the system by multiple disciplines. Clinical data from multiple sources are integrated and displayed to support multiple types of clinical decision making. This multiplicity of functions and disciplines also has implications for the language or terminology used and may well influence changes in how individuals practice their profession.

The application of cutting edge technologies pertaining to the computer, communication and information sciences has much to offer the health sciences. We are of the view that appropriate use of these technologies will result in improved health, lower costs and improved service delivery methods. To achieve this health professionals should be aware of the possibilities today and in the future and participate in this discipline's further development.

About 25 years ago Martin and Norman (1970) predicted that in medicine the computer promised revolutionary changes. Today the same may be said about communications technology. There is a convergence between com–munications, computing and television or broadcasting technologies enabling the merging of all types of data into integrated multimedia information, and providing rapid interactions between persons from any location. The speed by which these changes will impact upon health service delivery is determined by and dependent upon how quickly the health professions accept the role of these new technologies. It is they who need to identify the potential use of these new technologies within the health care industry. The international network of health informaticians is growing rapidly. There is evidence of an approaching critical number such that the process of change is now self sustaining. This network could be compared with what Marilyn Ferguson describes as an Aquarian conspiracy where conspirators (read health informaticians) collude to change social institutions, modes of problem solving and distribution of power (Ferguson 1980). Conspirators are characterised by their habit of rethinking everything, examining old assumptions, by looking differently at their work, relationships, health, political power, experts, goals and values. They are leading the way towards a paradigm shift. Ferguson (1980) notes that:

> New paradigms are nearly always received with coolness, even mockery and hostility. Their discoveries are attacked for their heresy. (For historic examples, consider Copernicus, Galileo, Pasteur, Mesmer). The idea may appear bizarre, even fuzzy at first because the discoverer made an intuitive leap and does not have all the data in place yet.

Many health informatics network members can no doubt identify with these sentiments. This book is dedicated to these pioneers who dared to be out of step with their peers and who have provided the building blocks for this paradigm shift. It has proved difficult for the discipline to gain acceptance from mainstream health professionals and recipients of health care, and enabling procedures and legislations have been slow to emerge (Mandil 1992).

In Australia the health informatics network is made up of a number of discipline, focus or geographically based health informatics groups brought together under the Health Informatics Society of Australia (HISA). HISA is a special interest group of the Australian Computer Society. It is a member of, and the official Australian representative to, the International Medical Informatics Association.

Health informatics is about data, information and knowledge and what we do with all this as health professionals. It is no accident that the advent of low cost easily accessible computer technology has occurred at the same time as the so-called information explosion that has affected all areas of modern life. The problem of managing the ever increasing volume of information and developing methods to help keep abreast of important changes in knowledge is particularly applicable to those of us working in health care.

It is becoming increasingly difficult to practice as a health professional without the use of information technologies. This challenge is going to continue as expectations of increasing quality of health care is demanded by the consumers of our services. Improved information management of health care data has become an accepted essential element of the infrastructure of all health care systems (Dick 1991).

The discipline of health informatics has arisen from the fairly recently established science of medical informatics (Shortliffe et al 1990, Hannan 1991, Coiera 1994). It is noted that the First World Congress on Medical Informatics was held in 1974 in Stockholm. Although the two disciplines share many concepts, and the terms are often used interchangeably, in this textbook we have chosen to focus on the use of information technology in all areas of health care, rather than just focus on a more traditional view of medicine. The term health informatics is all embracing and medical informatics could be viewed as a subset of health informatics along with nursing or dental informatics.

Those of you who have had little past experience in the use of computers may be reticent about approaching this text. Information technology can be a daunting challenge for those of us who missed out on being part of the 'computer generation' currently graduating from our high schools and tertiary institutions. Remember that you don't need to be a computer genius to use a computer effectively in your professional life. You just need to understand the basic concepts. It's like driving a car; you don't need to know exactly how the engine works but you do need to learn how to drive the machine, to identify when something is wrong and to understand the road rules so that you minimise the risk of getting into trouble.

The difference between information systems specialists and health information systems specialists is that the latter place a greater emphasis on the application of the technology in health care. They focus on solving very complex medical or health related problems using the information technology to the fullest extent as the tool to achieve that. This often means a change in work practices for health professionals. The use of information technology in health care permits greater accountability, leads to improved research to gain a better understanding of the inputs, processes, outputs and outcomes relationships which in turn should result in changes in practice and continuous improvement in terms of outcomes.

If you are already computer literate, you can enjoy applying your acquired skills to the health sciences and learn how to use information technology in the provision of high quality health care. The computer age poses real challenges for us all. We hope that you find this text useful in assisting you to meet the challenges ahead.

REFERENCES

Coiera E 1994 Medical informatics. Medical Journal of Australia 160:438-440

Dick R S, Steen E B (eds) 1991 The computer based patient record—an essential technology for health care. National Academy Press, Washington

Ferguson M 1980 The Aquarian conspiracy. Paladin Grafton Books, London

Graham I 1994 HISA—informatics enhancing health. Health Informatics Society of Australia, Melbourne

Hannan T 1991 Medical informatics—an Australian perspective. Australian and New Zealand Journal of Medicine 21:363-378

Mandil S H 1992 From 'EDP in Health' to Health Informatics. In: Lun K C, Degoulet P, Peimme T E, Rienhoff O (eds) Proceedings of the Seventh World Congress on Medical Informatics. North-Holland, Amsterdam

Martin J, Norman A R D 1970 The computerized society: an appraisal of the impact of computers over the next fifteen years. Prentice Hall, Englewood Cliffs, NJ

Shortliffe E H, Perreault L E, Wiederhold G, Fagan L M (eds) 1990 Medical informatics—computer applications in health care. Addison Wesley, Sydney

History of health informatics

BRANKO CESNIK

> Those who cannot remember the past are condemned to repeat it. (*George Santayana (1863-1952), American philosopher, poet*)

In considering a 'history' of health informatics it is important to be aware that the discipline encompasses a wide array of activities, products, research and theories. Health informatics is as much a result of evolution as planned philosophy, having its roots in the histories of information technology and medicine. The process of its growth continues so that today's work is tomorrow's history. A 'historical' discussion of the area is its history to date, a report rather than a summation.

As well as its successes, the history of health informatics is populated with visionary promises that have failed to materialise despite the best intentions. For those studying the subject or working in the field, the experiences of others' use of information technologies for the betterment of health care can provide a necessary perspective. This chapter starts by noting some of the major events and people that form a technological backdrop to health informatics and ends with some thoughts on the future.

History of computing

While thousands of individuals have been part of the evolution of computing in the last century, some perspective on the history of computing development is useful in understanding the current level of development and sophistication (or lack of it) in today's computing environment.

The desire to represent information in ways that allow real world issues to be more easily managed has been a common pursuit for centuries. As far back as in the 17th century Wilhelm Von Liebnitz was advocating the idea that it might be possible to represent the entire nature of human behaviour in some codified form. This principle still forms the basis on which many software developers, especially in medicine, view coding. That is, if we developed a fine enough coding system, then all things may be classified (not that Herr Liebnitz was in possession of tools that could assist in this desire).

The first example of how such tools might be created and the uses to which they could be put can reliably be ascribed to Charles Babbage in the 19th Century. It is generally agreed that Mr Babbage created the first computer, a mechanical device aimed at solving mathematical problems. The machine never succeeded in functioning as desired and he stumbled from funding source to funding source (kings, queens and heads of state). The issue of whether or not his 'analytical engine' could ever have succeeded is moot; however his machine not only still exists, but has also been recreated in an attempt to settle the argument. It appears that, if accurate enough engineering techniques had been available, his life work could have succeeded.

The above two historical figures highlight the fact that the principles underlying today's use of computers has been around for a very long time. The punch card system devised by Herman Hollerith in the 1890s to manage the United States census data demonstrates the effectiveness of technologies that do not use the microchip capabilities of today.

This system was so successful that it was still being used after World War II. It involved hundreds of workers developing the ability to punch cards and also to pass long needles through trays of such cards to perform data analysis. Even when digital (electronic) computers were developed, punch cards were still used as the major form of data input, as any computer science student of the 50s and 60s can verify. Despite the development of ever increasingly powerful computers over this time, it was not until the end of the 1960s that this technique finally was laid to rest.

Computers

The electronic computer

The need for information management during the Second World War spurred the development of electronic computers. The first digital or electronic computer was ENIAC, created in the 1940s. This device occupied a large room and ran on valves with enormous power consumption and remains at the Smithsonian institute as a reminder of the scale of change in this century. Following the Second World War computers continued to evolve in speed, capacity, sophistication and reliability, and they also continued to reduce in size. Due to the specialised environments, space and support needed to run these devices, the concept of mainframe computing developed.

Mainframe computing implies a central computer which supports users at distance through the provision of 'dumb' terminals. Note that the idea of computing at distance (via a terminal) only occurred in the late 1940s and early 1950s. This centralised form of computing services supported by an information management service (IMS) remained the norm until the early 1970s.

In the late 1950s Ledley and Lusted, living in a world of now powerful new computing devices, were among many who recognised the potential of computer-assisted medical decision making. While access, cost, and implementation were seen as limiting the ability to provide such support in a widely available fashion, the belief was evident that increasing computational power could be harnessed to model, assist and enhance health care. While the 'dumb terminal'-mainframe model of computing services was not able to adequately address this desire, the coming years would see the 'personal computer' become a reality, initially as the minicomputer.

The emergence of minicomputers in the late 1960s provided what were, in essence, stripped down mainframes with their own storage ability, aimed at supporting a small number of local users and promising a future of 'personal' computing. These were still very expensive but were a major leap forward from the distributed, 'dumb terminal' philosophy of previous decades. So enthusiastic were many of the proponents of minicomputers that ad–vertisements from the 1960s and 1970s described the desirability for medical practitioners to purchase them to improve their office and patient management. The promise that such technologies could so intimately assist health professionals at a personal level remains today. That promise is satisfied more often today than then but disappointment often remains even with current advanced systems.

Microcomputers arrive

The highly personal availability of computing technologies became more possible with the advent of the microcomputer. The Apple II microcomputer, released in 1978, with 6502 chip, monochrome display, and tape or floppy storage provided the first real personal computer. Whilst many other microcomputers existed such as Tandy, Commodore, Zenith the Apple II microcomputer was the first that encouraged average users to indulge in programming and the production of software on a large scale destined for personal use.

While these machines initially penetrated the home and hobby market rather than business, the introduction of the program VISICALC (the first, functional, spreadsheet program) altered the perception of microcomputers and their usefulness. The business world suddenly had a powerful new tool for financial modelling offering a familiar paradigm (an accounting sheet) with the power of microcomputer based technologies behind it. Such applications did not escape the attention of those responsible for the financial management of health care. As for all aspects of society, the personal computer found its way into practice environments, hospital systems, organisations working in epi–demiological work and a host of other health related areas.

In 1982 IBM released the IBM PC (640K, cassette or floppy storage, colour display). It appears that IBM did not consider this machine as a serious project and that the explosion of clones, acceptance by business and the massive secondary industry generated by software developers was completely unpredicted. Initial projections were for a few thousand sales. The currently installed base of machines with this architecture is well into the millions.

The release of the Macintosh computer (evolved from the Xerox PARC work and the Apple Lisa) offered a whole new principle in how users could interact with computers. Now called the WIMP interface (Windows, Icons, Mouse and Popdown menus), this was the first practical, commercially available, graphic user interface or GUI and its underlying philosophy can be attributed in large part to Douglas Engelbart, the inventor of the mouse as a pointing device.

As these microcomputers became increasingly powerful and popular through the 1980s IMS groups finally began to agree that these 'toys' should have some access to mainframes, usually with the proviso that they agree to behave as dumb terminals. Users also found the need to connect PCs together resulting in the development of local area networks (LANs).

Without an agreed standard for these endeavours we have the current situation with a wide (but reducing) number of ways to link PCs together. LAN structures now communicate with each other forming wide area networks (WAN) with links into mainframe services.

Overall, this progression of increasingly powerful, smaller and faster computing possibilities has resulted in the availability of the 'personal' computer. Ideally, technology should be an additional tool for individuals providing connectivity to resources far greater than personal experience, education or traditional paper based repositories of information could provide.

All of this is possible because of the development of the microchip or integrated circuit, predominantly developed by the companies Intel and Motorola. These 'chips' are evolving at a rapid pace providing more and more processing power. These 'hardware' advances are not matched by developments in software; processors spend much of their time doing nothing. The widespread adoption of the GUI interface, larger and more sophisticated software creations and the need to enhance the means whereby users interact with the computer means that the hoped for developments of handwriting and speech recognition in a highly interactive graphic environment are now occurring.

Computer languages—telling the computer what to do

The software programs have evolved along with the hardware base itself, although at differing rates. These languages range from telling the computer what to do at a very low level, such as assembly language, to much more abstracted means of representation provided by object orientated systems, natural language tools, artificial intelligence methodologies and a variety of others. In an inevitable progression, the increased hardware capabilities are used by developers to create more and more sophisticated means of 'communicating' with the computer to manage information in more and more natural ways.

While the above is promising, the actual tools we use on computers today are still in their infancy in many ways. The vast majority of computer human interaction is via the keyboard, itself an unfriendly legacy of the past. The QWERTY keyboard design aims to reduce typing speed so as to decrease the possibility of the letter 'hammers' jamming, despite the fact that such typewriters are now museum pieces.

Health care poses some of the greatest challenges for both the technologies and those seeking to apply them to patient care. Health care often deals with the most abstract of ideas such as 'well', 'pain', 'happy', 'sad'. Health care also generates enormous volumes of information regarding the community and its needs. Thus understanding health informatics requires not only familiarity with the technology but, more importantly, insight into the nature in which health care delivery occurs. These questions are not yet answered but health informatics lays claim to some of the possible directions and solutions most likely to be of benefit.

Health informatics—a discipline

Health informatics is often described as a new discipline. It has come to address the desires to apply and explore the uses of these relatively new tools for the better provision of health care. This is a bold claim with some merit. The successes of the field in living up to the claim have been less than expected and have, at times, disrupted the timely delivery of health care rather than enhanced it. This is not entirely surprising given the accelerating rate of change in technologies and the relatively 'young' nature of a discipline which is now examining itself to clarify its role. Health informatics began as medical and nursing informatics during the 1970s, a period described by van Bemmel & Shortliffe (1986) as undergoing exponential development due to the growing availability of steadily less expensive hardware, more powerful software and the advent of microcomputers.

A gradual change from electronic data processing in health, through the use of informatics in medical care, to health informatics, is discernable from the types of papers presented at the three yearly World Congresses on Medical Informatics (Medinfo), which began in 1974 in Stockholm. The use of computers to support medical decision making, including artifical intelligence, was strong during the 1980s. The linkage of systems emerged in 1989 when multiple disciplines began to work together to develop integrated systems utilising new database technology and the power of networks. This produced synergistic applications where the whole became greater than the sum of its parts. The most popular papers presented at Medinfo'92 in Geneva were those on knowledge based work such as concepts, methodologies, software and other tools, systems and evaluations of systems and experiences (Mandil 1992). These congresses were organised by the International Medical Informatics Association (IMIA), which began as a special interest group of International Federation of Information Processing (IFIP).

While health informatics aims to articulate its place in health care, other health care professionals continue to adopt the technologies into their own areas. For example, the use of computing systems in radiological imaging is extensive. Amongst the lessons to be learned from the history of health informatics is that health informatics as a discipline must be cognisant of, and involved in, the aims and activities of health care itself. Technologies are becoming ubiquitous in their availability with ever increasingly powerful tools allowing health care workers to readily create systems for their own benefit. health informatics should communicate to the health care profession the lessons of its past, just as health informatics needs to learn from the work and activities of this same community.

The benefits of the technology as well as the ability to demonstrate such benefits to others are becoming compulsory. The reasons for this include: the effect of computer usage by practitioners on patients themselves; the security of medical information; the need for new skills to be learned; and the price of the technology at a time when rising health care costs are an international concern.

Health informatics strives to enhance all aspects of health care at all times. If this is kept in mind, the lessons of history to date will be heeded and incorporated into the future of information technology in health care, rather than ignored.

REFERENCES

Mandil S H 1992 From 'EDP in Health' to Health Informatics. In: Lun K C, Degoulet P, Piemme T E, Rienhoff O (eds) Proceedings of the Seventh World Congress on Medical Informatics. North-Holland, Amsterdam

van Bemmel J H, Shortliffe E H 1986 In: Salamon R, Blum B, Jorgensen M (eds) Foreword to the Proceedings of the Fifth World Congress on Medical Informatics. North-Holland, Amsterdam

3

Health care services and information systems

EVELYN J S HOVENGA

Health care service delivery could be described as an information intensive industry. In contrast the banking industry is transaction intensive. Both are able to benefit greatly from the use of computing, information and com—munications technology, yet the banking industry is much further advanced in this regard. A transaction based system relies predominantly on data. These are observations or facts which when collected, evaluated and organised become information or knowledge. Data are computer input elements. Information on the other hand consists of data which are:

> processed, organised or classified into categories to serve a useful purpose. Nobel Laureate Kenneth Arrow defined information as 'a reduction in uncertainty'. Information as an intellectual construct is subject to constant change. Its importance depends on who makes any information based transactions and when. It is both resource and commodity but unlike matter and energy is not consumed by use. Communications is central to information flow and essentially subsumed in it. 'Information' depends heavily on 'information technology' (IT) but is a far wider concept, with educational, social, economic, employment and cognitive implications. Data, information, knowledge and intelligence ascend hierarchically. The concept of encoded data organised as 'information' is the common feature of genetics, biotechnology, language, communications, mathematics, electronics, computing and robotics (HRSCLTS 1991)

In the banking industry data consists of numbers whilst in the health care industry data takes many forms including numbers, text, concepts (coded data), graphics, images, physiological measures (signals), and sound. Health care professionals rely on all their senses, including smell to collect assessment data from individuals. These data are recorded in a person's medical history or health record. Now that technology has progressed to the point where all types of data, with the exception of smell, may be produced in digital form it has become feasible to develop fully integrated health information systems. This should assist greatly in meeting the functional needs for health information. Dick (1992) noted that 'we lack the evidence to make more informed decisions in health care today across the spectrum from the bedside up to the formulation of national health care policy'. He went on to say that 'most of the evidence needed to make more informed decisions remains embedded in fragmented, irretrievable, and often illegible paper-based patient records'.

To define the health problem one must be able to identify and describe the population or groups for whom the problem exists as well as various aspects denoting health status. These aspects range from incidence of disease, ill health, deaths, and quality of life, to the functional, emotional and mental aspects of health status. An understanding of the problem requires data which are identified as being determinants of health such as reasons for occurrence, predisposing factors, causes, access to health care services and risk factors. Arriving at solutions to the problem requires the identification of effective interventions provided directly to individuals and to communities, including management protocols, resource and service utilisation. All interventions must therefore be identified and described and linked to defined outcomes in order to determine effectiveness. In essence outcome measures are identical to problem identification measures. These then are the functional health information requirements irrespective of the economic, political, philosophical or organisational considerations of any country's health care system. These considerations will determine the health information systems detailed architectural framework, although in broad terms this should be standardised to suit any health care system.

The Australian Institute of Health and Welfare (AIH&W) has as its mission to inform community discussion and to support public policy making on health and welfare issues by coordinating, developing, analysing and disseminating national statistics on the health of Australians, and health and welfare services, and by undertaking and supporting related research and analysis. An important mechanism for improving Australia's health information has been the National Health Information Agreement between the Commonwealth, State and Territory health authorities, the Australian Bureau of Statistics and the AIH&W. This has resulted in a National Health Information Work Program (AIH&W 1993) which incorporates those health information activities that both meet agreed national priorities and have either a national focus or national implications. Projects cover data collections that describe health service institutions, primary care and community health, mental health, medical services, health service outcomes, pharmaceuticals, health insurance, national health expenditure, health labourforce, vital statistics, population surveys, surveillance, population health outcomes, national health information policy and infrastructure. In the process a health data dictionary has been developed and is expanding. This represents a major initiative towards the provision of an authoritative set of national definitions. The AIH&W is developing a national health information plan designed to overcome identified deficiencies in its data collections to support its mission (AIH&W 1994). For example Harper et al (1994) note that quality of life and most of the behavioural aspects of illness are very poorly described and not available for whole populations.

Similar activities are taking place in other countries. For example in the United States the Agency for Health Care Policy and Research (AHCPR) consists of several components one of which is the Office of Science and Data Development which supports and conducts activities designed to increase the amount and usefulness of data (such as that from health insurance claims data bases and computer based patient research) for outcomes and other health services research. The Computer-Based Patient Record Institute (CPRI) was established in 1991 following a report by the Institute of Medicine's committee for improving the patient record to provide a sustained, coordinated and concentrated effort to establish the widespread use of computer-based patient records (Dick 1992). One of a number of high priorities for the CPRI is the development of health data standards.

Three factors have determined the characteristics and development of health information systems. These are economic considerations, technological advances and changes in philosophies regarding health service delivery. The last decade has seen enormous change in all three areas. Various approaches aimed at controlling health care expenditure have emerged. Technological advances in medicine, computing, and communications technology can only be described as explosive. Global changes regarding social structures, attitudes and values are influencing and changing the expectations of recipients of health care services. In Australia and elsewhere a paradigm shift from a medical model with a physical ill health focus of health service delivery, towards a social and community based model is clearly evident. A state of health may be defined as a general sense of physical, social and psychological well being. Ill health on the other hand denotes a deficiency in well being in one or more of these aspects which may result in an inability to function at one's usual level.

The structure and type of health information systems developed and implemented tend to reflect a country's health care system. This is turn is greatly influenced by the philosophical, political and economic underpinnings of that system. The dominant value driving information system development in industrialised countries has been that of economic constraints, competing pressures regarding resource allocation whilst focusing on the treatment of ill health from a medical perspective. Thus systems have tended to support administrative and financial activities associated with the treatment of disease and physical ill health. Until more recently clinical management considerations did not feature in most health information system development efforts.

Economic and political influences

The Organisation for Economic Co-operation and Development (OECD) has noted that 'in recent decades, the growth in health care expenditures has exceeded the growth in gross domestic product across the OECD area' (OECD policy study 1992). This has resulted in a growing emphasis on and interest in efficiency and effectiveness of health service delivery. It is the concern about effectiveness which is finally stimulating the development of clinical information systems. To maximise the benefits of these systems they must link with other health focused systems to gain a thorough understanding of the many variables which influence the general health of a population and of the measures or circumstances which successfully improve health.

The Commonwealth, State and Territory health authorities have committed themselves to improving the health outcomes of Australians. Their aim is to achieve optimal individual and population health within available resources through this focus. The Australian Health Ministers Advisory Council (AHMAC) defined a health outcome as 'a change in the health of an individual, a group of people or population, which is attributable to an intervention or series of interventions' (DHS&H 1994). As a result of this initiative national goals and targets for making significant improvements in the health status of Australians were established. These focus on cardiovascular disease, cancers, mental health and injuries. These were chosen because they are of major concern as a result of their contribution to a high level of death, illness or premature loss of life. Furthermore effective interventions to improve health outcomes were perceived to be possible and the measurement of progress towards these were seen to be feasible.

Other components of the AHCPR in the United States include the Medical Treatment Effectiveness Program (MEDTEP); the Office of Health Technology Assessment which evaluates the safety, efficacy, effectiveness and where possible, the cost effectiveness of health care technologies; and the Office of the Forum for Quality and Effectiveness in Health Care. The latter arranges for the development, periodic review, and updating of clinical practice guidelines. This office also supports the development of performance measures, standards of quality, and medical review criteria for use by health care practitioners and others in reviewing health care quality and services. McCormick (1992) notes that the impetus for practice guideline development comes from identified practice pattern variations, concern with inappropriateness of care and high healthcare costs.

The United States implemented in 1983 output based funding based on patient classification, i.e. diagnosis related groups (DRGs), to control health care expenditures. Their prospective payment system using DRGs was mandated by the passage of the Tax Equity and Fiscal Responsibility Act of 1982 (TEFRA) (Shaffer 1985). In Australia the second round of Medicare Agreements negotiated in 1988 between the Commonwealth, State and Territory health authorities, included the introduction of the Casemix Development Program. Its purpose was to develop casemix (output) based approaches to hospital management and financing which was a component of micro-economic reform within the health care industry. The third round of Medicare Agreements negotiated in 1993 provided for the continued development of casemix related activities. Victoria was the first State to introduce casemix based funding in July 1993. New South Wales uses casemix as a component of its Resource Allocation Formula which is used to fund all health services. It is also a major component of the NSW Efficiency Index used to compare relative efficiency between areas and districts. Casemix based budgeting and funding models are used within NSW Area Health Services, districts and hospitals. South Australia introduced casemix based funding in July 1994 and the Queensland Government did so in January 1995. In Tasmania casemix information is used for program reporting and evaluation and as a component of the Tasmanian Resource Allocation Model (TRAM) used for the purpose of costing inter-regional patient flows. Western Australia uses casemix as a performance indicator to appraise and compare provider organisations as well as to monitor hospital performance.

In Australia a number of different casemix systems have been developed or are in use including the Australian National Diagnosis Related Groups (AN-DRGs), Australian Paediatric Ambulatory Classification (APAC), Australian Ambulatory Classification (AAC), Major Ambulatory Diagnostic Categories (MADCs), Major Diagnostic Categories (MDC), Non-acute Inpatient Classification System (NAIPs), Neonatal DRGs, Nursing home type (NHT), Paediatric modified DRGs (PM-DRGs), Patient Assessment and Information System (PAIS) which is a patient/nurse dependency system, Psychiatric Patient Classes (PPCs), Resident Classification Instrument (RCI) used by nursing homes and Urgency Related Groups (URGs) for emergency services. These casemix systems combined with their intended usage greatly influence the types of data collected throughout the health care system.

The United Kingdom initiated a series of projects designed to introduce business practices regarding financial control and budgeting following a management inquiry into the National Health Service (NHS) in the late 1980s. Recommendations included the use of classification systems such as ICD9, ICD9-CM, and DRGs to provide clinical workload information (Catterall 1988). This marked the beginning of major structural reforms within the NHS. Their Resource Management initiative introduced a new approach to resource management within the NHS aimed at demonstrating measurable im‐ provements in patient care (Department of Health 1989). The UK now uses Healthcare Resource Groups (HRGs) which represent a UK modification of DRGs. Other countries including New Zealand, Canada and Sweden have experienced similar major reforms to their health system. Canada uses Case‐ Mix Groups (CMGs) as its output measure. These and similar policy initiatives have had a significant impact upon health information system development and the discipline of health informatics.

Philosophical aspects

There is a growing realisation that social structures, the economic, social, occupational and environmental circumstances of individuals, methods of health service delivery plus public health measures, greatly influence the incidence of disease and ill health episodes and the quality of life experienced. Disease and ill health may be defined by the prevalence of physical, social or psychological problems experienced. Medical interventions are designed to respond to the physical aspect of ill health and to a lesser extent to the mental aspect of ill health. Health outcomes, as measured by the general health and well being of a population or the impact of disease or ill health upon daily living, are determined not only by the possible underlying disease or medical interventions but also by the management of the response to these problems within the context of the whole person in their environment. Thus a population's health is not a discrete domain of medical practice (Harper et al 1994). According to Harper et al (1994) health data serve three broad purposes: to define the problem, to understand the problem and to identify effective interventions, preventative and curative.

The political influences and financial considerations together with an underlying desire by governments towards a philosophy of a health service delivery system which has a primary health care focus, are driving health care services away from institutional care towards community based care. This reorientation of the health care system from a medical model of health care towards a social model began in 1977 at the Thirtieth World Health Assembly, followed by the 1978 Declaration of Alma Ata; the 1986 Ottawa Charter for Health Promotion; the 1988 Adelaide Conference Statement on Healthy Public Policy; and the 1991 Supportive Environments for Health: The Sundsvall Statement. Australia is a signatory to the Global Strategy for Health for All by the Year 2000, thus accepting international obligations (DHH&CS 1993). Thus increasingly more health services are expected to promote health and there is an expectation to involve the community in health care decision making. Health care services required for any one episode of care may be provided by any number and combination of community and institution based services. Consequently there is a greater need to inform the community about health related concepts and interventions and to make provision for the continuity of care. This has major implications for health information systems including data definitions and collections.

Technological advances

Advances in computing, communications and medical technologies are explosive. It is increasingly difficult to keep up with the enormous volume of new knowledge created by medical advances and needed for the purpose of informed decision making. Medical advances are forcing changes in attitudes and values regarding the sanctity of human life, creating many dilemmas associated with resource allocation. Much is possible but is it worth doing? Computing and com–munications technological advances on the other hand are making what wasn't realistically possible previously more feasible, cost effective and in some instances commonplace. High performance computing and networking technology plus advanced software technology and algorithms will provide enormous benefits to health care in the areas of research, imaging, telehealth and telemedicine. Communications technology needs to be embraced to ensure continuity of care as health care recipients move through the system and are serviced by any number of providers during any one episode of care.

Conclusion

It may be concluded that health informatics provides the most significant infrastructure needed to manage health care in the future. This infrastructure should not be dependent upon existing economic, political, or philosophical considerations. It should be capable of accommodating future changes at the lowest possible cost. Notwithstanding this requirement, it is noted that the developments in technology, philosophical transitions, and the desire to contain cost whilst improving the health of any nation, are all interdependent. They are the drivers of health information system specification, development, implementation and usage. The next chapter explores health information and its role in communication within the health sector in greater detail.

REFERENCES

Agency for Health Care Policy and Research (AHCPR) Fact Sheet November 1992. US Department of Health and Human Services, Rockville

Australian Institute of Health & Welfare 1993 National Health Information Work Program 1993-94. AGPS, Canberra

Australian Institute of Health & Welfare 1994 Australia's Health 1994, AGPS, Canberra.

Catterall J 1988 Resource management and the use of DRGs. In: Proceedings of the Second International Conference on the Management and Financing of Hospital Services. Sydney

Department of Health 1989 Case mix management system core specification. NHS Management Board Resource Management Directorate, London

Department of Health, Housing and Community Services 1993 Towards health for all and health promotion: the evaluation of the National Better Health Program. AGPS, Canberra

Department of Health, Housing, Local Government and Community Services 1993 Casemix: a new direction in health care management. The National Casemix Education Series publication A, AGPS, Canberra

Department of Human Services and Health 1994 Better health outcomes for Australians. National Health Goals and Targets Section, Canberra

Dick R 1992 A bold vision: the computer-based patient record institute. In: Ball M J, Collen M F (eds) Aspects of the computer-based patient record. Springer-Verlag, New York

Harper A C, Holman C, Dawes V P (eds) 1994 The health of populations, 2nd edn. Churchill Livingstone, Melbourne

McCormick K A 1992 Clinical practice guidelines. Health Progress December

Organisation for Economic Co-operation and Development (OECD) Social Policy Studies No. 7 1990 Health care systems in transition. OECD, Paris

Shaffer F A (ed) 1985 Costing out nursing: pricing our product. National League for Nursing, New York

HRSCLTS 1991 Australia as an information society: grasping new paradigms, report of the House of Representatives Standing Committee for Long Term Strategies. AGPS, Canberra

4

Health information science

DON C WALKER

The communication of information is fundamental to health care. In pre-history, knowledge and skills were passed from healer to apprentice by talking and example. Early cuneiform writing on clay tablets record some medical techniques and remedies. In more recent times, medical books have documented an accumulating human knowledge. Currently, journals, magazines, books, proceedings and pamphlets deliver a daily avalanche of written health care information, while audio and video tapes, radio, television, CD-ROM, video-discs and films produce a mountain of audiovisual material.

There is a well established communication between health care providers; such as between the nurse and the doctor, the doctor and the pharmacist, the radiologist and the pathologist, and so on. A health care system must also be managed and funded. This requires a flow of information from the health care recipient and the provider to various organisations for fund and resource allocation, and for management.

All the above information is small compared to that which passes between the recipient of health care and the provider. This intercourse contains the daily application of health care. In it, and too often hidden, are the clues to new diseases, complications and interactions. Some clues are recorded and they form actual or potential food for researchers.

Health care is about people and mostly one-to-one relationships between recipients and providers. However, the domain is steeped in information and its management. In this, technology will have an ever increasing role to play.

There is no point in applying information technology unless advantages result which outweigh any associated disadvantages. Let us briefly consider some of these and the building blocks required for advances to occur.

The communication of medical information and its management

Communication with literature

The overwhelming volume of printed health care information has, from the turn of the century, been indexed in libraries. In recent years, these indices have been created and stored on computers.

The key concepts within the text are identified and named according to a standardised list of terms. One controlled vocabulary used for this purpose by the National Library of Medicine (NLM) in Washington DC is called MeSH (Medical Subject Headings). It evolved for computer use from *Index Medicus*, the original list of terms used to index a catalogue of the publications in the US army medical library. It was compiled and published by Surgeon General Dr John Shaw Billings in 1879. Some medical and other health related literature is indexed using a different vocabulary, for example the Library of Congress Subject Headings (LCSH), and the Cumulative Index to Nursing and Allied Health Literature (CINAHL). These and others are discussed in greater detail in Chapter 29.

The volume of new written material has long been far beyond any one person's capacity to read, let alone learn and apply. The challenge for information technology is to present relevant information to the healthcare worker when it is needed. For example, if a combination of disease and medications have potential side effects, then the provider should be warned of these at the moment of prescribing. For this to occur, an up-to-date database of drug interactions must be provided to the computing industry. The electronic medical record must also record a person's details in terminology equivalent to that used by the database.

In the future, the literature may be searched (in a semi-automated process) according to the contents of a person's electronic medical record. This would save the provider compiling searches, and would thus save time and effort. The major obstacle to be overcome before this is a reality, is the difference in terminology used by the healthcare provider and the library indexing system. The UMLS (Unified Medical Language System, a research project sponsored by the NLM) is attempting to provide a solution.

All people will inevitably have greater access to current literature and databases. Searching will be easily done from the home computer or local library. Some more aware patients will result. An informed recipient of care is a two edged sword—more able to self-care, but more demanding of new investigations, therapies and procedures. To avoid increasing costs, co-ordinated education programs may be needed. Thus what is required for improved literature communication are:

- increased awareness of the existence of available resources
- wider use of computers
- unification of health care terminologies
- improved searching programs
- educational programs which improve user interpretation of the literature.

Communication between providers

Health care is very much a team game. Communication between players is constant—between general practitioners, physicians, surgeons, pathologists, radiologists, nurses, pharmacists, therapists, lawyers and many more. The essence of any communication should be recorded. The background history of the person concerned, and a summary appropriate to the provider is usually required. The management of a person seeking care can evolve into a complex round of repetitive forms and letters. With each communication, the risk of inaccurate information increases. If there is a coordinator such as a general practitioner, or a case manager from a hospital, or other health care agency who compiles and collates all documents into a person's record, then this record can become a confusing collection of difficult to find documents. Its usefulness declines as its thickness increases.

Electronic communication between members of the team such that each has a view of, and some access to a person's medical or health record, would save time, increase accuracy, and result in better management. In general terms, as the number of pieces of paper are reduced, so the efficiency increases. The pharmacist's prescription should be an electronic message sent directly by the doctor to the pharmacist. Likewise the laboratory and radiology requests and reports should not involve paper. For this to materialise:

- Providers must use computers.
- The terminology used by each provider should be consistent and universally understood.
- All involved should agree as to what will be transmitted.
- An adequate communications network should exist.
- Each network node should adhere to standardised message protocols.
- Adequate security, confidentiality and integrity safeguards should exist.
- Up-to-date information resources should be provided in a standardised form which are computer understandable.

Communication with organisations

Current communication with funding and resource management organisations involves a complex paper trail with an occasional interspersed computer. Medicare slips, discharge details and workers compensation forms are posted by the millions. Wishes, advice, warnings, demands, rules and regulations issue forth from administrative and professional organisations or associations to health care providers, on pieces of paper, brochures and books. Much of this traffic could be replaced if a health care network of provider computers existed, and each computer understood the concepts or facts used by the other. Wishes, advice, warnings, demands, rules and regulations could be composed in a computer understandable way, such that when appropriate, the provider would automatically be advised, prompted or warned. Electronic fund transfer is already well established (e.g. EFTPOS). It will inevitably be used by the health care industry. For these things to eventuate the same conditions listed previously as required for electronic communication between members of the health care team apply.

Communication between provider and patient

The role of the front line providers of health care involves listening, questioning, examining, provisionally diagnosing, investigating, confirming the diagnosis, caring, supporting, providing, educating and treating. The facts gleaned and the events which ensue must be recorded. These are required (a) for accurate management and resource allocation, and (b) for future reference by a person's current provider or future providers, and (c) for potential medico-legal requirements. Traditionally this record is the written medical record.

Medical records are certainly the hub of information management for each recipient of health care. They should form the hub of the entire health care system. However, in their written form they are generally speaking illegible, disorganised, inaccessible, mislaid, and impossible to digest quickly. They offer to the provider no timely, useful and current medical information. No prompts. No warnings. They cannot be easily communicated (in whole or in part) to others. On the other hand, they are as confidential as the inverse of their understandibility. They are cheap to initiate, and are created in a medium familiar to all.

There is a real potential for information technology, if applied to the medical record, to change the health service. The resulting electronic medical or health record (EMR) is the subject of Chapter 12 of this book. Its functional needs will be considered in this chapter.

Good information management demands that data are recorded once only, by the person best qualified and at its source. Thus, for example, the office secretary should enter administrative and demographic information; the doctor the medical history, examination and orders; the nurse the daily observations and events; the pathologist (or technician or automated analyser) the laboratory results; the radiologists the interpretation of X-rays. Transcription of data should not occur.

In the Australian environment of unconscripted and unregimented private health care providers, the EMR must be desired by potential users if it is to succeed. This means it must offer the provider advantages over the competing alternative pen and paper system. It must generate less tedium, more speed, timely and current clinical information and, diagnostic and management assistance. It should prompt the provider so as to avoid excesses and omissions. Automated case summaries and views of any aspect of a patient's previous records should be available. Form and letter generation should be semi-automated. It should manage financial matters. It should be accurate, secure, accessible yet confidential.

The following must come together to enable a significant improvement in health care information management:

- Health care terminologies: Consistent health care terminology, and standard coding and classification of concepts.
- Resources: Computer understandable, current, useful and useable information; data and knowledge resources.
- Computing: Adequate computing hardware, and software development tools.

- User interface and data capture: Optimised user interface and data capture methods.
- Electronic communications: Adequate electronic communications.
- Safeguards: Adequate security, confidentiality and integrity safeguards.
- Benefits: There must be benefits to all concerned—to the computing industry, the health care funding organisations, the health care providers, and to the patients.

Let us now glance at each of the components necessary for improved health care information management. Several of the topics will be considered at length in other chapters. This chapter is designed to offer an overview of the 'science' involved. This should help in the formation of a perspective of the subject.

Healthcare terminologies

Components of a terminology

As we have seen, there is a need to describe health care concepts in a consistent manner. We, as humans, are able to assimilate, without confusion, many variations of description. Computers on the other hand are very poor at recognising concepts from inconsistent descriptions. To manage this, a standard list of terms is collected and divided into *preferred terms* and *alternative descriptions* (or *synonyms*). For example, the preferred term 'subacute thyroiditis' could have as its synonyms 'de Quervain's thyroiditis' and 'granulomatous thyroiditis.' Within any terminology, the preferred terms should be unique; however each preferred term may have synonyms which are shared with other preferred terms. For example, 'cold' could be a synonym for both 'hypothermia' and the common viral infection 'coryza.'

The preferred term is an agreed short description of a *concept*. A concept is the image created by the words which describe it. A *definition* of the concept may be needed. Too often the wording of the preferred term means something different to different users.

As health care is ever-changing, the preferred description of a concept may change. For example, an international terminology has recently changed the preferred term 'maturity onset diabetes mellitus' to 'non insulin dependent diabetes mellitus.' The concept has remained unchanged (i.e. the disease is the same).

A unique identifier (or *code*) for each concept is required. Anything would do as long as it is unique and suitable. If the preferred term is used, its description should not change. As we have seen, this can happen. Thus the preferred term is not suitable as a code. In fact, words are not efficient ways to store identifiers in computers, as the computer may be required to store an identifier many times. The code should thus be reasonably compact—a 'number' of some sort. It need not be seen by users, as the computer can always display its equivalent descriptive words. The process of matching a health care entity to a term in a terminology and assigning a code to it, is called *coding*. The terminology may be called a *coding system*. Some terminologies or coding systems describe themselves as (a) a *'controlled vocabulary'* such as MeSH (National Library of Medicine 1994)); (b) a 'classification' such as the International Classification of Diseases 9th Revision (ICD9) (WHO 1977), ICD9 with Clinical Modifications (ICD9-CM) (Commission on Professional and Hospital Activities 1978), International Classification of Primary Care (ICPC) (Lamberts & Wood 1987)); or (c) a 'nomenclature' such as the Systematized Nomenclature of Medicine (SNOMED) (Cote & Robboy 1980).

Sometimes rules are offered to improve the accuracy of coding. These instruct the user to consider certain other concepts under various conditions.

Thus far we have seen that a terminology is composed of a *code*, a *preferred term* to describe each *concept* (ideally *defined*), and various *synonyms*. *Rules* may be provided to direct the user.

Classifications, hierarchies and terminologies

Knowledge enables us to refer to something and unconsciously all related things come to mind. Thus if we consider the concept of 'appendicitis' we think of those conditions which we have learnt are included, for example 'acute, subacute, chronic and relapsing appendicitis.' We also know that 'diseases of the large intestine' include appendicitis. This organisation of concepts into groups (or classes) such that one group includes others is called *classification*. The resulting structure can be visualised as a branching tree (perhaps turned up-side-down!), and is described as an *hierarchy* (for which the adjective is *hierarchical*).

When the concepts of a terminology are arranged to form a hierarchy, some concepts by their nature will be found to belong in more than one place. For example, 'tuberculosis of the lung' is both an 'infectious disease' and a 'lung disease.' Another finding when building hierarchies is that concepts belong in different classes depending on the *context* of the classification. For example, various types of apples can be classified according to their size, colour, or time of ripening etc.— and each grouping would be different. Many health care concepts can have *multiple hierarchies*. For example, 'bleeding disorders' include some diseases from 'congenital, infectious, allergic, nutritional and metabolic' conditions, and each of these groups of conditions belong to a hierarchy of their own.

The practical importance of classifications or hierarchies is in their ability to include all subordinate concepts. They can thus specify the detail (or *granularity*) of the data:

• An organisation may need to know how many operations were performed, while an association may be interested in the number of hysterectomies. If the obstetrician records the details of each type of hysterectomy, using an appropriate terminology, then the less detailed requirements of the association and the organisation can be automatically supplied by utilising the hierarchy of the terminology.

- Information resources which can be harnessed by health care computing systems should be able to include various groups of concepts. For example, if the indications for a blood test are required, and they are specified in the resource as 'bleeding disorders', the hierarchy of the terminology should be able to determine which conditions are included in the concept 'bleeding disorders'.

As computing systems become 'smarter', their internal use of hierarchies increases.

Specifying hierarchies in terminologies

A classification or hierarchy may be specified by a numbering system:

2	level one concept	(e.g. 'diseases of the large intestine')
27	level two concept	(e.g. 'appendicitis')
271	level three concept	(e.g. 'acute appendicitis')
272	level three concept	(e.g. 'chronic appendicitis')
273	level three concept	(e.g. 'relapsing appendicitis')

In this example there can only be ten concepts at any level. This method is used by ICD9 and ICD9cm systems.

Note: An hierarchy can be described in terms of parents, siblings, and children. In the above example, the *parent* of 'appendicitis' is 'diseases of the large intestine'. The *children* of 'appendicitis' are 'acute appendicitis', 'chronic appendicitis', and 'relapsing appendicitis'. The *siblings* of 'chronic appendicitis' are 'acute appendicitis', and 'relapsing appendicitis'.

By allocating several digits to a level, more space can be reserved (e.g. 200700100, where 100 concepts can occur at each level). The resulting string of characters may be inefficient and unwieldy.

Another method is to count using the base 16 (hexadecimal), and the numbers 0-9 and A-F. This compacts the string of characters, but lack of room between levels may continue to be a problem. This method is used by SNOMED-3 (Cote et al 1993).

Further compaction can be obtained by using the characters 0-9, A-Z, and a-z, making about 58 levels between each character (confusion between the numbers one and zero and upper and lower case 'o' and lower case 'l' (el), may need to be avoided). This method is used by the Read Code Classification system RCC-1 and RCC-2 (Computer Aided Medical Systems 1993).

Another approach is to use a series of numbers of any size each one of which is separated by a *delimited* character (e.g. 'D.12.98.21.7'). This method is used by the 'tree numbers' of MeSH (National Library of Medicine 1994).

It is possible to specify hierarchies in a computer file (or table). Two fields (or columns) are required. One for 'the concepts', and the other for 'the parent of each concept'. By *directing* the computer in its search of this file, the parents, siblings and children of any concept can be determined. Repeated searches allow the full hierarchy to be displayed. Multiple hierarchies can be represented. A concept is simply given more than one parent. Certain *cyclic* references must be forbidden (e.g. a concept cannot have itself as a parent). This computing structure (or *graph*) is called a *'directed acyclic graph'*. It is used by RCC-3 (Computer Aided Medical Systems 1993).

Single and multiple axes and terminologies

Health care concepts can be expressed by concepts from a single list (or *module* or *axis)*; however this list becomes extremely long as more clinical detail is coded.

Consider the diagnosis of 'acute infection of a bone'. The site of the infection will be required and will need to be coded. Thus, there needs to be a list of concepts for 'acute infection' of 'each part' of 'each bone' in the body. Now consider a diagnosis of 'fracture'. Again the bone will be required. An additional list of 'fractures' to 'each part' of 'each bone' will be required. Thus two complete lists of sites for two diagnoses results.

Another approach is to use *multiple axes*, and combine them. Thus, if there is a single list of 'site' codes containing the bones and their parts, then this can be combined with the code for 'acute infection' or the code for 'fracture' to form *compound codes*. Thus one complete list of sites can be used for all diagnoses.

The need to combine axes may be even more apparent when considering a laceration, an abrasion, a bruise, a rash, or an itch, to any part of the body.

The more *atomic* approach of combining *elements* from various axes to form *compound* codes requires the definition of extensive *rules* or *relationships* to avoid the possible generation of nonsense (e.g. a 'fractured eyebrow').

Qualifiers (or modifiers) and terminologies

Some systems offer *qualifiers* (RCC-3.1) (Computer Aided Medical Systems 1994) or *modifiers* (SNOMED-2) (Cote & Robboy 1980). These are modifying concepts which can be linked to a chosen concept. They enable increased clinical detail to be coded. In effect qualifiers are an additional axis. If they can be associated with only specified concepts they can be called *legal qualifiers* — otherwise *general qualifiers* would best describe them.

For example, legal qualifiers for bacterial agents using the SNOMED-2 terminology are:

'0 = not otherwise specified'
'1 = growth present'
'2 = growth absent'
'3 = growth contaminated', etc.

The qualifier code number (e.g. '1') is added to the concept code number. (For example, if the code for 'actinomyces israellii' is 'E10730,' then 'E10730-1' would specify 'actinomyces israellii growth present'.)

Mapping terminologies

There have evolved several coding systems and each has been designed for its specific purpose. For example ICD9-CM (International Classification of Disease, 9th revision with clinical modification) is used by health care managers to code hospital discharge diagnoses and procedures which may then be grouped to become diagnosis related groups (DRGs). This casemix class–ification system is discussed in further detail in Chapter 27. The Medicare Benefit Schedule (MBS) (DCSH 1994)) is used by doctors to code their procedures for payment claims. MeSH is used to code the contents in biomedical literature in the National Library of Medicine, Washington DC. There is often a need to *translate* or *map* or *cross reference* the codes from one system to another. If the above systems were mapped, a procedure identified by a MBS code could be also described in terms of ICD9-CM for the hospital manager, and MeSH for literature research. Some coding systems offer mappings to other systems. Maps to ICD9-CM are virtually mandatory for hospital coding systems in Australia and the US.

Mapping one terminology to another is not an easy task. Various types of cross references result. Terms are found which are exact matches, while others have the same meaning using different words; some are less specific, some more specific, other terms do not match at all.

The Unified Medical Language System (UMLS) (Humphreys & Lindberg 1989), as mentioned earlier, is an attempt to develop a terminology interface to biomedical literature, health care records, health related databanks and knowledge bases—in the US. The UMLS has developed a Metathesaurus (Sherertz et al 1989), a Semantic Network (McCray 1989) and a Resource Map (National Library of Medicine 1990). These enable a single query to obtain information from multiple data sources. The *Metathesaurus* is a large compilation of several terminologies which are mapped to MeSH. The *Semantic Network* consists of hierarchies of 'semantic types' which have heritable relationships. They form a network. Examples of these relationships are: 'is a ...', 'exhibited by ...', 'carried out by ...', 'forms ...', 'is an evaluation of ...' etc. The *Resources Map* supplies the information required to access various data sources.

Subsets and terminologies

Health care terminologies are large. Because they often exceed 100 000 terms their use requires a coding process. A few words, or beginnings of words, are typed into a computer and used to search the terminology. A list results, from which the user *picks* the most suitable preferred term. If the entire terminology is searched every time, the resulting list may be long and contain many terms which are obviously unwanted. For example, a medical practice is unlikely to require veterinary terms.

The contents of a terminology can be identified (by the use of a simple *scoring* system) to show the concepts more likely to be used in various *contexts*. Application programs (e.g. medical record systems) can then use the *context score* to reduce the size of *picking lists*. Thus, for example, if a terminology identifies its concepts for age, and the age of the patient is known by the computer, then only those terms appropriate for the age of the particular patient need be listed. To give a specific example, if the patient is an adult, and 'penicillin' is required, paediatric versions of penicillin could be omitted from the initial list of options. Likewise, female diseases and operations should be omitted from lists when the patient is a male.

The context scores applied to terminologies can include the type of provider (e.g. nurse, general practitioner, surgeon); the component of the task in hand (e.g. history, examination, diagnosis, investigation, procedure, medication, operating theatre reports, midwifery reports); and the race, age, and sex of the patient.

The scoring system can enable the picking list to be graded to show 'the probable', 'the possible', 'the improbable' and 'the lot, regardless'.

Usage frequency may dictate the picking list. Systems may thus *learn-as-they-go*. This is achieved by scoring the frequently used terms so they sort to the top (where they are more accessible). This process may be made *user specific*; that is, those terms most used by a particular user (provider) can be shown first.

The application program should consider the previous history of the patient, and attempt to present previously used terms.

Thus presenting lists of terms appropriate for the provider, the recipient of care and the task, can be a non-trivial undertaking. Some systems offer *micro-glossaries* (SNOMED) (Cote & Robboy 1980) or *specialty subsets* (RCC-3), *subject types* (RCC-3), *sorting numbers* (RCC-3) (Computer Aided Medical Systems 1993), and *sex* and *age groupings* (ICD9-CM) (Commission on Professional and Hospital Activities 1978).

Resources

Information resources are essential ingredients of any quality health care information management systems. It is generally beyond the scope of system builders and vendors to generate and maintain these resources. Bodies with the appropriate authority and domain expertise are required for their creation. They need to be supplied in a form that is both predictable and readily useable by the system developer, and potentially useful to the end user. Examples of resources include:

- library contents containing indexes of authors, and keywords and text of the contents (all or a summary) of each publication
- medicines data which enable items to be searched from several aspects (e.g. generic name, brand name, composition, indications, contra-

indications, interactions, side effects). Drug and disease interaction warning, description and explanation data files are required. Default values useful to the prescriber are essential. Prompts to remind the user of current rules and regulations are valuable.

- laboratory data, which provides information about available tests, their indications, alternatives, costs, requirements, availability, default values, prompts and warnings
- procedure data which describes each procedure in a manner suitable for the patient (using lay language), the provider (using professional language), and the account (a shortened form). Indications, contraindications, default values, prompts and warnings should supplement the usually extensive instruction text. These should enable the provider to be prompted and helped at the moment of recording a procedure. They would reduce the time spent on the study of organisational and health care rules, regulation, preferences, or advice.
- provider data, which list health care resources and providers, what they do and their contact details
- management guidelines which remind the user of the preferred management for a disease or situation.

The above resources can vary from simple *text data files* to *knowledge* which can be utilised by a computer. The representation of knowledge (*knowledge representation*) is a complex field, and is discussed later in this book. If the knowledge is mixed in with a computer program it is called *hard coded*, and maintaining it becomes impossibly difficult. The knowledge should be in a separate *knowledge-base*, where non-programmers who are *expert* in a field may create and change it. It may be presented in a *knowledge frame*. The knowledge is represented using a standard hierarchical terminology, and carefully thought out *rules*. These usually take the format of '*if* this, *then* that *or else* something'. The creation of these rules requires expert domain knowledge and the help of a *knowledge engineer*. Often the *logic* of the rules is expressed in terms of probability or likelihood, requiring a numeric scoring system (e.g. 0-4). It is thus somewhat *fuzzy*—hence the term *fuzzy logic*. A computer program (or *engine*) is specially designed to utilise the knowledge in the knowledge base. The required answer may have to be deduced or *inferred* from the rules and their fuzzy logic. A *knowledge base* or *expert system* is thus driven by an *inference engine*.

Health care providers are constantly making decisions about the management of an individual's health care. The numerous factors requiring consideration make the task difficult. Any system which aids in the decision process can be called a *decision support system*. For example the timely presentation of relevant information in an easily understood form can help — a graph for instance, or a case summary. Thus, the optimal organisation and presentation of data is a large component of a decision support system. These systems may also contain extensive expert knowledge and apply this to give results which rival that of a panel of experts. These concepts are discussed in more detail in Chapter 14.

Some *computer diagnostic systems* are designed to present a list of possible diagnoses based on a given history, examination and results of investigations. The differential diagnosis is shown in order of probability. An explanation as to why each diagnosis is included is available. Some of these systems are able to tell the user what is the best thing to ask or do next. They may consider the risks and the costs. They are useful training systems, but are no match for an experienced clinician. Their future may be to run in the background of a system, and provide helpful messages when it is appropriate, or when called upon. Examples of diagnostic systems include Iliad (Warner HR et al 1988), DxPlain (Hupp et al 1986), and Quick Medical Reference (Miller et al 1986).

The electronic medical record is destined to evolve from a relatively simple database of coded events and facts, to an information resource centre and decision support system. As its complexity and expert knowledge increases, its ability to be created and maintained by one author or organisation will decrease. It may have to be built from *modules* (or be *modular in design*). Each module would be created and maintained by an organisation which has the necessary expertise. Modules could 'plug into' a basic database system. They could be called, have messages passed to them, and return results to the calling system i.e. the basic database system. For this to occur, agreed communication protocols and message standards must be established. These may be *proprietary standards*, or a *national standard*. The latter is preferable, but usually later in coming. Each of the above resource examples could be a module.

Computing

Adequate computing *hardware* (the boxes and touchable parts), and *software* (the programs) must exist before computers can be used to their potential. The hardware manufacturers provide computers which can do many things. An operating *system* is used to make the hardware 'go.' A *programming environment* which contains *development tools*, allows the system designer and programmer develop *application programs*. These are sold to the public.

The evolution of programming environments and development tools have enabled complex programs to be written in a relatively short time and at little cost. This evolution will effect health care information management. It is a reasonable thought that doctors create their own simple electronic medical record systems using a modern database environment. Doctors and nurses in hospitals are now able to create their own prototype systems. The development and demonstration of their requirements is invaluable to the system designer.

User interface and data capture

The appearance of the computer screen, where things are, how they function and what happens next, can be described as the *human machine interface*, or *user interface*. It is a vital part of quality software, and is, in a way, an art form and a science. If all else is equal, the interface sells the product. The design should be such that things are where expected, and happen as expected. This is called *intuitive* design. It involves human dynamics, taste and consistency of presentation. A well designed interface can greatly reduce the time taken to learn how to 'drive' an application program. Help is usually provided in a manual. The better the software, the less the manual is used. Helpful instructions on the use of the program are provided by *on-line help*. This should be *context sensitive* (i.e. the help changes in accordance with the computer screen or screen object).

Computerised health care information management requires that data be captured by the computer. This is traditionally done via the *key board* by typing. This can be fast, accurate and quiet. However it does require keyboard skills. A *pointing device* is helpful and enables (by a 'point and click and drag' action) the selection of an object or a part of the screen. Pointing devices include the *mouse, trackball, drawing pad, joy stick* and *touch sensitive screen*.

The chore of typing can be greatly reduced by the automatic entry of 'what is probably required' (e.g. 'today's date' in a date field). These probable answers are called *defaults*. Complex and intelligent defaults may be provided. These can greatly improve data capture accuracy and speed. For example, the list of medications used by a particular patient would make sensible defaults for the medications possibly required at each consultation (as a repeat of a previous medication is a frequent event).

Complex management guidelines can be designed to improve data capture, reduce typing, improve accuracy, and improve management. *User defined guidelines* and *resource guidelines* should be (or will be) a feature of any electronic medical record system.

Data may also be captured by the computer analysis and recognition of *handwriting* and the spoken word (*speech recognition*). These methods require much computing power, are inaccurate, and are currently in their infancy. Some systems however show promise. The smaller the vocabulary, the better the result. Systems can be designed so at any time only a small vocabulary is required, yet the total vocabulary is large.

Bar-coding is widely used in non-medical arenas. It is very easy to create the bar-code equivalent of any text. Reading the printed bar-coded text back into the computer, with the use of a *wand,* is just as easy.

Printed text may be captured from an electronic copy of the document (via a *scanner*) and the application of optical character recognition (OCR) software.

Electronic communications

Adequate electronic communications are necessary. More details regarding data communications, standards and privacy issues are provided in Chapters 10, 5 and 8 respectively. Some basic requirements are listed here:

- physical connection between hardware apparatus. Cables are commonly used (telephone lines, twisted pair, coaxial, optic glass fibre transmitting laser light). Rays are not uncommon (infra-red, radio and microwaves).

- organisation and infrastructure. Hardware joined together forms a *network*. If the area involved is *local* (e.g. a hospital), then a *local area network* is formed. If the connections involved a *wide area*, then a *wide area network* is the result. Some times the data involved resides on a central computer to form a *central database*. It is possible to *distribute* the data so parts of it reside on many different and widely separated computers. A *distributed database* results. Provided the computer knows the whereabouts of the required data, a distributed database can be made to behave very much like a central database. The creation, organisation, regulation and maintenance of complex national networks represents a major infrastructure. Expansion of these networks or *data highways* to carry vast quantities of information (e.g. a moving picture to every home) has coined the phrase *super data highways*. Nations are currently negotiating their construction. They will have the capacity to carry all the required medical and educational data for the nation's health care.
- standards. An electronic message must be *packaged* so the network knows who sent it and where it is to go. On arrival, the message must be correctly processed. This requires that specific instruction be included within the message. Standard *message formats* and *transmission protocols* are the essential ingredients.

International and national organisations are devoted to the creation and maintenance of standards. Without them much of our complex civilisation could not function. In the health care communication field, the following standards may be encountered:

- OSI or Open Systems Interconnection standards. This specifies a seven layered structure with many options. Options may be specified to form an optimised profile for a specific purpose. One example is GOSIP.
- GOSIP, or the Government OSI Profile, has been specified for public sector use in Australia, Europe, and North America.
- EDI, or Electronic Document Interchange is a standard for message transmission. Currently EDIFACT standard messages are evolving.
- EDIFACT, or EDI For Administration, Commerce and Transport is a message standard adopted by the UK and of interest to Europe, New Zealand and Australia. It has a well defined set of message structures and rules for the development of new messages. Standard health care messages are largely undefined at this stage.
- MEDIX, or MEDIcal data eXchange is a language specification for the output of hardware used in healthcare. It has North American origins.
- HL-7, or Health Level-7 refers to the seventh level of the OSI standard. It is a language specification for the output of hardware used in health care. North America has widely adopted HL-7. It is of interest to Australia and New Zealand.
- MIB, or Medical Information Bus is a defined data exchange protocol to enable laboratory equipment and computers to be interconnected.
- ASTM or American Standards for Testing and Materials which has a Clinical Data Interchange Standard (E1238).

Safeguards

Adequate security, confidentiality and integrity safeguards must evolve with improved information management. *Security* refers to the ease with which non-authorised people can access data. *Confidentiality* refers to the anonymity of the patient or health care provider. *Integrity* refers to the accuracy of the data.

As the data held within a system become more secure and more confidential, the less accessible it becomes to those who have authority to access it. Any system is a compromise.

Security is attained by *locks* (on doors, windows and computers) and *user identification* (by the use of passwords, magnetic stripe badges, smart keys and PIN numbers, security beams emitting badges, thumb print recognition and voice imprint recognition). Once a system has granted access, only that information and those actions allowed by the access code will be made available to the user. Thus an accountant may see all financial data, but no clinical data. The data itself can be disguised by *encryption*. This process jumbles the data according to a formula which contains an access code supplied by an authorised user. The unjumbling process (*decryption*) can occur only if the access code is supplied. A system of *smart keys* (using 'smart card technology') and personal identification numbers (PIN) can be used to encrypt and decrypt data for secure transmission.

Confidentiality may appear to result if only authorised people access data, and patient and provider identifying information has been removed to create anonymity. However, it is possible to electronically *cross match data* from several sources and determine with a possibly high degree of accuracy, the name of the provider or patient. *Legislation* is designed to prevent government authorities unlawfully cross matching data.

Integrity of data involves the accuracy of the data received (e.g. from the patient), and the accuracy of its interpretation (e.g. by the doctor), and the accuracy with which it is entered into, and stored and transmitted by the computer. Elaborate mathematical data integrity checking occurs as a computer manages its data. During processing, the hardware is unlikely to change data by error without notifying the user. However the program (software) may be instructing the computer incorrectly. To ensure a program acts correctly it must be tested. It is not possible to test a complex program in all combinations of circumstances. Thus, no program is absolutely error free.

Benefits

As stated earlier, information technology should not be applied to health care information management unless all concerned benefit—the computing industry, the healthcare funding organisations, the healthcare providers, and the patients.

The computing industry should benefit by the increased sales of computer hardware, software and communication resources.

Funding and administration organisations should benefit by an improvement in the education of and information available to the public, students, providers, administrators and epidemiologists. If it is known what is happening and what is needed, resources can be better allocated. A better quality and less costly health service is a potential outcome.

The provider should benefit by a saving of time, by a reduction of tedium, and an increase in the quality of care. Because continuing health care education becomes less time consuming and tedious, a reduction of errors, excesses and litigation should result.

The patient should benefit from a quality health care service which offers efficient communication between providers, organisations and patients. A better informed patient is more equipped for self-care.

REFERENCES

Commission on Professional and Hospital Activities 1978 International Classification of diseases, 9th revision, clinical modification (ICD-9-CM). Edward Brothers, Ann Arbor, Michigan

Computer Aided Medical Systems 1993 Read codes system developers' guide. CAMS, Leicestershire, UK

Computer Aided Medical Systems 1994 Read codes version 3.1 system developers' guide addendum. CAMS, Leicestershire, UK

Cote R A, Robboy S 1980 Progress in medical information management, Systematised Nomenclature of Medicine (SNOMED). Journal of the American Medical Association 243(8)

Cote R A, Rothwell D J, Beckett R S, Palotay J L, Brochu L 1993 The systematised nomenclature of human and veterinary medicine: SNOMED, international introduction. College of American Pathologists

Department of Community Services and Health 1994 Medical benefit schedule book. AGPS, Canberra

Humphreys B L, Lindberg D A B 1989 Building the unified medical language system. In: Kingsland L C (ed) Proceedings of the Thirteenth Annual Symposium on Computer Applications in Medical Care. IEEE Computer Society Press, Washington

Hupp J A, Cimino J J, Hoffer E F, Lowe H J, Barnett G O 1986 DX-plain: a computer-based diagnostic knowledge base. In: Proceedings of the Fifth World Conference on Medical Informatics (MEDINFO 86). Amsterdam

Lamberts H, Wood M (eds) 1987 ICPC International Classification of Primary Care. Oxford University Press, Oxford

McCray A T 1989 The UMLS semantic network. In: Kingsland L C (ed) Proceedings of the Thirteenth Annual Symposium on Computer Applications in Medical Care. IEEE Computer Society Press, Washington

Miller R A, McNeil M A, Challinor S M, Masarie F E Jr, Myers J D 1986 The INTERNIST-1 QUICK MEDICAL REFERENCE project: status report. Western Journal of Medicine 145

National Library of Medicine 1994 Medical subject headings, annotated alphabetical list. NLM, Bethesda, Maryland

National Library of Medicine, US Department of Health and Human Services and National Institutes of Health 1990 General description of META-1. In: UMLS knowledge sources experimental edition September 1990, documentation draft

Sherertz D, Tuttle M, Cole W, Erlbaum M, Olson N, Nelson S 1989 A hypercard implementation of meta-1: the first version of the umls metathesaurus. In:

Kingsland L C (ed) Proceedings of the Thirteenth Annual Symposium on Computer Applications in Medical Care. IEEE Computer Society Press, Washington

Warner H R, Haug P, Bouhaddou O, Lincoln M, Warner H Jr, Sorenson D, Williamson J W, Fan C 1988 ILIAD as an expert consultant to teach differential diagnosis. In: Greenes R A (ed) Proceedings of the Twelfth Annual Symposium on Computer Applications in Medical Care, IEEE Computer Society Press, Washington

World Health Organization 1977 International classification of diseases: manual of the international statistical classification of diseases, injuries, and causes of death, 9th revision. WHO, Geneva

2

Basic informatics concepts

5

Standards in health informatics

EVELYN J S HOVENGA

Standards are the key to facilitate the sharing and exchange of information between departments, health agencies and health workers. They are needed for the information content, language used, database and system architectures to facilitate linkage between systems through an apparently seamless integration of highly distributed systems. This is often referred to as *interoperability*. Electronic medical or health records require standards to index and to catalogue health related information effectively for rapid retrieval and to obtain uniform clinical data for research purposes. Without standards, classification and coding systems we are unable to compare the health status, processes of health care, costs and outcomes between various treatment options, health agencies, regions or countries in a meaningful way.

In industry generally the adoption of standards has resulted in an increase in market opportunities and lower costs for equipment and services to users. In health informatics the widespread adoption of standards is expected to improve the health of the nation's population at a lower cost by improving the ability of health professionals, public and health service administrators to share and make better use of the information generated.

What are standards?

A standard may be defined as a prescribed set of rules, conditions or requirements concerning definitions of terms, classification of components, specifications of materials, performance of operations, delineation of procedures, or measurement of quantity and quality in describing materials, products, systems, services or practices. Standards are benchmarks. Effective standards are needed to guide conditions of data access and data usage and to make it technically feasible to exchange data electronically. This is a prerequisite to cost efficient and accurate data collection and storage, which enhances the retrieval of quality health information needed to obtain the correct knowledge on which to base decisions. Information exchange requires standards which provide a mutual understanding of the meaning of the data used. That is, a standard language is needed and the context within which health data or other related information, such as a personal identifier, date and time which are related to clinical observations, are collected must not be lost. Standards may be mandated or be adopted voluntarily.

According to Megargle (1991) the quality of the knowledge thus obtained is dependent upon three factors: reliability, relevancy and responsiveness. High quality can only be delivered when standards dealing with issues such as electronic compatibility, character encoding and message structuring are adhered to by the many different computer environments and software programs which may need to be connected to make for example one hospital network. Standards development for health informatics requires input from discipline experts; that is, those who need to use the information and knowledge provided by a system. Much of this knowledge now resides in medical records and the health related literature.

Who develops standards?

Various health and related professional groups, both public and private organisations have established standards for paper based health records, for health information systems, for health service delivery and for the health professions. Many such organisations have also implemented mechanisms by which compliance with these standards could be measured. As the automation of health information and communication technology is progressing it has become more apparent that standards for documentation and electronic data interchange within the health care sector are urgently required if we are to maximise the benefits offered through the use of these new information and communication technologies. The health care sector has special communication needs.

Several organisations nationally and internationally are addressing this issue from various perspectives. Many standards applicable to information and communication technology generally need to be adopted within the health care sector. But additional standards are required specifically to meet the unique needs of the health care sector especially in the areas of data specifications, data integrity and security. Increasingly these are being developed through the well established standards organisations such as Standards Australia, the European Standardisation Committee (CEN), the Institute of Electrical and Electronics Engineers (IEEE), the American Society for Testing Materials (ASTM), the American National Standards Institute (ANSI), the European Strategic Program for Research and Development in Information Technologies (ESPRIT), the International Standards Organisation (ISO), and many others or through ad hoc groups such as Health Level 7 (HL7). In 1991 Mandil (1991) noted that 'despite progress in recent years, the lack of standards remains a major impediment to technical and international collaboration in health and health informatics'. He went on to say that standards 'tend to liberate cornered clients but (that) they also increase uses of the technology and hence its clientele'.

European standardisation activities for health informatics began in 1990 when the CEN established Technical Committee 251. Standards Australia established its IT/14 committee on health informatics early in 1991. A Healthcare Informatics Standards Planning Panel (HISPP) was established by ANSI late 1991 to bring together the many standards groups which had been developing medical informatics for nearly a decade. Since then many more activities have taken place. In 1993 CEN's Technical Committee 251 published a directory of the European standardisation requirements for health care informatics which includes a program for the development of standards. Also in 1993 CEN/TC251 and ANSI/HISPP produced a publication detailing the worldwide progress made in standardisation in health care informatics (De Moor, McDonald, Noothoven van Goor 1993). There is considerable collaboration between the various standards organisations. Priorities for standard development are guided by considerations regarding feasibility, user requirements, medical benefits, and economical impact (CEN/TC 251 1993).

Which standards should be developed?

Individual needs for standards are being identified daily and concurrently with activities such as the Advanced Informatics in Medicine (AIM) project (Rossing 1993) and the Health Care Information and Communication Network (RICHE) in Europe, the Australian Health Communication Network (HCN), the development of systems to support electronic health records, and with the introduction of new government policies which aim to provide greater accountability and contain costs. There is consensus that ultimately there will be a desire to have longitudinal (from birth to death) electronic health records to overcome the problems and costs associated with a highly mobile population, increasing specialisation within the health sector, duplication of data collection, incomplete and inaccurate medical histories and incomplete data for research and policy development purposes. Three years ago Murphy (1991) reported that a standard description for the content and structure of an automated longitudinal health record was under development. European countries and the United States of America have allocated millions of dollars towards standards development in recognition of this need. It is postulated that accurate and complete information will lead to improved knowledge, better decision making, improved quality of care, less cost and better use of available resources.

Gabrielli (1991) identified three reasons for why the medical record was slow to be automated: the extensive use of narrative text; a lack of a standard medical terminology; and the lack of a medically useful taxonomic code scheme. As a result he notes that clinical experiences are available to others only via expensive research studies. Manual monitoring of the quality of care is labour intensive, and health care policies are more intuitive than fact driven.

Adoption of standards

The adoption of standards may be mandatory or voluntary, and various types of standards exist. The type of standard is determined by who has developed or adopted the standard or by the purpose for which the standard was developed. For example many activities are directed towards the development of a common medical (health) language which is the subject of Chapter 4. There are corporate standards developed and used by one company alone, and industry standards which represent the standards used by an entire industry. There are government standards such as GOSIP (Government Open Systems Interconnection Profile), and there are consensus standards. The adoption of consensus standards are the result of input from all stakeholders and are the most useful, but they may take years to develop.

The adoption of standards is achieved more rapidly when users or potential users insist that suppliers comply with consensus standards. One of the reasons the health care industry in Australia and possibly other countries, is so far behind other industries in this regard is because purchasers have continued to acquire proprietry systems. As these vendors are unable to satisfy all health information needs, there is a proliferation of disparate systems and an industry devoted to connecting them with tailor made solutions (interfaces). On the other hand a generic and ultimately more cost effective solution providing faster connectivity, is to adopt the what is referred to as the *open* solution, which requires only minor adjustments to link machines.

Open systems are those with which other systems can communicate via highly distributed systems. However the extent of such 'openness' appears to vary. Bakker (1994) identified five different meanings for the term. Open systems may be characterised by:

- the possibility to communicate with other systems
- extract data for external use
- import data from external systems in the database
- run the system on different hardware platforms
- extend an information system with modules from another supplier.

The ability to extend an information system is possible only if different suppliers produce identical modules. Bakker provided an analogy with cars. Both cars and health information systems are made up of many parts; however the engine meant for one car does not necessarily fit another. He notes that for some of the essential aspects of openess, consensus of users and standardisation are indispensable. Chapter 10 discusses data communications in more detail.

Although open systems are highly desirable, the degree of openness, or rather access to various components of such connected systems, must be controlled to maintain patient privacy. Standards are required specifically to ensure that systems enable adherance to privacy and freedom of information legislation, where applicable for system security, and to deter unauthorised access to information. Chapter 8 is devoted to this topic.

From a user perspective, standards are also required for the user interface. These are emerging slowly. The aim is to allow users to quickly navigate and use any system with minimal training as users within the health sector often need to access a number of different computer applications.

Conclusion

The development of standards for use in health informatics is pivotal to more and better use of information and communications technology in the health industry. Considerable progress has been made to date; however the widespread adoption of standards has been slow. Purchasers especially need to include the need for standard compliance in their system specifications.

REFERENCES

Bakker A 1994 Open systems: perspective or fata morgana? In: Grobe S J, Pluyter-Wenting E S P (eds) Nursing Informatics: an international overview for nursing in a technological era. Elsevier, Amsterdam

CEN/TC 251 1993 Directory of the European standardisation requirements for health care informatics and programme for the development of standards version 1.7, Gent, Belgium

De Moor G J E, McDonald C J, Noothoven van Goor J (eds)1993 Progress in standardization in Health Care informatics. IOS Press, Amsterdam

Gabrielli E R 1991 Need for standards in medical communication. Topics of Health Record Management 11(4)

Mandil S H 1991 Health Informatics should influence, and be influenced by, its key components: the example of Nursing Informatics. In: Hovenga E J S, Hannah K J, McCormick K A, Ronald J S (eds) Lecture Notes in Medical Informatics Volume 42, Proceedings of Nursing Informatics '91, Springer-Verlag, Heidelberg

Megargle R 1991 Role of ASTM in computer information standards for medicine. Topics of Health Record Management 11(4)

Murphy G 1991 Standards for automated patient records. Topics of Health Record Management 11(4)

Rossing N 1993 Health Care Telematics in the European Communities. In: De Moor G J E, McDonald C J, Noothoven van Goor J (eds)1993 Progress in Standardization in Health Care Informatics. IOS Press, Amsterdam

Conclusion

REFERENCES

6

Basic applications and expectations

TREVOR LORD

Most health professionals would agree that computer technology could help with many aspects of their work. The problem lies in using the computer. The focus of undergraduate and post graduate training is on delivering health care and information management and information technology have had a low priority in this process. Many health professionals complete their tertiary education with little or no exposure to computers.

We are all busy and keeping up with our professional work and continuing education takes time. Developing computer skills requires a commitment in time. However gaining a short term benefit from a simple useful computer application will enable a new user to maintain interest. From this point skill can be developed further into more serious use of the technology.

The first problem is communicating with the computer. In the past learning to type was a skill reserved for those moving into clerical tasks. Keyboard skills are required to use a computer well. This is rapidly changing. Speech will soon be the major form of communication between the computer and its user. This will break down many of the barriers faced by health professionals in the past. The next problem is: what immediate use do you have for a computer? If we look at surveys of computer usage amongst medical practitioners the major usage is in the simple tasks (Wynekoop 1994). This chapter looks at these simple tasks to ask: What are they, what do you need and what are the benefits?

Communicating with the computer

The keyboard and screen are still the major communication vehicles between us and the computer. In the early 1980s we all thought we would be talking to computers before the end of that decade. The task of identifying all the variations of human speech proved more difficult than first anticipated. The computer has problems with our accents, and with words that are phonetically similar. Further problems arise when minor illness affects our pronunciation. It takes a great deal of processing power to incorporate these variations. Despite the rapid advance in hardware technology it took some time to deliver sufficient power in a low cost personal computer format. Even with speech recognition and touchscreen technology now well established in the personal computer world, keyboard skills are still an essential element.

The keyboard

The design of the original QWERTY keyboard is to slow down the user. Letter placement defies logic to a user faced with the keyboard for the first time. In fact the frequently used letters are relatively inaccessible.

The computer keyboard has added complexity. There are at least twelve function keys labelled F1-F12. These have different roles in different software packages. F1 has an almost constant role: it will generate the help information in most software packages.

In addition to the SHIFT key there is an ALTERNATE (ALT) and a CONTROL (CTRL) key. These are relatively easy to use. Like a SHIFT key, they are used with letters, numbers or the function (F1-F12) keys. They differ from the SHIFT key in that they generate commands to the computer instead of simply placing characters on the screen. The commands vary depending on what computer software package you are using. For instance in a common word processing package CONTROL + A generates a command to format all the characters as capitals. In a common database package CONTROL + A means locate the next field in the database.

In addition to a numeric keypad and arrow (direction) keys there are usually eleven other keys. These are easier to understand. The ENTER key is the most important. It tells the computer to accept what the user has typed or to run a particular task offered by the computer. ESC is a favourite key—it means escape out of here. It is particularly important to the new user when exploring the unknown. Pressing ESCAPE will return the user back to the previous step or out of the programme. PAGE UP, PAGE DOWN, DELETE, INSERT, HOME and END mean what they say. PRINT SCREEN, SCROLL LOCK and the pause or break are little used.

Combining the CONTROL + ALTERNATE + DELETE key generates a command used often by the new user. This restarts the computer erasing the current tasks. This resets the computer back to the state it was in when it was initially switched on. The major disadvantage is that one loses any new work that has been created but not filed. All the keys beyond the standard typewriter keyboard generate commands not characters and most computer programs give guidance on how to use the extra keys.

The mouse and the graphical user interface (GUI)

Older design software relied on the user learning or at least becoming familiar with the command keys and when to use them. This added greatly to the barrier for the new user. Unfortunately most of the common medical record software has retained this system. With the advent of the mouse it has become much easier to drive modern software.

The mouse and a screen layout called the Graphical User Interface changed the face of personal computing. A Graphical User Interface (GUI) is where the computer software produces pictures and pull down menus to indicate the choice of commands available to the user. A mouse (or other pointing devices) controls a moving arrow on the screen. The user points at the command and presses a button on the mouse or presses the computer enter key to request that the computer runs the command.

No longer does the user have to learn which keys to press to generate a command. Instead it is available on the screen. 'Point and click' reduced the learning time for new users. The GUI made it easy for anyone to learn to use a computer.

Touch screen technology was available prior to the common use of the GUI and the mouse. Hardware technological development usually precedes software innovation. A sophisticated computer screen can provide input to the computer. When the user touches the screen, the screen identifies the location of the touch. The software processes the location of the touch and uses this information to generate a particular response. The computer can then use this information to respond to a command or the input of information.

This is particularly good for situations where non-computer users need to communicate. Shopping center location maps and automated post offices provide good examples of the use of this form of interface. The disadvantages include the slow speeds, the cost of the screens and the limitations of size in defining the location of the touch point. Modern electronic diaries have taken this technology to the next stage. They have combined touch screen technology with the Graphical User Interface.

Apple was the first to effectively market the GUI. It did not take the IBM and compatible personal computer world long to see the benefit of the GUI environment. Microsoft designed Windows to fill the role. This is now the major GUI interface around the world.

The real advantage of GUI is that the command format is the same across a wide range of computer software applications. For instance a user will find that a word processing package, a database, a cashbook and a spreadsheet all look much the same in a GUI system. Pull down menus for filing new and finding old material are the same. Common tasks such as Cut, Copy and Paste are requested from the same pull down menus across different packages. Once a user has learned basic commands in one package they find that they can easily drive others.

The GUI controls the printer and printing initiated by any software package. The process of printing is standard from any application running under the GUI. The Help screens are standardised. In any application Indexing and Searching are the same. Learning new software becomes a matter of understanding the principles of what it can do rather than learning yet another detailed set of commands.

Having learned to drive a word processing package one can move easily into driving a database or spreadsheet. It is simply a question of understanding what a database is and how it can help you. Prior to the GUI it would take many weeks of use to learn to drive a database even when the concepts were understood. Today it may take one to two days to get to a level of reasonable productivity.

The medical software industry has been slow to develop within the GUI environment. This has contributed to the slow implementation of medical records in practices. This situation is rapidly changing and most major suppliers have or are developing software for the GUI.

The GUI allows the user to drive the commands. The user still has to type to enter information and data. In medical records and other health applications there is a great deal of information and typing skills to some level are still essential.

Typing

The computer itself has proved a useful tool in teaching people to type. One can run any number of typing tutor programs on a computer and learn to type without taking the time to travel to lessons. Few health professionals however take advantage of these programs. Most prefer to hunt and peck. This is using one finger on each hand and hunting around the keyboard looking for letters in the manner of a chook in a yard. Gradually their speed improves. They start to learn where the keys are and use more than the two index fingers. Eventually one can slowly progress to typing without looking at the keyboard (touch typing).

There is good evidence that learning to touch type from the start is more efficient. Health professionals spend most of their time consulting and communicating with other people. A computer can be a tremendous barrier in this communication. Most write notes as they go and loose eye contact with the patient or client. To type can be even worse. A health professional skilled in touch typing can maintain eye contact and still generate notes.

Typing tutor programs make reasonable claim to teach basic touch typing with less than a day of user time. In learning to type the user needs to be in a situation where they can continue to use and build on the skill immediately. Moving straight into word processing can be an easy way to accomplish this. Having someone skilled in word processing build the format for a letter or document to allow the user to enter text is a productive way to build skill.

Voice recognition and notepads

Voice input has been available in various forms since the late 1970s and it is now available at reasonable cost for the average user. The current programs are useful in word processing, but they are only just starting to be useful for commanding the computer and running other software programs.

English has a large vocabulary. In addition, many words with different meanings sound the same. To complicate matters we have many quite different pronunciations within the English speaking world and minor upper respiratory illness further alters the pronunciation. Extraneous noise compounds the problems.

We can speak quite rapidly and as we speak the computer has to compare each word with its own phonetic list. The computing power required to do this at reasonable speed is enormous. It is only in the last few years that the average personal computer user has had access to the power required to run voice recognition. Many companies are developing in this area. Voice recognition programs draw heavily on the computer power and the memory storage. A typical example requires a computer with 12 megabytes of Random Access Memory (RAM) to run and occupies 22 megabytes of hard disk space with an additional 5 megabytes required for each individual user.

Most voice systems come with both software and hardware. The software consists of the programs to run the system and the dictionary. The hardware includes the voice card to fit inside the computer and the headset microphone. This raises another issue for the health professional—a headset microphone is a definite intrusion into the consultation. New directional microphones are now being designed that attach to the computer terminal. These are likely to be more acceptable to patients.

Currently these systems are still less efficient than learning to type. Typing is still required for difficult words and one still needs to learn to use the normal computer applications.

Notepads are another mode of entry. A notepad is a small hand held personal computer. The user can print or write using a special pen on the notepad and it will respond to a command written with the pen. The software then interprets that writing and converts it to text. This is slower than moderate typing speeds. This technology is designed for the electronic diary type application

For the new user a GUI as seen in the Apple or Windows environments is an essential starting point. One can then focus on understanding the concepts and functions of the software application. Gone is the need to spend endless hours learning the complex commands to drive the computer.

Specific applications

Health professionals have found a number of basic software applications important to their everyday needs. The relative importance depends on the nature of their work.

Word processing

This is still the major software application of the personal computer. Old typewritten and handwritten letters no longer fit the image of the modern health professional. Who has not seen the occasional referral letter written on prescription stationary? 'Dear doctor herewith Mrs Jones, chest pain, please take over her care.' To promote a confident professional image modern health communication needs clarity, detail and legibility. Word processing meets this need.

A word processor is a software package that combines a text editor with sophisticated formatting and page layout tools. Fifteen years ago to be able to bold, center and underline were the new important features. Today the modern programs can format and produce a full text book ready for the printer.

For health professionals there have been further changes to word processors that are important. Take producing a letter. When comparing word processing for yourself with dictating to a clerical person you may conclude that the dictating consumes less time. The time consuming task for the professional is the formatting and layout of the document, particularly a letter. Modern word processors solve this with document templates and intuitive help tools.

The program already contains basic formats for letters, memos, faxes, agendas, reports presentations, résumés and any number of other basic office documents. The user can choose the appropriate layout and simply fill in the details. The software automatically creates the page and document layout. The software can also produce the envelope information and send it to the printer.

Some of the help tools will take a user through producing their own version of a letter or other document. By asking the user a series of questions the software designs the appropriate document format. This further expands the flexibility of the program. The user can focus on the content and forget the extraneous formatting detail.

The programs retain mailing names and addresses. One can quickly recall these details for use in future letters. This includes merging one letter with an address list sending out any number of personalised letters from one typed letter.

An average typing speed and working knowledge of the word processing package enables the health professional to match the speed of clerical personnel when producing documents.

The GUI has made a big difference to the word processing software. Altering a margin is simple. Point and grab at the edge of the margin and then drag it to the new position. A page layout view is available when editing a document. The screen then provides the same layout on the page as will be seen on the printed document. Called What You See Is What You Get (WYSIWYG) this tool has enhanced the ease of using a word processor.

One can use many different fonts and sizes of fonts throughout one document. One can place lines, drawings, tables and graphs anywhere in the document. Tools such as spelling checkers, grammar checkers and on-line thesaurus add to the value of using a word processing package. A spelling tool can go through and check the document. It will learn new words or names from the user's response to corrections. One can add a medical dictionary to the word processing dictionaries.

In addition the word processor can trap common spelling errors as the user types. It can then be set to correct these errors automatically. It can also retain common abbreviations converting them to the full version (e.g. type

'GP' and the computer responds with 'general practitioner'). It will keep track of documents retaining the most recently used documents on a simple list for recalling.

With the advent of the fax one can now set the computer up to fax straight from the word processing package into the telephone.

The current major packages include Word and Wordperfect. Both are available in a Windows and an Apple format. Each one leaps the other with additional features in the new versions. Using a word processor even at a sophisticated level is easy. A few hours of training and the new user can expect to feel comfortable with most of the tasks described. For the health professional a word processor is an essential tool.

Spreadsheets

For the organised and mathematically minded the spreadsheet is a creative tool. In its simplest form it is a table of columns and rows. The intersecting space is a cell. A cell can retain text, numbers, formulas or a macro. A macro is a small program that performs a simple task. Formulae and macros can be combined to make the spreadsheet one of the most powerful basic computing tools.

The spreadsheet program builds a large number of functions around this basic table structure. A single cell can contain a large amount of information. The user controls how much is displayed and in what format. A cell may contain a formula to average the contents of a number of other cells. One can set the cell to display either the formula or the resulting number. The user can then manipulate the formula and assess the result.

A large range of mathematical, statistical, logical, date/time, special and financial formulas are available for use in a cell. These vary from simple sum, average and standard deviation to complex financial tools. Each formula can include data from a range of other cells in the table. Formulas can be combined to achieve a vast range of functions.

In addition spreadsheets can be used to calculate 'what if' solutions to research, financial and other mathematical problems. 'What If' functions allow the user to build up a set of information and then use the computer to model the outcome of different sets of conditions or events.

The problem for the new spreadsheet user is comprehending the power and flexibility. It takes time to build up more than a basic range of formulas and functions. Often there are short cuts in handling a problem that the user will not know. Modern spreadsheet software actually monitors what the user is doing and will offer these short cuts as an alternative. This allows the user to build skills as they use the tool.

There are unlimited ways to use a spreadsheet. The most common use is for financial tasks—building budgets and financial models. In the health area the uses extend to research (data collection and statistical analysis), graphing information and analysing data direct from databases (medical record software).

It is more difficult to learn to use a spreadsheet than most other computer tools. For the non-computer user it is difficult to understand the concept of a spreadsheet. There is no equivalent non-computer based tool. The range, size and complexity of spreadsheets defy our capacity to conceptualise them.

A single sheet table can be eight thousand rows by two hundred and fifty-six columns. This is two million cells. One can expand this by having more than two hundred such tables in the particular spreadsheet file. One can use a formula or macro to build a relationship between one cell and any other cell in the whole file of more than four hundred million cells. In addition one can relate the information in a cell or range of cells to a completely separate spreadsheet file. Consider that for a multi-dimensional mathematical puzzle.

In large organisations a number of people will build a particular spreadsheet. They will share their spreadsheet over a computer network. They can use information from sections of the file created and updated by another member of the team. One needs to foster true team management in these circumstances. Issues such as data security and back up of data are of paramount importance.

The current major spreadsheet tools available are Microsoft Excel for Windows or Apple, Lotus 123 for Windows and Borlands Quattro for Windows. Like the word processing programs the newest version of each of these will leap frog the other two in terms of function. For the health professional interested in research, administration or practice management learning to use and working with spreadsheets is challenging, productive and fun.

Database applications

At a conceptual level a database is easier to understand than a spreadsheet. We have a non-computer equivalent. It is a filing cabinet. Each drawer contains a set of information. Within each drawer is a set of files. In each file are pages of information relevant to that file.

The computer based filing cabinet is more rigid. The drawers are similar. At the file level there is a defined structure. The term for the individual file is a table. The table consists of columns and rows. Each column defines the nature of the information (e.g. surname, initials, date of birth). Each row is a record in the table (e.g. Bloggs, J H, 24 January 1952).

A database program allows the user to build their own tables. The user defines the fields of information. What will go in the field (e.g. a number, a date, text), its length and any special properties (e.g. default to female, default to today's date). Once a table and the information are defined, the user can enter the data. This data then forms the records in the table.

The most startling difference between a filing cabinet and the computer database is in the way the computer can handle the information. The computer can quickly sort the table into any required order. The user may want to sort by postcode or by date of birth. Knowing the structure of the table one can quickly determine the field containing postcode. The computer can then sort the whole table by that field. It can sort by more than one field (e.g. list the patients by the field age and then by the field sex).

One can ask the computer to pull out a subset of the information. One defines the field and type of information required (e.g. in the table of patients, list all the patients where the field sex contains the term female). This process is filtering of the information. By sorting and filtering one can manipulate and analyse the information in a computer database to an extent not possible in the paper equivalent.

There is an additional concept not so evident in the paper filing system. One can link tables. In the paper world we do this by making a reference (e.g. see file on medication, page 25 paragraph 2). In a computer database this is much more powerful. We can relate one table to another table through a common field of information. This field will need to be present in each table. In a medical record system we may wish relate the table containing patient medication records to the table containing the patients' details. To do this we would need a common field or fields. The easiest common field would be a patient number. By having the patient number in the table of patient details and in the table of medication records one can relate the two tables.

A database program with this facility is a relational database. A single table is limited. Consider a medical record. Defining fields for the name, address and date of birth is easy. How do we incorporate the need to have a medication list or a list of allergies? The table becomes very large with a field each for one medication, one allergy, one health problem, etc. What if the patient is on two medications?

When one can build relationships between tables then a table can be small and simple with a limited number of fields. Medications, allergies, health problems and patient details would each be in their own tables. The relationships between the tables allow the computer to put the information together.

The sorting and filtering functions can be added to this relational database. This produces a powerful information management tool. List all the female patients over forty with hypertension and on medication is a massive task in a paper medical record filing system. In a relational computer database it is simple and fast.

There is a vast range of database tools. A medical record system is usually based on a relational database. Companies developing this type of software use these database tools and often programme a great deal of the database themselves.

The average health professional does not always need that level of performance. There are now simple modern database tools that are easy to use and will service most needs. Dbase was the original major personal computer based tool. There is now a range of easy to use Microsoft Windows and Apple based databases. They combine all the simple Windows based functions with a full relational database.

The graphical user interface has made a big difference to the ease of use. One can see the relationships between tables on the screen. A table is a physical table. The fields can be moved and re-defined by pointing with the mouse and dragging them across the screen. The relationships are seen as graphical lines between fields in the tables.

There are help tools that take the user through building a query or report. No longer does the user have to type a carefully prepared sentence in a strange version of English to retrieve information.

One could build a medical record system using the 'over the counter' database tools. It takes some time and considerable skill with the chosen product to do this. It is the design, layout and relationships of the tables that causes the most problems. A poor initial data structure will diminish the efficiency of the system. As the system develops this underlying weakness will become more obvious. This is a major frustration for amateur medical record designers. Another problem is the speed of the software when under the loads of large complex medical record tables. Poor design will reduce the speed of the program. In health care the speed of information management is a key feature.

Not all health professionals want full medical records. One may wish to create a subset of a medical record. For example an infant health nurse may wish to track some aspect of children's health. Building a data collection and reporting for this type of application is now quite easy with the modern tools. A three day course on a typical relational database would allow the average user to build such an application.

A new feature of the modern programs is the ability to integrate with other databases. This includes mainframe systems. A user with a commercial medical record system could attach tables from the medical records to tables in their own database. By building relationships between the tables from both systems they have access to composite data. For example one may build a simple table containing information about diabetic patients in a personal computer database. One could then attach the patient names and address table from the main medical record system. The personal computer can now use the address information combined with the list of people with diabetes to mail out a letter to all diabetics.

Care must be taken when connecting different databases. Firstly confidentiality may be an issue. Who has access to what information? How will it be used? In a commercial medical record package the designers have usually thought through these issues and set safeguards. By networking one database to another one can bypass some of these safeguards.

An additional problem is in the potential to corrupt data in the host database. If one uses a personal computer database to alter data on the main medical record computer then it is possible to seriously damage the medical record information. One needs to understand the structure and function of both databases before using one to alter information on the other.

It is relatively safe to use different tools to read and report on information. For changing or adding information it is important to use the original product that created and is responsible for maintaining that data.

Object linking adds an extra benefit in using a modern database. Object linking is where information created and stored in one application is used in another. For instance one may create a Diabetic mailing list in a database. With object linking that information can be linked to a letter in a word processing tool. When the letter is created, the word processing package can open the database and retrieve the latest mailing list.

Another example of object linking is creating a budget in a spreadsheet. One can link the tables from that budget to a financial planning document in word processing. An alteration to the figures in the spreadsheet appears the next time the word processor prints the financial plan document. These features add a great deal to productivity in the administration, practice management and research areas. They are an important function within the Windows environment. Most major software producers are taking advantage of this object linking feature.

Presentation software

Health professionals have to communicate well. Modern presentation software provides some real solutions. Take the typical presentation to a group of people. One needs an outline, speaker's notes, slides or overheads and a handout. Modern presentation software allows the user to create all these with a minimum of duplication.

The modern laser and the colour ink jet printers can create overhead templates direct from the software in colour. The computer can place the images on a disk for colour slide production. The tools that automatically process the computer image on to 35mm slides are now relatively inexpensive.

The software can correct spelling. It can use object linking to grab charts from the spreadsheet or text from a document created in the word processor. Large files of diagrams and illustrations come with the software. These can be quickly incorporated into the overhead. The software comes with tutorials on the computer and on-line help. A course is not necessary but is more efficient. A half day will assist the average user to generate simple and effective presentations.

The modern software will produce miniature copies of each overhead. It then places speaker's notes beneath these. These can then be used as prompts during the presentation. The software can produce a handout by combining two or three overheads on one page, printing them out for photocopying. The time taken to generate a full quality presentation is reduced considerably. With all the information on the computer, updating and modifying the presentation is easy.

The slide show is another feature. Most presentation packages can link direct to video projection units. The presentation is transported to a notebook computer. The presenter then connects this to a video projection unit. The overheads run on the notebook as a slide show. The presenter uses a mouse to change slides as the presentation proceeds.

Financial tools

The simple financial tools have led the way in ease of use. The computer is particularly good at manipulating numbers. When this is combined with a graphical user interface one can change the face of small business management. There is a proliferation of all the financial tools. From simple cash books to full accounting and payroll tools, the choice is enormous. For less than one hundred dollars, users can finally bring some order to their personal finances.

Some of these tools act as cheque books. They can print cheques ready for you to sign. They keep track of all income and expenditure. They can then provide reports. One can group expenditure under tax deductible and non-tax deductible. All accounts and credit cards are entered and reconciled within the package.

In addition they can take the user through the process of producing a budget. One can build this from the preceeding years figures or from scratch. The computer will then convert this to a quarterly, monthly or weekly budget. Information entered during the year is reported alongside the expected budget figure. One can immediately see the variance and take corrective action. In addition to personal finances these packages are adequate for small companies such as medical practice, health care centre and community service agency.

More sophisticated packages are available for the larger business. These carry additional features such as general ledger facilities, accrual accounting and payroll. With increasing sophistication there is an associated increase in price. Ease of use is inversely proportional to sophistication. It is often tempting to go to these higher level packages.

The new user should choose a product however that suits current needs. Such a product is likely to be easier to use. With the development of one's own business there is usually a parallel development of the selected computer software.

The cashbook is a good application for the novice computer user. It provides immediate tangible benefits for little learning time. The tutorials in the manuals and on-line are usually adequate to get a good grasp of the product.

Payroll products have been slow to develop. They are specific to Australian conditions and it has not been easy to revise a popular American product as is the case with cashbooks. Payroll is a difficult area to manage for most small business. Many health professionals practice through small business structures. The modern medium to high end cashbooks are adding payroll tools. For any business with more than a few employees this tool is easy to set up and can save considerable time.

REFERENCE

Wynekoop J L, Finan J A 1994 A survey of office computing in medical practices. MD Computing 11:107-113

Establishing user requirements

JEFF COOKE

There are several ways to go about establishing user requirements. One could just ask the users because they should know what they need— right? Or, one could ask the system analysts. After all, system analysts or managers are the ones with the requisite knowledge of information systems and the charter to define what their system should do — right? Isn't it really only a sprinkling of computers, spread sheet software and database? How difficult can that be, it's done all the time these days. Just hook them up, provide some training and— Voila!—we're in business. Well—not quite.

Recent experience suggests that both of these approaches end in catastrophic failure. First of all, in spite of our training or self education in *systems* methods and techniques, each scenario is different to various degrees. A 200 bed hospital is certainly different than a 50 bed hospital. What about the neighbourhood or small town surgery? Surely their needs and requirements will be different. In fact, aren't needs and requirements the same thing?

Objective

Getting slightly more serious now: the primary goal and responsibility of the leader of a systems development team is to establish a formal process and to manage this process toward a successful conclusion. What this chapter is about is to review a process, or methodology, which works.

To start with, one must carefully establish the difference between *needs* and *requirements*. Then, some tools are 'needed'. (The 'requirement' which partially satisfies this need are some forms to collect data and information). Also 'needed' is a structured methodology (the 'requirements' of which are described herein) which supports the collection of meaningful data through an interview technique. These forms are then collated, grouped, and prioritised into need categories. Once the top six or so need groupings have been identified, then and only then are we in a position to establish user requirements.

The methods for establishing user requirements which are believed to be most useful have a basis in project management, software development, and system specification 'standards' developed over some time by consulting firms, government agencies, and prestigious companies. These methods are regularly applied with various degrees of success. The material to follow is an integrated compilation of many different methods which have been applied and modified by experience gained in actual industry practice over many years. Although exposure here is necessarily brief, it is sufficient to get one on the way toward delivering quality results on time and within budget.

Terms and definitions

Before continuing, some definitions are in order:

AS-IS: the existing system or enterprise at the time of initial analysis. The current state of the system, warts and all.

Cost drivers: all of the financial factors influencing the enterprise. Examples include, but are not limited to, expense items e.g. surgical supplies, revenue, profit, capital, endowments, and labour.

Enterprise: the management, staff, buildings, infrastructure, support facilities and operations, all working in concert to provide cost effective and quality health service to the community. However, the degree of quality and cost effectiveness may vary considerably from enterprise to enterprise.

Income drivers: financial factors, including funding formulae and occasions of service, which determine revenues.

Information: data which have been organised to support the enterprise to function in an integrated manner, such as schedules, reports, policies and directives, and budgets.

Information resource management (IRM): the processing, organisation, and management of information associated with all functions affecting the quality of operations of the enterprise.

IS: information systems

NAD (Needs analysis document): The NAD is utilised 1) as a record of system needs and 2) as an analysis tool to determine system requirements.

Needs: needs define the baseline from which all improvements are measured for determination of effectiveness. They provide the primary input for establishing and defining user requirements.

Needs analysis: the process for identifying the AS-IS needs.

NISF: needs identification survey form

Requirements: identified characteristics, procedures, or specific improvements which satisfy a need previously identified in the needs analysis. It is important to understand that a requirement defines the degree of improvement necessary to satisfy a need and does not identify specific equipment or details.

RDR: requirements definition report. The RDR is based on the NAD and documents the requirements. It collects and presents alternative requirements and is linked to the needs in an easily traceable way.

SD: scoping document. The SD is the foundation document to establish user requirements. It is based on, and congruent with, the enterprise strategic plan and its contained mission statement. We can think of the SD as a contractual requirement, which states the purpose for and general results expected from the improvement analysis effort. It focuses our activity on a specific area of interest and establishes the boundary of what we hope to achieve. For example, a statement which requires us to 'identify and perform a complete review of all current operational deficiencies' is a project of far greater scope than one which says 'identify the ways and means to establish a computerized patient record system'.

SSR: System specification report. The SSR is beyond the scope of this chapter. It is included only to complete the picture of the entire system development life cycle as represented in Figure 7.1.

TO-BE: The AS-IS system with its enhancements and improvements applied which correct deficiencies identified in the needs analysis

TSR: Technical specification report. The TSR is beyond the scope of this chapter. It is included only to complete the picture of the entire system development life cycle as represented in Figure 7.1.

Users: managers, decision makers, medical practitioners, employees, and other health sector staff that use computer based information systems to their benefit. Their benefit, is of course, to help them work smarter rather than harder in delivering quality and cost effective health services.

Methodology overview

The proven methodology described in this chapter is simply the first phase of a structured approach to problem solving. Note again Figure 7.1, which a) describes four phases, each containing two steps; b) superimposes major documentation products; and c) superimposes a functional timeline mapped to the AS-IS and TO-BE models. It is a generic description which can be used for most system development, i.e. improvement projects of any size with very little modification. Note that this chapter concentrates on understanding the problem. In so doing the reward is documentation of the *needs* as well as the *requirements* to satisfy those *needs*. Necessarily then, the remainder of our focus in this chapter is only on Phase I of Figure 7.1.

At this point it is recommended that the reader review the definitions of the SD, NAD, RDR, TSR, and SSR. Each of these documents or reports is clearly identified in Figure 7.1 as outputs of a four phase program. It is re-emphasised that we are only focusing on the 'understand the problem' phase with its two major steps of performing a needs analysis and the requirements definition.

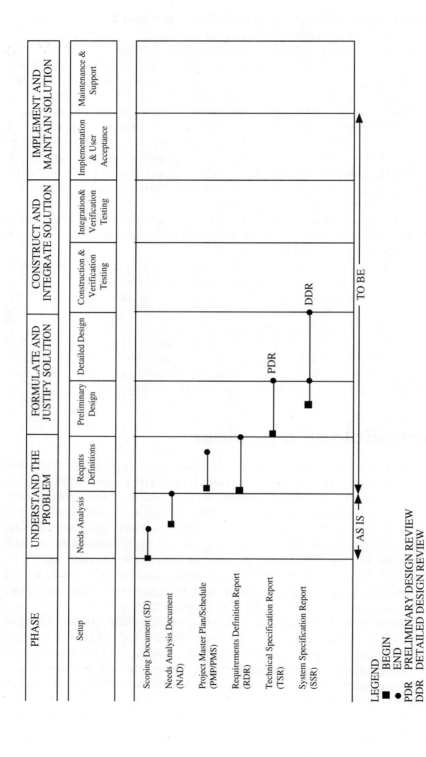

Fig. 7.1 System development life cycle (Documentation schedule)

Phase I: understand the problem

This first phase consists of two steps. These are:

1 Needs analysis step
2 Requirements definition step.

Needs analysis step

The SD is updated during the needs analysis step and the NAD is produced. The SD deals primarily with understanding the existing AS-IS system environment. The NAD is the transition document to the improved TO-BE system environment and identifies system needs.

Requirements definition step

Utilising the NAD, the RDR is produced. The RDR contains requirement categories derived from the NAD which describes and views the system in terms of specific system requirements definition, and provides sufficient criteria to enable system conceptual design, test and subsequent system evaluation. The RDR provides a breakdown of requirements in sufficient detail to enable subsequent conceptual design. The RDR is not expressed in terms of solutions, but rather is expressed in details of functional performance, physical and interface characteristics.

Establish the systems development team and project scope

Let's think about this title a minute. Why is it called the systems development team? First of all, we may not intend to literally develop anything! But to be complete, refer back to Figure 7.1. It makes sense to formulate a team which is broad enough to see the whole project to completion. The membership of the team can always be modified as appropriate, but for now, let us think in terms of a core or cadre of key players. For project continuity it is better that the same core follow the whole exercise through all four phases to its successful conclusion.

So who should these players be? Keep the number low. Include one individual from top management. After all, if top management is not involved, then they will not be committed. Without top management support and commitment the effort is most likely headed toward failure. Better save one's energies for something else.

Next, the team requires key users depending on the projected scope: how many major functional areas do we intend our system development to include?

Finally, the team should include someone from our IS functional area. If we don't have an IS functional area as such, surely at least one individual can be identified with the appropriate experience, training, or educational background in the discipline. Typically, this individual is also the project leader, so must have appropriate organisational 'stature' as well as leadership skills. Since you are reading this section of this book, it could even be yourself.

At this point a team has been formed to investigate the current system in order to understand the 'AS-IS' state or condition. Specifically the team is to

- build a functional model
- establish user needs
- define the requirements which satisfy those identified needs.

At the completion of Phase I, the team is in a position to present its findings to top management with rough estimates of costs. Then, dependent upon cost, schedule, feasibility, and estimated benefits and the team's recommendations, appropriate decisions can be made to determine what will be focused on for Phase II.

Develop a functional model

A functional model is very easy to produce (Fig. 7.2). This figure is based on a health services model and was chosen in order to show that we must concentrate on functionality, not organisational structure. Notice that each of the nodes (boxes) is uniquely identified e.g. A2, A21. The super node id for A21 is A2. Likewise one sub node id for A46 is A463, and so on. This is so that we can tie our results from the needs analysis exercise back to the model. By functionally modelling the entire enterprise (down to what ever level of detail we wish) we are assured of not missing any needs.

Determine the needs

While developing the functional model, we determine the scope of the interview process. In other words, is this to be a complete needs analysis across the entire enterprise, or are we going to focus on a particular area? Figure 7.2 shows the functional model expanded in the two areas of 're-engineer business processes' (node A2) and 'provide health services' (node A5).

The methodology of performing the needs analysis will be outlined in another section.

Define the requirements

Once we have completed the analysis of needs, we are then in a position to define various alternatives which have the potential to satisfy those needs. These alternatives may suggest

- a simple change in policy or procedure
- the application of some form of advanced technology
- a change in personnel capability.

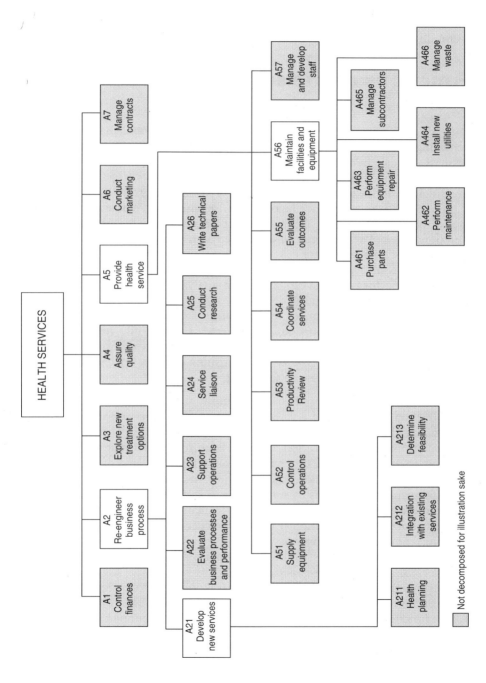

Fig. 7.2 Functional model

Obviously advanced technology can include, but may not be limited to, computer hardware and software. However, it is important to realize that there may be numerous alternative requirements which do not embrace technology.

Functions of the systems development team

Our systems development team, consisting of 4–5 people, has the task of achieving the 'understand the problem' phase of our systems development project. These people include top management representation; users representing all functional areas to be included in our baseline or AS-IS investigative effort; and a leader, typically with IS background.

If our task is to collect needs for the entire enterprise, across all functional areas, we do not need, in fact we do not desire, to have a user from each functional area. The team can be structured with appropriate individuals who can represent all appropriate functional areas. Firstly, experience has proved that a small team will get the job done more efficiently. Secondly, if it takes too long to perform the investigation and analysis, project enthusiasm may wane and jeopardise its completion.

An encapsulated version of the execution steps, which is also a project plan, is to be presented to top management. After all, you want their endorsement for the project, and you prefer the project to be made known to the entire organisation in advance of the ensuing activity. Specifically, lay out a schedule for and carry out the following:

1 Put together a short brief to all organisational managers stating that a collection of needs and subsequent analysis is to be performed in each functional area. This brief states the goals your team hopes to achieve and structures your activity. Solicit needs from functional managers and ask them to provide a list of other individuals within their area of responsibility whom your team should/could interview. It is also the responsibility of management to explain to staff the process as well as benefits expected from the exercise in order to allay any fears or misconceptions.

2 Distribute and assign the list of interviewees to appropriate members of your team (the interviewers).

3 Complete the interviews (6 or 7 a day per team member) and transfer to the NISFs (Fig. 7.3) in concise format.

4 Develop the enterprise functional model. This model is constructed through structured interviews of key personnel who have requisite knowledge of the functional areas. This begins at the top management position and flows down through the enterprise. (The section on 'Needs Identification' to follow presents the basic interview technique and associated questions.) Needs are also collected and later included on the NISF.

Author:	Date:	Working	Reader date
	Revised:	Draft	
		Recommended	
		Publication	

Sub node ID number:
Sub node function title:

Source:
Organisation:

Problem: _____

Need: _____
_____
_____
_____

Encompassing need category title: _____

Cost drivers: _____
_____

Human Factor considerations (positive & negative): _____
_____

Benefits tangible: _____
_____

Benefits intangible: _____
_____

| Super node ID: | Super node function title: | Need sequence number: |

Fig. 7.3 Needs identification survey form

67

Interview comments should be written up, sent back to the interviewee for validation or correction, used for model creation, then filed for audit trail. Note also that subsequent analysis of the AS-IS functional model should identify:

- redundant or overlapping functions
- functions that should be performed but are not
- possible incorrect emphasis on particular functions
- functional interdependence deficiencies.

5   Present the functional model to management for endorsement of correctness and authenticity. Re-work the model as required until it is endorsed officially.

6   Collate and categorise the NISFs. Determine the most pressing needs. Try to limit your focus to a manageable set, say half a dozen.

7   Develop and produce the NAD.

8   Analyse the needs categories and apply alternate requirements which satisfy the needs groupings. Develop and produce the RDR.

9   Brief top management and offer recommendations for Phase II.

Needs determination

Needs are associated with the AS-IS environment problems and voids. They are defined to establish a basis for improvements and provide the primary input for defining the TO-BE system. (The complete TO-BE system is not described in this chapter.) The determination of needs includes, but is not limited to, background information about the need and what problems are involved. The needs definition also looks at human factors, cost drivers (so we can get an insight into potential cost savings), and benefits (both tangible and intangible.) An examination of human factors considers the impact on staff if the need were addressed. Cost drivers and benefits are associated with the costs that drove the need assessment and further identifies what could/should be improved. From the determination of the costs we can estimate expected savings associated with meeting the needs with appropriate requirement alternatives.

The output of this activity is the NAD, which is a record of system needs, and is an analytic tool to determine system requirements. Based upon the objectives stated in the SD, the TO-BE system needs will be determined. These needs will address improvements to functions that are partially performed, incorrectly performed, or address non-existing functions that should be performed.

Needs identification (and functional model development)

The structured interview allows us to develop the functional model and simultaneously identify needs. From the AS-IS functional model we are able to specify and identify all functional areas of the enterprise which the SD has defined. Each of these areas will have specific individuals which we interview using structured interview techniques. Questions should be standardised for the whole team and typical questions may include the following:

- What occupied most of your time in the last week, month, and quarter?
- Describe the functions which you perform, or have direct authority over.
- What prevents/enables you from/to accomplish your tasks?
- What objectives are you measured against?
- With no restrictions on resources, what would you obtain to help ensure the completion of your tasks?

Note that the NISF provides for the model sub and super node identification as well as the name and organisational affiliation of the individual interviewed. The sub or super node is NOT the interviewee's organisation. Remember, we are developing a functional, not verifying an organisational, model.

It is recommended that the NISF be filled out from your rough notes upon the completion of the interview. This allows your full concentration on the information content of the interviewee response. Then, later, but before you forget the intent of your notes, allow yourself sufficient 'replay' time to formulate a tight response and develop a concise and informative data collection instrument. Don't forget that the team is to interview appropriate representation of the entire enterprise, from top management down.

The key information of the NISF is as follows:

- Model sub-node id number and function title
- Source of the information, i.e. the interviewee and their organisation
- Problem as the interviewee sees it
- Need identification as the interviewee sees it
- Encompassing need category title. This is determined later. See below.
- Cost drivers
- Positive and negative human factors
- Benefits (if corrected), tangible/intangible
- Model super-node id number and functional title
- Need sequence number

Needs classification

The data gathered from the interviews including the interaction with experts, management, and other enterprise knowledgeable associates, has been used to determine the AS-IS needs. Each of these needs and a) their associated benefits such as real cost savings, b) intangible issues, c) human factors, etc. is on a separate NISF. We must now classify or group the large number of needs into 6 to 8 encompassing categories.

The key to successfully grouping our needs is to carefully choose the words representing a needs category title. This deliberate choice of consistent words allows requirements to be determined systematically. The needs listed may be identified as residing in more than one needs category. This indicates the scope or breadth of a specific need. The functional model node, together with an encompassing need category title, provide the information to specify a functional area of the enterprise. The sequential need number is required to provide traceability back to the original needs identification survey form (NISF).

Needs cross reference

Basically at this point we have lots of data (NISFs) which can be organised by spreadsheet or database by simply sorting in the following useful ways:

- by sequence number
- by sub-node id number, and
- by super node id number.

Once we have accomplished the above sorts we are in a position to analyse and determine meaningful groupings which can be identified by 6 or 8 encompassing need category titles (see Fig. 7.3). We can then develop a needs category titles table, sorted by needs category title. It is this table which can be analysed for tightening up the needs groupings.

Figure 7.4 displays a basic example of what a needs cross reference table might look like. Other needs categories may include a) facilities and equipment, b) information availability, c) housekeeping, or d) staff training. The idea is to sort on the needs category titles in order to see the needs patterns evolve. As this evolution continues, we can ultimately re-classify all of our NISFs into a more manageable grouping of 6 to 8 inclusive categories which will focus our attention on the most pressing problems.

Further sorting can be made to help us analyse the data to be able to prioritise our needs.

Needs prioritisation

Once we have sorted and cross referenced all our needs in meaningful ways, our attention can be focused on prioritisation. We determine what is most important to improving the enterprise. Perhaps it is patient service, cost containment, labor efficiency and process streamlining. It all depends on our mission. Since our NISFs contain data regarding potential tangible and intangible benefits, we can quantify costs and benefits by needs categories. In other words, in order to establish a prioritised list of needs it may be necessary to establish estimates of the potential benefits for each of the 6 to 8 (encompassing) needs categories.

Whatever reasons may be driving our analysis, the needs are prioritised to determine which encompassing need categories should take precedence over others in the implementation of the TO-BE system. Figure 7.5 shows another example of a category matrix.

The next step is to look at the methodology of determining requirements.

SPECIFIC NEEDS/PROBLEMS	NEEDS CATEGORIES		
Seq Needs Model No. Title Functional Node	Operations	Information Resource Management	Other

Fig. 7.4 Needs cross reference Example 1

NODE		NEEDS CATEGORIES			
Number	Function	Opns	IRM	Facilities	Training
A21	Develop New Service	1,17,21	2,43		
A22	Evaluate Bus. Process				
Super Node		**Functional Title**			
A2		Re Engineer Business Processes			

Fig. 7.5 Needs cross reference Example 2

Requirements definition

This is the second step in the Understand the problem phase of the System development life cycle (see Fig 7.1). One report, the RDR, is produced at the completion of this step. Using the NAD, the transition to the RDR is achieved. The RDR contains requirement categories derived from the NAD which:

- describes and views the TO-BE developed system in terms of specific system requirements definition
- provides sufficient criteria to enable system preliminary and detailed design.

Stated another way, the RDR provides a breakdown of requirements in sufficient detail to allow solutions to be formulated and justified. The RDR is not expressed in terms of solutions, but rather is expressed in details of functional, performance, physical and interface characteristics.

The RDR is used:

- to present needs in a form that first identifies a system, and then presents a more detailed view of a specific system by listing functional characteristics
- to generalise system costs and then support system cost estimates
- to serve as a tool for determining that all major TO-BE system functional improvements have been addressed
- to provide sufficient criteria to enable the Formulate and justify solution phase of our system development.

The requirements result from assessing of needs in terms of categories with the added insight of determining how much of an improvement should take place to fulfil the needs. Furthermore, the determination of system requirements is the initial statement of major requirements for the TO-BE system expressed in terms that can elucidate solutions.

The methodology

The approach is to translate each grouping of needs categories from the NAD in terms of characteristics. This process uses lists to present a grouping or categorisation of needs at a top level and then further break down each category to a finer grained level of characterisation. The output of this process is a requirements list which contains sufficient supporting data to permit an understanding of the requirements. These requirements will provide a basis to develop a design that is responsive to the needs of the enterprise.

Requirements will state what should be done, not how it should be done which Phase II addresses. The requirements are mapped to the needs categories, and at the more detailed level of needs breakdown categorisation, to the specific need statements from which they originated. One need may stimulate several requirements; one requirement may encompass several needs; or a need may equal a requirement.

Requirements definition based on need categories

At this point it is probably best to look at an example. Our goal is to provide a list of system level requirements that will be further detailed in future reports (the TSR and the SSR) of the TO-BE system. To accomplish our goal, our format should present each of the major needs categories as a list of summarised needs statements. A list of requirements is then presented for each needs statement. The presentation of these requirements retains the same prioritisation of the need categories already determined. For example, from Figure 7.4 we had the needs categories of Operations and Information resource management. In an actual enterprise we would have strived for and achieved about 6 to 8 categories. Here we will only work with one to illustrate the process.

Needs Statement	Needs Sequence No.
1) To provide adequate and timely patient information in the wards	3, 6, 16, 101
2) To provide sufficient surgery procedure planning which raises the utilization level of facilities and staff.	121, 130
3) To provide for timely communication between administration, surgery scheduling, and patient billing.	11, 14, 76, 83, 104, 112, 127
4) To provide for periodic staff training.	3, 151, 170
5) To reduce excessive time spent in determining patient drug therapy requirements.	1, 16, 124

Fig. 7.6 Summary of operations needs statements

Needs category: operations

Problem statement: This needs category emphasises that deficiencies exist with policies and procedures regarding the internal functions and communication between departments of patient scheduling, planning, and support.

Five needs statements encompass the Operations needs category and are summarised to indicate the direct mapping to the original NISF (see Fig. 7.6).

Let us focus on need statements 1 and 2 above and map our requirements to them:

Needs statement 1: To provide adequate and timely patient information in the wards.

Requirements:

• Implement automated computer based information workstations that allows access to all systems which provide patient details, therapy requirements, procedure schedules and test results at the nursing station.
• Eliminate the shift control log. This function will be compensated for by the computer based workstations.
• Institute the procedure that doctors provide appropriate level of detail to the computer based information system regarding the outcome of their daily rounds.

Needs statement 2: To provide sufficient surgery procedure planning which raises the utilisation level of facilities and staff.

Requirements:

- Circulate current process and procedure instructions.
- Group like surgery procedure categories to reduce facility set-up and turn-around times.
- Co-ordinate facilities to account for specific support staff skills and availability.

We continue in this manner until all need categories and associated NISFs have been accounted for. The document generated from this exercise is the RDR.

Thus we have by these steps established user requirements. Hopefully the reader will find the material useful and applicable to their needs. However, we can see that there is much remaining work to be accomplished in implementing a system, training users, and monitoring the system for further improvements, and the last section of this chapter outlines the final stages of the systems development project life cycle.

Closure

Referring again to Figure 7.1 we see that the next phase of the systems development project life cycle is the Formulate and justify solution phase. This second phase consists of the two steps: Preliminary design culminating in the TSR; and Detailed design culminating in the SSR. Both of these reports deal with the TO-BE development effort.

Technical specification report (TSR)

The Preliminary design step is documented by the TSR, which is written at a conceptual level to define how the system requirements (as detailed in the RDR) will be satisfied. The Preliminary Design Review (PDR) is conducted during this step.

The TSR is the transition report from the system requirements definition design and forms the foundation for the remainder of the development process. The TSR documents the TO-BE conceptual system design by addressing how each requirement definition stated in the RDR will be satisfied and incorporated with the existing system. The TSR is not a report from which items will be directly constructed, but rather it is a design strategy report from which subsequent detail design will be based. It conceptualises how the system requirements will be satisfied by providing a preliminary design to include system characteristics of system architecture/hierarchy; communications/networks/data flows; and information processing.

System specification report (SSR)

This is the second step in the Formulate and justify solution phase. The SSR is produced during this step. This report contains sufficient detail to produce vendor bid packages. The Detailed design or critical design review (DDR) is conducted during this step, concluding this phase.

The SSR contains sufficient detail such that the characteristics of function, performance, and physical and logical interface may be seen. This may help to produce vendor bid inquiry packages including vendor software availability surveys. System implementation planning is also conducted during this step to establish the transition to the Construct and integrate solution phase of the project life cycle.

REFERENCES

Cost Modeling and Technology Assessment (Costech) Software Users Manual, 2 January 1990

Integrated Computer-Aided Manufacturing (ICAM) Function Modeling Manual (IDEF0), Materials Laboratory, AF Wright Aeronautical Laboratories report UM110231100 June 1981

US DOD Directive 5000.44, Industrial Modernisation Incentives Program (IMIP), 16 April 1986

8

Privacy, security and confidentiality

JO LUCK

When describing the important assets of a health care facility, people list the buildings, equipment, finances and personnel. But rarely do people think of the information held by the hospital as being an asset. Yet the information is a very valuable asset. Hospitals would not be able to function for very long without access to the data held in their health information systems. The value of the information is equivalent to the amount of money it would cost to recreate the health information system in the event of the computer files being completely corrupted or destroyed. If the system had not been backed up adequately, it may mean that the files could never be fully restored. No hospital would be able to afford such a loss. In the event of clinical systems the non-availability of information could place a person's life in jeopardy.

The concepts of security and privacy in health information systems are distinct but inextricably linked, like Siamese twins. The distinction can be expressed as follows: security is the protection of computers from people, and privacy is the protection of people from computers. The maintenance of privacy and security are two of the goals of a health informatics system (Robinson, 1994). They can be achieved through the adoption of various policies and procedures. This chapter discusses various policies and procedures which will serve to protect the computers, data and people associated with health information systems.

Security of health information systems is an important issue because information technology (IT) has removed many of the inherent erstwhile safeguards. The consequences of a breach of security have become more serious. Hospitals have become more highly dependent upon their information processing and communications systems. Ultimately, management carry the legal responsibilities for computer security.

The major security concerns are the impact on the hospital of security events which will affect:

- availability of data and services: the extent to which the ability of the organisation to provide a service will be affected by the loss or degradation of a given information processing or communication facility or the loss of a given set of data
- authenticity and integrity of data: the extent to which the ability of the organisation to provide a service will be affected by the accidental corruption of a given set of data or the malicious corruption of a given set of data or the acceptance of a given set of data which did not originate from its purported source.
- confidentiality of data: the extent to which the ability of the organisation to provide a service will be affected by the disclosure of a given set of data to an unauthorised person.

One can never reduce the risk of these security concerns to zero. But as the clinical information in health information systems is so important to the health care process, one must find a balance between the risks and medical effectiveness. This chapter will outline the basic steps to take to try and preserve the availability, integrity and confidentiality of data stored in health information systems. The bibliography contains a list of books and articles that will give you a more detailed examination of the security process.

Physical security

Physical security is 'that part of security concerned with physical measures designed to safeguard personnel, to prevent unauthorised access to equipment, facilities, material and documents and to safeguard them against espionage, malicious damage, theft or interference' (Caelli 1992).

The physical vulnerabilities to security can be disasters (both natural and artificial), human vandals, interception by an outsider and unauthorised access and use. A natural disaster can be defined as any event that is an act of God or the result of environmental or natural causes that are not predictable or avoidable. While it is virtually impossible to prevent natural disasters from affecting computer centres, measures should be taken to assess the potential risk. By proper planning damage and destruction can be lessened. Some of the disasters to be considered include floods, water, fire, power loss, power surges, heat and humidity (Forcht 1994) and earthquakes or cyclones in some locations. It is also advisable to insure the computer centre against such disasters.

Floods generally are the result of natural causes such as storms, cyclones, tides and waves. Floods can also be the result of artificial (or man-made) disasters, such as broken water pipes, sewerage pipes or sprinklers. The damage to the computer system may result from rising water, from flood water rising up through the floor or it may result from falling water, caused by overhead sprinkler systems being activated or water pipes breaking. If located in a flood prone area, the computer centre should never be located below ground or even on the ground floor. To prevent damage from falling water, large plastic sheets should be kept in the computer centre to allow employees to cover the computers quickly if needed. It would be advisable to have a policy that stated that all computers should be covered when not in use.

Fire is a much more serious problem than flooding, because it usually happens much more quickly than flooding and is a bigger threat to human life. It is important to devise a fire drill for the computer centre and to practise to ensure that the plan is up to date and effective. The placement of the computer in the building is important. A windowless room with fire-proof doors and nonflammable walls may prevent the fire from spreading into the room. The building should also be fitted with fire and smoke detectors and ideally they should be linked directly to the fire service (Forcht 1994).

Computers need a constant, pure supply of electricity. After a direct power loss, all computation needs to cease immediately. The information systems also need to be able to recover from a premature shut-down, and back-up and recovery procedures should be in place. For certain time-critical applications, such as systems that monitor a patients' vital signs, loss of service may be intolerable, and may even result in the death of patients. For such applications alternate complete power supplies must be available. One protection against power loss is an uninterruptible power supply.

Another problem is the 'cleanness' of the power. Instead of the voltage on the line being constant, it may have many brief fluctuations such as drops and spikes or suges of current. These variations in the voltage can be destructive to sensitive electrical equipment. Simple devices called surge suppressors can filter the electricity supply to the computers (Pfleeger 1989).

Excessive heat or cold can also be destructive to sensitive electronic equipment. The only effective way to deal with extremes in temperature is to turn the system off. Changes in temperature are usually gradual therefore there will be adequate time to take evasive action. It is desirable to house computing equipment in rooms that enable the temperature, humidity and airborne pollutants, such as dust, to be controlled.

What do you do after a crisis? The key to successful recovery is adequate preparation before the event. The most important asset is data; physical items can be more easily replaced, therefore be prepared, make a backup of your data and programs regularly. A backup is a copy of all or part of a file to assist in reestablishing a lost file. Computer centres should make a complete backup regularly; for example, once a week at the same time every week. In a complete backup, everything on the system is copied. During the week the computer centre should do selective backups. In a selective backup, only the files that have been changed or created since the last backup are saved. The backups should be stored in a fire and water resistant safe. A copy should also be stored off-site to allow the information systems professionals to recreate the system if the centre were to be completely destroyed.

It is important that data and programs stored on personal computers are backed up as well as the data and programs stored on maniframe computers. Personal computers tend to be overlooked when preparing a backup schedule for the computer centre.

Organisations should also guard against the physical presence of people who are not users. Unauthorised visitors can cause three problems, namely, theft of machinery or data, destruction of machinery or data, and viewing sensitive data. Three approaches can be taken to prevent theft, prevent access, prevent portability or detect exit.

The oldest access control is a guard; the second oldest access control is a lock. Both of these still provide simple effective security for access to computing facilities. But there are also various authentication devices that are available to control access to a computer centre. Users can be identified by what things they know (for example, passwords), what objects they possess (for example, smart cards), and what characteristics they have (for example, fingerprints). The best authentification procedures will combine all three. A password is a code word or phrase assumed to be known only to the user and the system. A smart card is a plastic card, about the same size as a credit card, that has an embedded microchip. These cards can be used to restrict access to authorised individuals at specific entrances, during specified hours of particular days. Biometric devices or personal characteristic recognition devices are used to detect some personal (physical) characteristic of the user. There are systems available that will recognise voice patterns, the blood vessels of the retina, palm prints, finger prints and handwriting characteristics.

The disposal of sensitive media is important to prevent it being read by unauthorised personnel. Data should be destroyed so that it cannot be read after disposal. This can be done by using shredders, disintergrators and incinerators.

Computer systems accessible by dial-in modem ports represent a major vulnerability in your system. The system should be protected by security controls such as dial-back connections. These are complex authentication schemes handled before connection to the computer and silent modems.

Cryptography

When information is transmitted along a communications line there is a need to protect it. The most common method used is encryption. Encryption is the process of encoding a message so that the meaning of the message is not obvious and decryption is the reverse process. The terms encode and decode or encipher may be used instead of the verbs encrypt and decrypt (Pfleeger 1989). You also need to be able to authenticate the source of the data and authenticate the data itself.

Cryptology is the science of disguised or secret communications. Cryptology is divided into two main areas, cryptography and cryptanalysis. Cryptography means hidden writing, the practice of using encryption to conceal text. Cryptanalysis are the methods used to break down or solve the encrypted message (Pfleeger 1989). The problem in sending messages is that the message can be interrupted, intercepted, modified or fabricated. Figure 8.1 shows a message being intercepted.

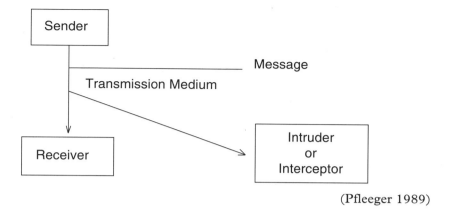

(Pfleeger 1989)

Fig. 8.1 Interception of a message

The two basic methods used in encryption are transposition, where the letters of the plain text (original, intelligible message text) are jumbled; and substitution, where the letters of the plain text are replaced by other letters, numbers or symbols.

The encryption key is the cryptographic key used for encrypting and decrypting the data. The decryption key reverses the process at the receiving end. The encryption algorithm is a sequence of rules or steps, generally expressed in mathematical terms, used to encrypt a message. If any of these components are compromised during the transmission of the message, the protection of the message being protected is severely weakened (Forcht 1994). The encryption process is illustrated in Figure 8.2.

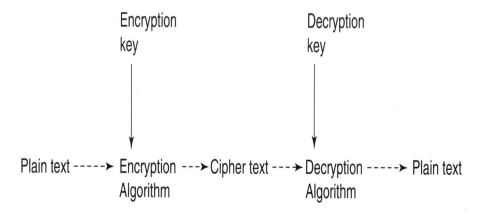

Fig. 8.2 The encryption process

Encryption is used to ensure the secrecy (privacy) of messages, and interceptors will not be able to read the message unless they have access to the encryption key and algorithm. The integrity of messages sent along tranmission lines can be checked by decrypting the message. If the message cannot be decrypted then some corruption of data has occurred and the message should be sent again.

Message authentication is ensured by the use of digital signatures. Documents are normally authorised by somebody signing the paper. In computer systems you don't have a tangible object on which to sign your name, only electronic signals. A digital signature is a protocol that produces the same effect as a real signature. It is a sequence that only the sender can make but other people can easily recognise as belonging to the sender. Like a real signature, a digital signature is used to authorise agreement to a message. They must be unforgeable and authentic. It is also desirable that they be unalterable and not reusable. These conditions can be met using a cryptographic sealing function that includes a date stamp to prevent reuse (Pfleeger 1989).

Computer viruses

Computer viruses are a special kind of threat to the health information system. The definition of a virus is a piece of code present on the system without consent of the owner. It is capable of moving from one computer to another, has the potential capability of destroying or altering files and has the capability to deny services to legitimate users.

Viruses are written for a number of reasons:

- viral code published in books
- virus construction software is available
- virus exchange bulletin boards
- greater awareness and understanding of computers
- cost of equipment decreasing
- standardisation of equipment
- challenge
- intrigue
- fun
- malicious intent
- recognition
- financial benefits

There are three types of malicious code: a virus, trojan horse and a worm. A virus is a propagating program that attaches to files and programs and may have time/logic bomb functions. Examples are: Stoned, Brain, Friday the 13th, and Michelangelo. There are several types of viruses, namely, boot sector virus, program attaching virus, data virus and source code virus. Viruses with time bomb/logic bomb features are triggered by specific circumstances; for example, the Friday the 13th virus is triggered when the system date is the

13th of the month and is a Friday. There are several different activation methods for viruses with time/logic bombs; for example, time, date, percentage of disk space used, number of executions, and programmer's name removed from payroll file.

A trojan horse is an apparently useful program that has hidden functions. It can hide something within its code that can be destructive to the user. For example, a trojan horse program could use the owner's file access privileges to copy, misuse or destroy data, format disks, overwrite files or cause the system to crash.

A worm is a propagating program that propagates through a network. It does not require a carrier program, as the program is self-contained. It may contain a malicious code; for example, the internet worm. The internet worm infected thousands of SUN and VAX machines on a UNIX network in the United States in 1988.

All operating systems are susceptible to viral attack. Only complete isolation provides complete protection from virus attacks. It is important to find a balance between the level of protection and inconvenience to the user. There are three types of anti-virus programs: virus specific products, detection programs, and prevention programs.

Virus specific products locate and remove *known* viruses. They may be able to restore damage or changes done by the virus but they need to be updated regularly to be effective and they should contain a list of viruses detected. An example is Mcfee Associates scan program. Detection programs detect damage done some time after it occurs. Notification occurs only when the detection program is run. Prevention programs are memory resident programs; that is, they are active in the computer's memory whenever the computer is turned on. Potential viral actions are brought to the user's attention, and the user may allow or disallow the action. They are useful against trojan horse programs but they need to be configurable to the user's environment. Users must be aware that they can be bypassed by clever programming.

Is there a cure for computer viruses? It is possible to detect known viruses, but it is impossible to guarantee that a section of code is not a virus. A virus may spread faster than it can be destroyed. It is possible that reinfection will result if any instance of virus remains. However there are a number of steps you can take to limit the risk:

- Keep a series of regular backups.
- Write protect all floppy disks.
- Archive all original software.
- Assign one boot diskette to each machine.
- Never boot from a floppy disk.
- Obtain public domain and shareware software from reputable sources.
- Always scan new software *before* using it.
- Reboot machine correctly; that is, do not use <ctrl-alt-del> or the reset button.
- Initiate security procedures to reduce risk.
- Be alert to system changes (Caelli 1992).

Risk analysis and security planning

Risk analysis is the study of the risks of doing something. Every computer user accepts the risk that a storage device will fail, losing all the stored data. Controls can reduce the seriousness of the threat. For example, banning all food and drinks from the computer room can reduce the threat of damage to the computer by food being spilt. A large organisation such as a hospital cannot easily determine the risks and controls needed for their computing facilities. For this reason, an organised approach to analysing risks is required.

Following such a study safeguards would be recommended which would reduce the likelihood of a security event, for example, fire proofing; or reduce the impact of an event, for example, fire extinguishers; or reduce the cost of the event, for example, disaster recovery insurance. Note that the emphasis is not on protecting against all possible mishaps but rather concentrating on those which would have the most impact on the organisation.

Some of the steps in performing a careful risk analysis are to determine exposures to risk, to assess the potential harm of risks, and to identify possible controls and the cost of installing these controls. Risk management involves developing and implementing a security plan (see Fig. 8.3). The reasons for performing risk analysis are to improve awareness of security issues, to identify assets, vulnerabilities and controls, to improve the basis for making decisions and to justify expenditures on security (Pfleeger 1989).

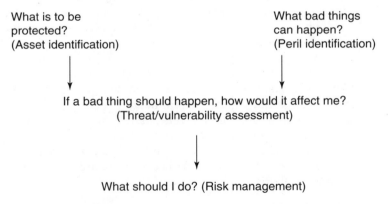

Fig. 8.3 Risk analysis and management

The basic steps in doing a risk analysis are as follows:

1   Identify assets: carry out an inventory of the system i.e. hardware, software, data, people, documentation and supplies.

2   Determine vulnerabilities: what are the effects of natural and physical disasters? effects of outsiders? effects of wilfully malicious insiders? effects of unintentional errors? One vulnerability can affect more than one asset or cause more than one type of loss. See Table 8.1 for an example of how to organise the consideration of threats and assets.

3 Estimate likelihood of exploitation: how frequently an exposure could be exploited.

4 Compute expected annual loss: the cost of each incident is difficult to determine. You will have to rely on data collected by insurance companies and observed data for a specific system. Talk to other people experienced in the field. The annual loss expectancy is calculated using the following formula:

Annual loss expectancy (ALE) = Loss of incident × the number of incidents per year.

5 Survey applicable controls and their costs: new controls are required if expected loss is too high. Identify new controls on per exposure basis.

6 Project annual savings of control: compute true cost/(savings) from implementation of new controls. The effective cost of new control = actual cost of new controls minus reduction in annual loss expectancy.

Table 8.1 Assets and vulnerabilities

Asset	Confidentiality	Integrity	Availability
Hardware			
Software			
Data			
People			
Documentation			
Supplies			

The types of controls that are available are:

- cryptography
- secure protocols
- program development controls
- program execution environment controls
- operating system protection features
- identification
- authentication
- secure operating systems
- database: access controls, reliability controls and inference controls
- network controls
- physical controls

There are a number of packages available to automate the risk analysis process. One of the best known packages is CRAMM (CCTA Risk Analysis and Management Methodology); it is the preferred risk analysis method of the UK government (Barber & Davey 1992).

A security plan is a document that describes how a company will address its security needs. The plan should be subject to periodic review and revision as the security needs of the organisation change. It should identify and organise the security activities for a computing system. The plan should contain the following: the security policy for the organisation, a description of the current status of security, recommendations for security controls, a listing of who is responsible for each security activity, a timetable identifying when security functions are to be done, and a statement of intention for periodic review of the security plan (Pfleeger 1989).

Privacy and confidentiality

The previous sections of this chapter have discussed matters dealing with the security and quality of data. This section looks at issues such as data content, access, control and ownership of data. Recent developments in medical information technology are putting enormous strain on the ability of existing standards, laws and regulatory mechanisms to deal with these issues in respect of the ethical handling of sensitive medical data. Existing standards, laws and regulatory mechanisms are suited to a material based data-technology. The advent of electronic data storage, handling and processing has significantly altered the way data is collected, stored and distributed and the changes involve more than technology alone. There has been an alteration in the role and function of patient records in health care delivery as well as in the ontological and epistemic status of the patient records themselves. This has serious implications for the ethical use of medical data (Kluge 1994).

In Australia the Commonwealth government has legislated on privacy and confidentiality through the *Privacy Act 1988*. This law is applicable to all Commonwealth government departments and their agencies. Pivotal to the Privacy Act is the concept of Information Privacy Principles (IPPs) which are set out in section 14 of the Act. The IPPs are set out in the same order as the information is likely to be handled by the keeper of the records. IPPs 1 to 3 deal with the collection and solicitation of information, IPPs 4 to 8 broadly relate to the storage, security and access to information, IPPs 9 and 10 look at the use of information by the keeper of records and IPP 11 focuses on the limitations placed upon disclosure of information (Tucker 1992). For a discussion of the IPPs and Health Information systems see Hardie (1994).

A number of statutory provisions relating to confidentiality in health information systems can also be found in the *Health Services Act 1991* and the Commonwealth government's *Freedom of Information Act 1982*. Some Australian States also have their own Freedom of Information Acts. For further details regarding this topic refer also to Chapters 21 and 22.

REFERENCES

Caelli W 1989 Information security for managers. M Stockton Press, United Kingdom
Caelli W 1992 Lecture notes for ITN502 Computer Security. Queensland University of Technology, Brisbane
Forcht K A 1994 Computer security management. Boyd & Fraser, Massachusetts
Kluge E H 1994 Health information, privacy, confidentiality and ethics. In: Barber B, Bakker A R, Bengtsson S (eds) Caring for health information: safety, security and secrecy. Elsevier Science, International Journal of Bio-medical Computing, Ireland
Pfleeger C P 1989 Security in computing. Prentice-Hall, Englewood Cliffs

Robinson D M 1994 Health information privacy: without confidentiality. In: Barber B, Bakker A R, Bengtsson S (eds) Caring for health information: safety, security and secrecy. Elsevier Science, International Journal of Bio-medical Computing, Ireland
Tucker G 1992 Information privacy law in Australia. Longman Professional, Melbourne

FURTHER READING

Andrews G, Wilkins G E J 1992 Privacy and the computerised medical record. Medical Journal of Australia 157
Barber B, Davey J 1992 The use of the CCTA Risk Analysis and Management Methodology [CRAMM] in health information systems. In: Lun K C, Degoulet P, Piemme T E, Reinhoff O MEDINFO '92 Proceedings of the Seventh World Congress on Medical Information, Geneva. Elsevier, Amsterdam
Bayne PJ 1984 Freedom of information. Law Book, Sydney
Bengtsson S, Solheim B G 1992 Enforcement of data protection, privacy and security in medical informatics. In: Lun K C, Degoulet P, Piemme T E, Reinhoff O MEDINFO '92 Proceedings of the Seventh World Congress on Medical Information, Geneva. Elsevier Science Publishers North-Holland, Amsterdam
Borovits I 1984 Management of computer operations. Prentice-Hall, Englewood Cliffs
Guidebook to Commonwealth freedom of information 1984 . CCH Australia, Sydney
Chadwick P 1985 FOI How to use the freedom of information laws. The Age, Melbourne
Freedom of Information Act 1982 (Commonwealth)
Freedom of Information Act 1992 (Queensland)
Hardie D 1994 Health information and the information privacy principles. Informatics in Healthcare, Australia 3(2) May
Harrison K, Cossins A 1993 Documents, dossiers and the inside dope. Allen & Unwin, Sydney
Hughes G 1991 Data protection in Australia. Law Book, Sydney
Kallman E A, Grillo J P 1993 Ethical decision making and information technology: an introduction with cases. Mitchell McGraw-Hill, New York
Knight P, Fitzsimons J 1990 The legal environment of computing. Prentice-Hall, Englewood Cliffs
Microcomputer control guide 1987. EDP Auditors, Sydney
O'Connor K 1993 Information privacy issues in health care and administration. Informatics in Healthcare, Australia September 2(4)
NSW Health Department (undated) Code of practice: privacy and confidentiality of data collection. NSW Health Department, Sydney
OECD 1980 Guidelines for the protection of privacy and transborder flows of personal data. Organisation for the Economic Co-operation and Development, Paris
Privacy Act 1988 (Commonwealth)
Queensland Health Guidelines for Information Technology System Security 1992 Information Systems Strategy Unit, August
Robinson D M 1992 A legal examination of format, signature and confidentiality aspects of computerized health information. In: Lun K C, Degoulet P, Piemme T E, Reinhoff O (eds) MEDINFO '92 Proceedings of the Seventh World Congress on Medical Information, Geneva. Elsevier Science Publishers Amsterdam
Standards Australia Draft Guidelines 1993 Information security and personal privacy protection in health care information systems. Standards Australia, Sydney
Storey H 1973 Infringement of privacy and its remedies. The Australian Law Journal 47, September
Waller A A 1991 Legal aspects of computer-based patient records and record systems. In: Dick R S, Steen E B (eds) The computer-based patient record. National Academy Press, Washington DC.

9

Database

RORY R MCNEILL

Basic database concepts

Database is a term that has entered common language as a result of the information revolution and the age of technology. As such, the term is often used incorrectly, even abused, and has taken on many connotations quite different from its original meaning in the information systems domain. Simple facts by themselves are of little value. When these facts are organised into a consistent, flexible framework they can be used to prove or disprove an hypothesis, substantiate or refute a claim, and indicate preferable alternatives for decision makers.

In a broad sense, a database is such a collection of simple facts, or data. The value in a database comes from the organisation of the data as much as from the data itself. This view of a database can include both manual data storage (such as an organised filing cabinet), and data storage on a computer.

For our purposes we will take the narrower view of databases and require that they be based on computer-accessible media. Furthermore, given the emphasis on organisation, this discussion is restricted to databases that are part of a database management system: a set of computer programs and files designed for the management (acquisition, organisation, storage, distribution, use, protection, archiving, and removal) of a data resource. Such a system is customarily purchased as a package with a number of options from one major software vendor. The common acronym for database management system is DBMS.

Typical features of database management systems

Most, but not all, database management systems will exhibit all of the following features: a set of data (database) stored on files; a data dictionary

89

describing the format, structure, and location of the data stored; a user interface allowing interactive query and update to the database; a set of utility programs for monitoring what is happening on the database, re-organising the database, backing up and recovering the database; and an application program interface allowing programs written in one of many computer languages to access the database. Slightly less common features include a system for managing concurrent use of the system by many people; security and access control features; and higher level languages suitable for developing entire applications. A system is not complete without the people involved with it: in the case of a database management system we usually see a database administrator, software developers, and end-users. A database management system rarely allows access to the data by any means other than its own software. In many cases this software implements a security system restricting access to authorised use. By forcing programs to use the database management system software, data independence is achieved. Changes to the database may be made with only minimal changes required to application programs. Database management systems are often concerned with the sharing of data, and this requires the ability to manage many users accessing the database at the same time. Database management systems often provide protection against the failure of the system, with periodic backups made automatically, and with recording of all activity that changes values in the database.

What is it about database management systems that make them important?

Database management systems are perhaps the primary mechanism for getting control of the organisation's information resource. By design, the data within a database can be shared; it has a logical, meaningful structure, and it can support the strategic and tactical goals of the organisation.

Data analysis and modelling

Even if the data needed for a new strategic thrust of the organisation is already captured by some part of the organisation, it is not likely to be of much use unless it has a form and structure that can be used by other parts. To ensure that this form and structure is correct, new and re-written applications must take a close look at the underlying reality. If the data model used is an accurate representation of this reality, the chances are good that the data will be able to be used in the future in ways that cannot be foreseen. Data analysis is the practice of examining the data and information requirements of an information system, and using one or models to represent these requirements in a systematic way. The most common approaches for modelling database requirements are the entity relationship data model and the object-oriented data model.

Why model?—the modelling process

A model is an abstraction of reality, representing those features that we consider important for the purposes of the model, and ignoring those that we consider unimportant. But what is the purpose of a model? By focusing on the important features, the model helps us to a better understanding of the underlying reality. We can use the model to make generalisations, to categorise and classify, to simplify, to organise, and to predict. Models help us to clarify our grasp of the subject modelled, and help us communicate our ideas to other people.

Models can take many forms. They could be clay models intended to show the shape of a novel aircraft, and used in wind-tunnels to test the aerodynamic characteristics of the proposed shape. They could be dummies with realistic facial features, mouth construction and body size, used to teach Cardio-Pulmonary Resuscitation (CPR) techniques when practising on live people would be dangerous and unsanitary. They could be financial models in the form of a spreadsheets, where the interaction of many financial variables can be estimated and the results used to help decide for or against investing in a project. They could be a large set of mathematical equations, used to understand and predict the behaviour of atoms, molecules, or galaxies under certain circumstances. They could be anatomical models in the form of diagrams and charts, used to teach the identification of body parts and functions.

Models can be static, used to represent existing form, structure, and relationships, or they can be dynamic, used to represent effects and interactions over a period of time.

Models may be created and used once for their purpose, or they may be reused time and time again. Models may be permanent, reflecting the area of reality well enough for continued use, or they may change and evolve as the understanding of the underlying reality changes and evolves.

Models are often composite or layered. A composite model may consist of a number of interrelated sub-models, each of which highlights a different aspect of the reality being modelled. A layered model has a sequence of similar models, with the top level showing only the most significant features and generalities, and the subsequent levels, each introducing features and details less important than shown on higher levels.

The modelling process begins when somebody realises there is some facet of reality that they need to understand better or to communicate to others. An initial model is constructed showing a few of the more important features that we are interested in. The model is checked against our understanding of the situation being modelled, and additional features are slowly added to make the model more complete. Modelling is typically an iterative and evolving process, starting with very simple, basic models that are well understood but tell us little, and gradually changing through progressive refinement into more complex models that are somewhat harder to understand but tell us much. Details and features needed for better understanding are gradually added, and errors and unnecessary complexities are removed when discovered. Each

91

stage of the model is tested against what is already known, and sometimes experimentation is used to verify implications of the model. Although models can be developed by individuals, their strength, robustness and applicability are improved if tested, verified, and validated by groups.

The entity relationship diagram

The model of most value in understanding databases is arguably the *entity relationship model* first introduced by Chen in 1976. This modelling approach has since been modified by Chen and others, and is used and understood by nearly all in the database management field. The model is principally a diagrammatic (although often augmented, in a composite manner, with text and other material) representation of the static structure of the sphere of information under consideration. Putting it more simply, the entity relationship diagram is a picture showing the most important classes of things (entities) we are interested in, and how they are associated with each other (their relationship to each other), at a particular point in time. The entity relationship model explicitly separates data and process, and completely leaves untouched the design of the functional parts of information systems. These functional aspects of information systems are typically designed using data flow diagrams and other structured design methodologies.

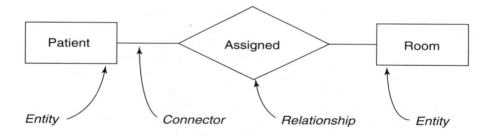

Fig.9.1 Basic entity relationship diagram symbols

In its simplest and original form, the diagram uses three symbols—a box for entities, a diamond shape for relationships, and lines connecting the entities and relationships (see Fig. 9.1).

The box shape for entities is used to represent classes of people, places, events, and 'things'. 'An entity may be an object with a *physical* existence—a particular person, car, house, or employee—or it may be an object with a *conceptual* existence—a company, a job, or a university course.' (Elmasri & Navathe 1994), (italics added). These entities are, in the real world, associated with other entities. The associations that are considered important for our model are represented by the diamond-shaped relationship symbol. In our example box we show that an entity patient has a relationship assigned with an entity room. Such a relationship is of interest to the hospital's admissions department, to its nursing staff, and to its food service department. We have made a satisfactory start in modelling the information requirements of our hospital.

It is likely that the different departments of the hospital are interested in different aspects and characteristics of the above entities and the relationship between them. For instance, we would like to know the patient's name, address, next-of-kin, special dietary requirements. We would like to know exactly what room the patient is assigned, whether or not it is a private room or a large ward, whether or not it has a telephone number, and which wing of the hospital it is in. We would like to know when the patient was assigned the room, and when the patient is expected to be discharged from in-patient care. Most of these aspects and characteristics are *attributes* of the entity or relationship. Of particular interest are those attributes that identify the entity, that serve to distinguish that entity from all others. In our example, patient-number and room-number are likely to be the *identifiers* for the Patient entity and the Room entity respectively (the identifier of an entity is also known as the *primary key* of the entity). In the entity relationship diagram, attributes are shown with ellipses, and identifying attributes are underlined (see Fig. 9.2).

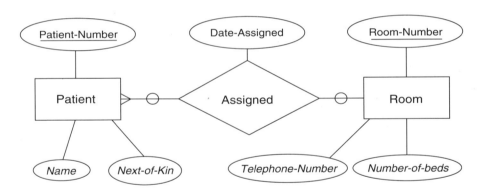

Fig. 9.2 Entity relationship diagram symbols: attributes and identifiers

Also important for us to model is whether or not a patient must be assigned a room (out-patients may be of interest), whether or not a room must have a patient, whether a patient may be assigned to more than one room, and whether a room may be assigned to more than one patient. These issues are important in designing reports and forms to be used, and in estimating the space required by the database. The term used for these issues is *cardinality*. The example entity relationship diagram shows that a patient is assigned to zero or one room (indicated by the circle next to Room), and that each room may have zero, one, or many patients assigned to it (indicated by the circle and the 'crows feet' next to Patient).

The object-oriented data model

Early examples of object orientation can be found in the development of object-oriented-programming-languages (OOPL). Largely contemporary with the development of the entity relationship model, object orientation is a more comprehensive modelling approach that embodies both data and process, and is not as inherently compatible with conventional information systems as is the entity relationship model. For that and other reasons, although the promise of the approach has been recognised for some time, it is only recently that the object-oriented model has gained both widespread acceptance and use. However, this acceptance and use is growing at a tremendous rate, and the object-oriented model for information systems development may well become the standard approach in the near future.

As an approach for developing new information systems, the object-oriented model is a radical departure from previous practice. There is no quick and easy way to convert a traditional process designed with data flow diagrams, flow charts, and conventional programming languages to the object oriented model, and even the reverse (converting an object-oriented design into a conventional design) is difficult. The object-oriented approach requires a whole new way of thinking for the information systems developer. Despite these differences in modelling process, the object-oriented model is remarkably compatible to the entity relationship model, as we shall see.

Like the entity relationship model, the object-oriented model is a reflection of a view of reality. Whereas the entity relationship model looks at 'entities' and how they are 'related', the object-oriented model looks at 'objects' and includes in this analysis behaviour as well as attributes. From this perspective, the object-oriented model can be viewed as an extension of the entity relationship model.

Central to the object-oriented model is the concept of *encapsulation*. Encapsulation is a 'packaging' of the various characteristics of objects, both descriptive and behavioural. The object has public, or external, characteristics that can be seen and affected by the outside world by means of *messages* sent to it. It also has private, or internal, characteristics that embody the implementation mechanisms that are not needed by the outside world and cannot be directly affected by it. The descriptive characteristics in the object-oriented model are called the *attributes* of the object, with the word having much the same meaning and use here as in the entity relationship model. The behavioural characteristics are modelled by means of *methods*, with the only means of accessing and modifying the attributes being via the object's methods, often requested by other objects by way of a message.

One major contribution of the object-oriented model is its explicitly formalised use of generalisation. Object *instances*, or occurrences, are members of a *class* of similar objects, with similar attributes and methods. Object classes can in turn be grouped into more general classes, or subdivided into subclasses. A subclass will *inherit* most of the attributes and methods of its more general class, and will introduce other attributes and methods specific to it.

Objects can be assembled into more complex objects, complex objects may be subdivided into more simple ones.

One important characteristic of object classes is that each instance of an object is distinct and distinguishable from every other object instance, and this differentiation is maintained no matter what changes are made to its attributes. Each object instance thus has its own *identity*.

The relational data model

Both the entity relationship model and object-oriented model above are useful in the earlier stages of design for a database. Both models express some high level ideas that are important for getting the design done correctly. However, neither model can be directly implemented. With the entity relationship model we need a conventional database management system; with the object-oriented model we need an object-oriented database management system or at least an object-oriented programming environment. The relational data model may be used to attach the extra detail needed to the entity relationship model to allow the implementation using a relational database management system.

Tables of rows and columns

Conceptually, the relational model consists of nothing more than tables of rows and columns, and operations on those tables. The relational model would represent the entity relationship diagram above using the following tables (see Fig. 9.3)

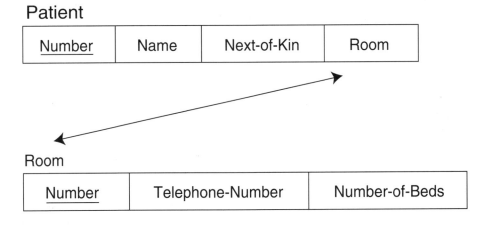

Patient

Number	Name	Next-of-Kin	Room

Room

Number	Telephone-Number	Number-of-Beds

Fig. 9.3 Relational data model

Note that the relationship 'assigned' is modelled by including a reference to the room in the patient table (called a *foreign key*).

Information resource management

Information resource management is a concept that first became popular in the middle 1980s. At the time there was a growing dissatisfaction by the senior management of many organisations with the performance of their information systems departments. These departments were seen to be costing more and more, yet were consistently falling behind on delivering what the organisation needed. A few organisations were spectacularly successful in using their information systems investment for strategic advantage in competitive markets, more organisations were still waiting for developments promised as much as three years previously. The information systems professionals responded to the criticism by noting that the development of appropriate information systems was a critical factor in implementing the organisation's strategies. Prior to this period, information systems development tended to operate in a reactive manner, with the squeaky wheel being greased. Planning was often limited to guessing what new hardware would be required, with little thought to what development projects should be undertaken. Information resource management starts with the premise that the information used by the organisation is of strategic value, and should be managed with the same care and attention as other corporate resources. Corresponding to the important role played by an organisation's chief financial officer, the zealots of information resource management suggest that the function of chief information officer be created and vested with similar powers and responsibilities.

The strategic role of databases

By taking a broad view of the organisation's information resources, future uses of information technology can be anticipated and accommodated, without needing to replace or discard the existing investment in information systems. It has been observed that the data used by an organisation is relatively stable, whereas the processes that use this data, and the structure of the very organisation, is not. Separating the design of databases from that of the organisational units and structures that use the data gives a high degree of independence, stability, and value. Databases that have been designed with modern, well-developed concepts can be used to lever the effect of new technology and innovation, and not hold these effects back.

Planning for databases

'The goal of the planning phase is to align information technology with the business strategies of an organisation' (McFadden & Hoffer 1994). Even with workbench technologies, prototyping, and other rapid information systems development approaches, it still can take a substantial amount of time, effort, and expense to create the databases needed to fulfil the strategic needs of the organisation. Organisations cannot afford to spend these resources unless by doing so they are furthering the goals of the organisation as a whole.

Organisations that can respond quickly to changes in their environment will outperform those that cannot. How can expenditures be managed and quick responses facilitated? By having a plan for the future, and working to it. The planning for databases is a fundamental part of strategic information systems planning, and needs to be closely integrated with the strategic planning of the entire organisation. Databases which support the critical success factors of the organisation must receive the highest priority.

Planning for databases is a process involving modelling the organisation, identifying and prioritising the information needs of the organisation, and developing a plan to progressively develop and improve the provision of critical information to the decision makers of the organisation. The plan itself is flexible, with regular review and provision for modification. Distant targets are provisionally sketched in, with detail increasing as the time horizon shrinks.

Distributed databases

Most organisations that might be interested in database technology are dispersed to a fair degree, occupying at least several buildings, and often having offices separated by hundreds of kilometres. To such organisations, the ability to share information quickly and easily across the organisation is important or essential. Mail systems, couriers, telephones and facsimile machines are all used to enable this dissemination. With computer networks, the computer-based information resources of the organisation can be easily on tap wherever needed.

Approaches to distribution

McFadden and Hoffer (1994) list four basic strategies for distributing databases:

1 Data replication, where some or all of the database is copied to different locations.
2 Horizontal partitioning, where the database is segmented according to the value of one or more of each record's attributes. (For example, patients listed with a Rockhampton postal code would have their patient data stored in Rockhampton, those with a Brisbane postal code would have it stored in Brisbane.)
3 Vertical partitioning, where the database is segmented according to the different functions using it. (For example, a hospital's detailed budget information may be kept in computers within the hospital, but the higher level budget information may be kept in computers within the regional offices.)
4 Combinations of replication, horizontal and vertical partitioning. (For example, where tables of valid pharmaceutical items may be copied and kept in all hospitals, pharmacy inventory kept by each pharmacy, and drug use statistics maintained monthly in Brisbane.)

Reasons for distribution

A database may have a number of reasons why it should be distributed. These reasons are usually based on cost, performance, or both. Compared with a centralised database, distributed systems offer the potential for greatly reduced communication charges, since the data resides closer to where it is actually used. Control of costs can be devolved, and local autonomy and accountability increased, with distributed databases. Response times for the more common transactions should improve considerably, since the bottleneck of the central computer has been removed. Parts of the network may be able to keep operating when the central site or network is malfunctioning. Some sites may be able to operate at different hours from others, they may not be constrained by the needs of others. Growth may be accommodated gradually, without the need for drastic spurts.

Implications of distribution

Whatever the approach used for distribution, the software and hardware required will likely be more complex than for a centralised system. This will make it more expensive, and could cause it to have more problems. Queries that span the data from several sites may be considerably slower. Data replication implies a greater risk for database integrity, inadequately implemented replication could both increase transmission costs and reduce the security and integrity of the database. Devolution without adequate resourcing can place a significant burden on the operating departments, without yielding the benefits promised.

Database security and integrity

Standard features with larger database packages are systematic and largely automated *backup* and *recovery* mechanisms. These features should be implemented to ensure that the database is adequately protected from the failure of either hardware, software, or the network.

The power and value of databases comes from being able to share the data. *Concurrent access* by many users must be enabled in order to maximise this value. Some database management systems that grew from personal computer programs may not have adequate performance and protection in this area.

Data kept in a medical database is often confidential. Damage to this data may threaten lives, whether the damage is intentional or accidental. A characteristic of good database management systems is the ability to identify who should have access to what parts of the database, and *restrict access* to the remainder of the database or to unauthorised people. Of particular concern is data distributed over a network.

We have argued that the organisation's database is a valuable, strategic resource. Plans should be in place, and exercised, to avoid the worst damages that might be caused by a disaster.

REFERENCES

Chen P 1976 The entity relationship model: toward a unified view of data. Transactions on Database Systems 1(1): March

Elmasri R, Navathe S B 1994 Fundamentals of database systems. Benjamin/Cummings, Redwood City

McFadden F R, Hoffer J A 1994 Modern database management. Benjamin/Cummings, Redwood City

REFERENCES

10

Data communications

GRAHAM IVERS

This chapter provides the reader with the ability to have a general appreciation of hardware and software, and data communication hardware and software in particular. It will raise an awareness of the need for networks to conform to international standards and for strategies to be developed to allow this transmission to be made. The importance and use of local area networks (LANs) and wide area networks (WANs) in any business environment, but particularly the health sector should be recognised. Finally the reader should gain an understanding of the importance of network management, especially for the health sector.

There is a vast array of information technology in the market today. Many think of this simply as hardware or software. In most instances, there is a need for the hardware devices to be linked together by a network.

This chapter discusses mainly the technology itself, but does mention applications using the network. It does this by conveniently initially dividing networks into LANs and WANs. Options available within each of these are explored. Technology to allow the interconnection and interoperability of LANs and WANs are also discussed.

It emphasises that it is necessary to utilise information technology to provide solutions for the applications—in this case within the health environment. Attention is also drawn to the need for privacy and security.

Some definitions

To provide a general framework, some definitions (Reynolds 1992) are first provided.

Hardware: physical devices that make a computer system.
Communications hardware: special class of hardware associated with transmission of data over a network.

Software: programs or instructions that tell the computer what to do.
Information system: a special class of goods whose components are people, procedures, and equipment that work interdependently under some means of control to process data and provide information to users.

The above definitions are broad enough to show that they apply in any particular sector of the economy. All sectors are seeking access to information technology, to achieve some specific purpose. As an example, the electricity industry requires the technology to bill electricity accounts (and other functions). The health sector has its own particular requirements. The important thing to note however is that most sectors use the same base hardware and software to allow information systems to satisfy the business requirements, be they a need or an opportunity. Whilst most of the technology is common, the application being run to satisfy the information requirements is often different. As an example, the health sector would not require access to packages for building power lines. Some of the possible applications used by the health sector are considered below.

Some basics

Under hardware, items such as personal computers, mini computers, mainframes, printers and other devices are normally considered.

The software can range from operating systems to database management software, application packages and other specialist software.

The definition of an information system highlights that it is necessary for the components of the system to work cohesively together to establish a quality system. The best computer hardware in the world is not enough, desirable though good hardware is. If the software is full of errors (bugs), then the system is no good to anyone. Similarly, good software is not sufficient on its own. If the hardware is faulty, then the presence of good software is wasted. The definition also shows that people are an important component in an information system. In recent times, particular attention is being paid to user interfaces such as can be achieved through Windows, menus and other common interfaces. It is also necessary to recognise that without the full support of people, even the best hardware and software will be not used to its full advantage.

One piece of computer hardware does not operate solely on its own. For example, a personal computer usually has a printer attached. The printer is attached using a printer cable. It is controlled by the operating system such as Windows95. This principle can be extended to a larger system such as a mainframe where the disk drives and tape decks are separate devices linked by some type of cabling method. Similarly, these devices are controlled by the operating system. There usually would be a large number of terminals attached to the mainframe. In some instances, mainframes at various locations might be linked together.

From the above, it can be seen that data communications needs to be considered specifically. Little happens in information technology without data communications. In its simplest form, it consists of special hardware, software and medium. The hardware might be a modem, a multiplexer, a concentrator or other communications hardware. The mix of these will be dependent upon the type of network installed. This is explored later. The data communications software consists of protocols. Formally, these can be defined as 'a set of codes to be transmitted and received in the proper sequence to guarantee that the desired terminals and computers are linked together and can send intelligible messages back and forth' (Reynolds 1992). So it can be seen that it is the protocol that faithfully ensures that what is transmitted is what is received at the other end—even if garbage is transmitted.

Before discussing data communications in more depth, attention is turned to consideration of the direction for selecting the appropriate technology.

A direction for selecting technology

With such an array of information technology available, the question that is often posed is 'How does an organisation identify what is required to satisfy its particular requirements? This question is even more relevant when the pace of changing technology is considered. It is important to recall that *if you fail to plan, you plan to fail*. No one is going to pretend that the planning process will be easy. But that does not mean that the process should not be attempted. The planning that should take place in organisations when considering information technology is the development of an information technology strategy and it is necessary for the information technology strategy to be supportive of the functional goals to allow the corporate strategic goals to be realised (Fig. 10.1).

Ahituv and Neumann (1990) advocate that policies need to be developed (and then implemented) in a number of key areas for the information technology strategy. Details are shown in the following list.

1 Hardware policies
   • Determination of computer capabilities
   • Computer system selection
   • Financing of equipment (rent, purchase, lease)
   • Use of service bureaus
   • Equipment deployment (integrated or distributed processing)
   • Standardisation of equipment
2 Software policies
   • Financing of acquired software (rent, purchase)
   • Acquisition of software packages
   • Software standards and languages
   • Employment of external contractors
   • Centralisation or decentralisation of software development

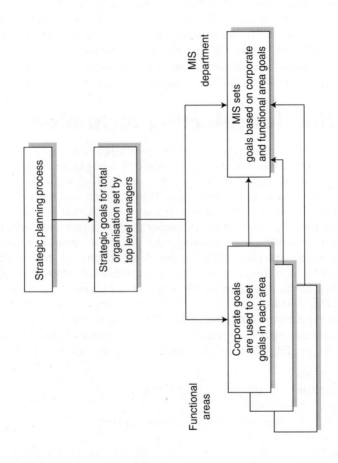

Fig. 10.1 Relationship among strategic goals, functional departmental goals and Management Information System goals
Source: Parker & Case (1993)

3 Personnel policies
   - Training and education
   - Recruitment and displacement of employees
   - Career development practices
   - Centralisation or decentralisation of human resources
4 Organisational policies
   - Committees (information system, steering, audit)
   - Location of the information system unit in the organisatiion
   - Organisational structure of the information system unit
   - Security practices
   - Information system unit responsibilities
   - Interface between information system unit and users
   - Auditing the information system function
5 Application development policies
   - Employment of external assistance (consultants, software houses, computer manufacturers)
   - Development approach (top-down, bottom-up, etc.)
   - Initiation, approval, and release of applications
   - Documentation standards
6 Planning policies
   - Information system planning responsibilities
   - The planning process.

In developing the policies, it is not only necessary to consider present requirements, but to have some regard to possible future requirements. The policies might result in a staged implementation. As an example, a medical practice may purchase a personal computer initially, but it would ensure that the one purchased could be networked later.

In recognition that models of hardware are continually changing and new releases of software are becoming available, any prospective purchaser needs to give strong consideration to what is known as open systems architecture. Reynolds (1992) defines this as 'one in which software can easily run on hardware from different vendors, and hardware from different vendors can be linked together in a multi vendor Telstramunications network.'

Of particular importance is the choice of operating systems such as Windows95 or UNIX, the choice of application software that can run on several platforms and also the choice of communications protocols such as those that fall under the umbrella of osi. The open systems are important as they are compliant with international standards and allow different vendors' hardware and software to work in harmony with one another. Strange as it might seem, this has only been a fairly recent development in information technology. Until recently, vendors simply developed to their own standards, and did not pay major attention to interconnection and interworking with other vendors hardware or software. The pressure from users has brought about this change in attitude by vendors.

Data communications

In recent times, it has become convenient to ignore some older technology used for connecting terminals and printers. Thus, as mentioned in the introduction, networks can conveniently be broken into LANS (local area networks) and WANS (wide area networks).

It would be very unusual to run word processing on a WAN, but is very common to run it on a LAN. On the other hand, a bank would not consider running its main banking system for customers on a LAN, but would run it on a WAN. The main determining factor is the nature of the application. In the above examples, customers want to be able to make bank transactions from any branch, so a WAN is necessary to support the application. On the other hand, where the bank simply wants to write to its customers and uses word processing, a LAN is suitable for this purpose. However, in many instances, businesses (including the health sector) have applications that need to be supported by both a LAN and a WAN. Methods of doing this are discussed later.

Local area networks

There are now few businesses of any size that simply operate a stand alone computer to satisfy their information requirements. At a minimum, there are several personal computers. Rather than operating each on a stand alone basis, consideration can be given to having these linked to form a local area network (a LAN).

A formal definition provided by Stamper (1994) states that a LAN is 'a communications network in which all of the components are located within several kilometres of each other and that uses high transmission speeds, generally one million bits per second or higher'.

In any LAN there is a need for specialised hardware. The definitions below provide a base introduction to hardware associated with LANs:

Server: the routine, process, or node that provides a common service for one or more other entities (Stamper 1991).
Multi station access units: a device used to interconnect workstations (Stamper 1994).
Bridge: an interconnection between like networks, for example ethernet to ethernet (Stamper 1991).
Gateway: the interface between two different networks (Stamper 1991).

The particular hardware required in any particular LAN will depend upon factors such as the facilities required, the size of the LAN and the type of LAN.

To operate a LAN, it is necessary to have LAN management software. Some of the more common packages in use are Novell, Lantastic and Pathworks. This software performs additional functions to the operating system as discussed below.

106

The terminals on a LAN are usually connected by a wire of some type. This is known as the *medium*. The choice of medium can range from coaxial cable to twisted pair to fibre optic. The particular medium type chosen for the implementation depends upon a number of factors such as level of security required, flexibility for alteration of the route later, the particular LAN implementation type and response time required. Although the distance that can technically be supported by a LAN is 'several kilometres', there are restrictions on this. As an example, a LAN cannot cross a public road.

LANs are required for purposes such as the need of several users to share data and the need to share resources such as a printer. Thus, two receptionists in a practice could have access to accounts, to word processing and other office environment software. Unlike stand alone personal computers where there is a need for example for word processing software to be installed on every personal computer, one copy of the software is installed on a server. It can be made available for use by all personal computers on the LAN. The site is required to attend to copyright matters by purchasing a licence for the number of copies that are to be made available concurrently. Under this arrangement, the number can be less than the number of terminals, but all terminals can be provided with access. As an alternative to negotiating a licence for a number of copies, a site such as a hospital can negotiate a site licence so that the software can be used on as many terminals as there are on the site.

The facilities required for LAN management are more comprehensive than those that exist under plain MS DOS. (LANs also are available for personal computers and workstations that do not use MS DOS; an example is Appletalk for Macintosh microcomputers.) This is because MS DOS was designed for a single user, whereas LANs are about multi users sharing data and resources. Some of the extra requirements include control over who can access what applications; if access is given and whether this is simply retrieval only or if update is allowed; and the need to control the resources such as sharing printers. As an example, a receptionist might not be given access to medical details, whereas that person would be given access to accounts.

There are three common types of LAN implementations and these are ethernet, token bus and token ring. Under ethernet, any user has the right to transmit data at any time. The protocol overcomes the possibility of two or more users transmitting at exactly the same instance by means of 'carrier sense multiple access with collision detection'. Users would only be aware of the collision when slightly slower than normal response times occur. On the other hand, under the token implementation, each user receives a turn at transmitting. Again, the user is not aware of this. The protocol passes a token to each user to allow the message to be sent.

It is important to note that these architectures are supported by international standards. The international standard varies according to whether the network is implemented using a bus or a ring architecture. The ethernet standard for a bus implementation is ISO 802.3. International standard ISO 802.4 applies to a token bus implementation. Where the LAN architecture is a token ring, international standard ISO 802.5 applies. Figures 10.2 and 10.3 show an example of a ring and a bus implementation respectively.

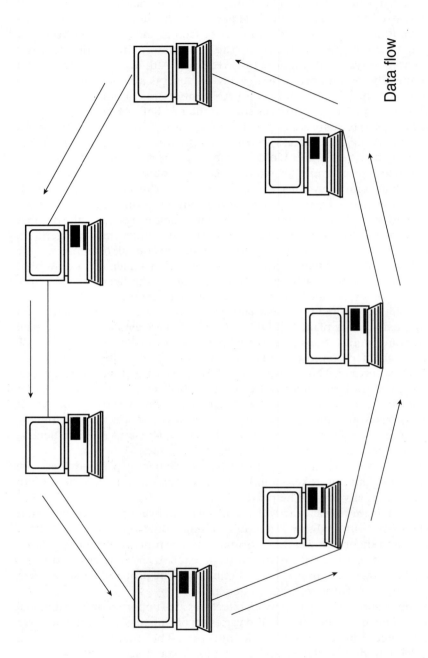

Fig. 10.2 A ring configuration
Source: Stamper (1991)

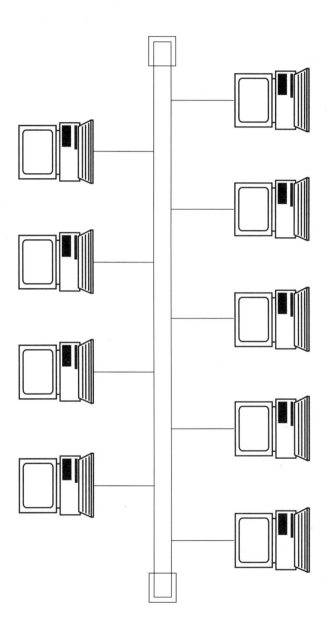

Fig. 10.3 A bus configuration
Source: Stamper (1991)

Now as there are several suppliers of LAN management software, it is necessary for the network manager to determine which management software is appropriate for the site. This can be done by setting up criteria and evaluating each supplier's software against the criteria. The criteria can be weighted to give recognition to those criteria deemed to be more important. The importance of the weights is vital, particularly where imaging data is to be transmitted over the LAN. For example, a LAN may be used to transmit images from the source to where the medical practitioner is located.

Criteria that are often used to evaluate LAN network management software include the following:

network architecture
applications required to be run
number of users
distances
expandability
vendor support
number of workstations
speed
device connectivity
cost
interconnectivity with other networks

The network manager needs to consider these criteria carefully and choose one that supports international standard protocols. As an example, the network manager might conclude that Novell is appropriate as it conforms with IEEE 802.3 or ethernet standard.

Alternatives to a LAN

With the vast array of technology that is available, it is possible to satisfy a particular requirement by more than one means. Two examples are provided below.

Suppose a hospital has an inventory system or a patient system. It might implement these systems on a central host computer (Fig 10.4).

Here the terminals are not connected via a LAN. Rather, they are connected via a communications controller. This implementation method is often used when dumb ASCII terminals are used. With the reducing price of technology, this implementation method is fast giving way to the LANs. Terminals on a LAN can be used to perform all processing under this method, but in addition offer extra processing options. Nevertheless, dumb ASCII terminals are appropriate when used for central processing such as creditors payment systems for a hospital.

In a small practice, initially, it might be decided to have only a couple of personal computers. Rather than purchase a printer for each or install a LAN, the option exists to simply use a switch. The switch can be manually operated or be a coded data switch allowing the program to select automatically the appropriate printer. The printers might be set up with different types of

110

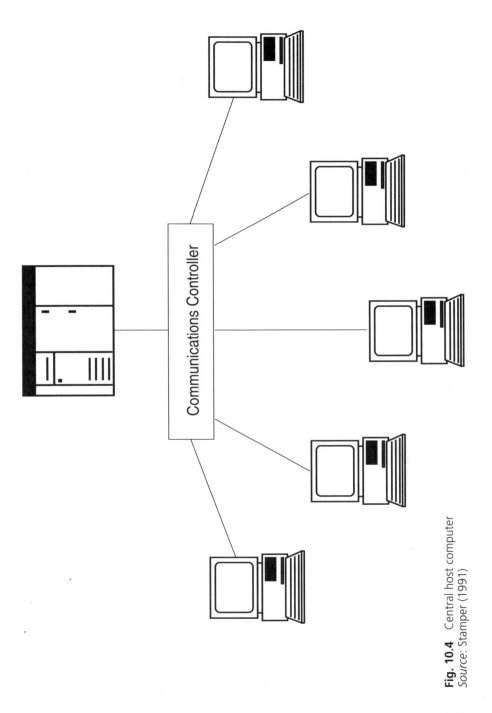

Fig. 10.4 Central host computer
Source: Stamper (1991)

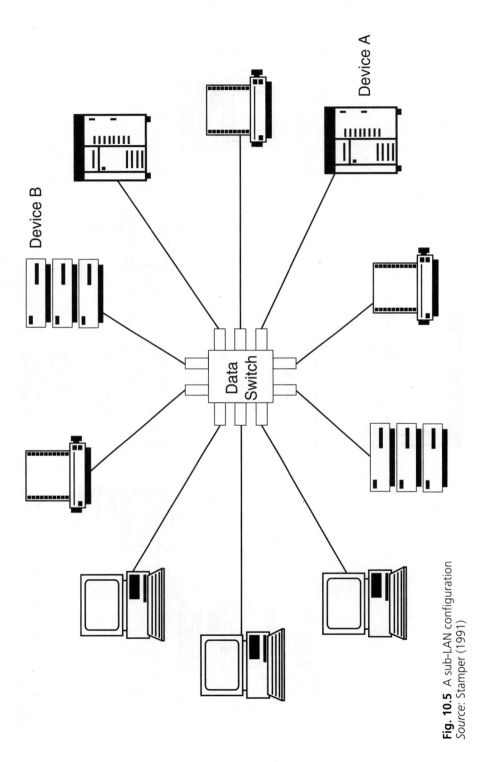

Fig. 10.5 A sub-LAN configuration
Source: Stamper (1991)

stationery. For example, ordinary stationery, account stationery, letterhead or Medicare forms. Each personal computer has access to whatever printer it requires (Fig. 10.5).

In general terms, the above has considered the use of conducted media. However, radiated media is now emerging. The use of wireless LANs, microwave and satellite are becoming more prevalent in the health sector. Whilst radiated media does have the advantage of not requiring the installation of cables, the use of radiated media needs to be carefully considered. This is because unless special measures are put in place, it is possible for the message to be intercepted. With privacy being such a major issue in the health sector, the network manager needs to give strong consideration to the use of encryption techniques when radiated media is used.

Wide area networks

Whereas a LAN provides communication over a relatively short distance, a wide area network (a WAN) provides communication over vast distances. This might be between suburbs, between cities, between states or countries. If the sites to be connected are different organisations, in most cases, it is necessary to use a WAN. Even if the communication is between different parts of the same organisation, then it is determined by distance.

For use of a WAN, it is only necessary to consider an electronic mail system. In the health sector, it could be used to send messages between doctors in different cities. Another example is the transmission of diagnostic imaging where a doctor seeks the opinion of a specialist in another location.

Another distinguishing feature between a LAN and a WAN is that whereas the LAN is privately owned, it is necessary to use a common carrier for a WAN. In Australia, Telstra is an example.

Both LANs and WANs require specific technology. The definitions below provide an introduction.

Analog: measurable physical quantities, which in data communications take the form of voltages and variations in the properties of waves. Data is represented in analog form by varying the amplitude (voltage), frequency (hertz) and/or phase of a wave (Stamper 1994).

Digital: where data is (are) represented by a series of distinct entities. In data communications equipment this series is almost always a binary digit, or bit—either 0 or 1 (Stamper 1994).

Packet distribution network: a network that divides messages into packets for transmission at their source and reassembles the packets into messages at the destination (Stamper 1991).

Asynchronous transmission: the method of transmission where each character is transmitted individually with its own error detection scheme, usually a parity bit. The sender and receiver are not synchronous with each other (Stamper 1991).

Synchronous transmission: the method of transmission where the sender and receiver are synchronised. Data is generally transmitted in blocks, rather than a character at a time as in asynchronous transmission (Stamper 1994).

Half duplex transmission: the method of transmission where the data travels in both directions over a link, but in only one direction at a time (Stamper 1994).

Full duplex: the method of transmission where data can be transmitted over a link in both directions simultaneously (Stamper 1994).

Bandwidth: a measure of the amount of data that can be transmitted per unit of time. The greater the bandwidth, the higher the possible data transmission rate (Stamper 1994).

Data compression: the method used to reduce the number of characters or bits in a message (Stamper 1991).

Not all users of a WAN have the same requirements. Traditionally, most sites only required connection to allow voice transmission. However, in recent times, this has been extended to text data and image.

Some users require dedicated access because of the large volume of communication required to be done. Others require access to numerous different sites on an occasional basis. Telstra offers a wide range of choices for sites requiring access to a WAN. Thus, Telstra provides offerings that allow analogue, digital and packet switching communication. Within these, there is a choice of asynchronous and synchronous. Further, Telstra provides a choice of speeds in half duplex or full duplex modes. The selection of the particular offering is entirely up to the site.

As the health sector moves to take advantage of communication technology (be it through the health communication network (HCN) or simply privately between medical practitioners), it will use WANs.

Suppose for example that a rural hospital requires permanent access to an application installed on a computer in its base hospital, it could choose between offerings such as Telstra's ISDN, Digital Data Service, Austpac or Datel. If a practice wanted occasional access to a pathology practice, it might select Austpac. Clearly, if patient information is to be available between practices, then WANs will become an important feature. Consideration might be given to optional facilities available within offerings. As an example, a closed user group might be established under Austpac for practices sharing the patient information. A further example involves a large hospital that might desire to have its voice, facsimile and data communications controlled in one system. Alternatively, a general practitioner might want an opinion from a specialist. To do this, it might be necessary to transmit diagnostic imaging. Here, the choice would be Telstra's ISDN. Even with the bandwidth available under ISDN, as Hovenga (1994) points out, to reduce the amount of data to be transmitted, it is desirable to employ some type of data compression.

So it can be seen that the offerings by Telstra differ in a number of respects. Different offerings support the use of different protocols. Some provide dedicated services whilst others provide non dedicated to numerous sites. Speed of transmission is another factor that differs between the services. Some offerings provide optional facilities. The different offerings also have different pricing structures ranging from fixed irrespective of volume to others that are variable including according to the time of transmission. Thus it will be recognised that it is necessary to have a detailed knowledge of Telstra's offerings and the applications that will operate on the WANs to select the most appropriate offering.

Just as it is necessary to manage every function in business, so it is necessary to manage a network. The network manager is responsible for the design of the network and its day to day running.

Expansion of the network or planned changes to the network can be performed in a controlled environment. The new equipment can be ordered and changes to the network management software and/or applications software can be planned in advance. By being able to plan in advance, the network manager can also plan the upgrade so that in the event of major unexpected problems, the network can be restored to its original condition.

On the other hand, some day to day matters require the immediate attention of the network manager. Often the network manager is contacted with the message 'The network is down'. On investigation, it might be found that only part of the network is down; that the network is all right but the users application is not working or that only a certain terminal is not working. So the first step in the fault finding is to establish the nature of the fault and working from there to establish the cause of the fault. With the cause of the fault established, the network manager can then carry out the changes to overcome the problem. Ideally, this should be an immediate permanent fix. However, on some occasions it might be necessary for the network manager to provide a temporary circumvention of the problem and then to provide the permanent solution at a later stage.

LANs have become reliable, so that it is the exception rather than the rule for them to be non operational. On occasions when a LAN does go down, it can be due to a hardware fault such as occurs on a personal computer. If the LAN is absolutely critical, it is possible to incorporate design features into the LAN to provide redundancy and to minimise the extent of the problem. One simple example is where the LAN extends over several floors such as in a hospital to split the LAN into sections and use bridges. If the cable is faulty in the top floors, the lower floors of the LAN can continue to operate. In this situation, staff can temporarily use the terminal on the other floors to gain access to the information in the emergency situation. It is possible to have terminals connected to a LAN so that even if the network does go down, the terminals can operate in a stand alone mode, thus allowing a reduced service.

It needs to be recognised that a LAN does not remain static. There are always new users, new applications, new hardware and changes of requirements that require the attention of the LAN Manager. One person should be responsible for the LAN management. The details of the LAN should be documented. Just as in any other position, there should also be a back up.

Many sites contract out the management of their LAN, in recognition that their staff do not have the necessary expertise nor is there the volume of work sufficient to warrant their development of the expertise.

The management of a WAN depends upon the Telstra option that is being used on the WAN. Where the service is a Digital service, the network manager has more capacity to perform diagnostics before contacting Telstra. Similarly, Telstra has better fault diagnostic equipment. The network manager requires access to tools for performing the diagnosis. These tools can be hardware or software.

The network manager requires access to at least a network line monitor and a break out box. The network line monitor can be 'attached to a communications circuit so that bit patterns being transmitted over the link can be captured and displayed to detect transmission or protocol violations' (Stamper 1991). On the other hand a break out box is a diagnostic tool that 'checks that signals being transmitted and to change the leads on which the signal is transmitted. A breakout box may also have features allowing cable testing and generation of bit test patterns' (Stamper 1991). Other hardware tools are also available.

The network manager also can make use of the trace facility often available under the operating system. Other specialised software to assist in fault diagnosis is also becoming more prevalent.

Security and privacy are also important matters, particularly in the health sector. These need to be considered in the design of the LAN. The LAN implementation can be made so that a particular terminal can be used by any user. On the other hand, it can be made restricted. The security and privacy measures available within the LAN should be only one part of the full security and privacy measures. It is highly desirable that several layers of security and privacy be incorporated. Examples of further layers are the use of passwords, restriction on users having access to applications and database access restrictions.

In general terms, a network carrier such as Telstra does not provide security and privacy features. However, new initiatives such as closed user groups under Austpac are beginning to emerge.

Communications in general

LANs and WANs are not mutually exclusive. A LAN can connect to another LAN. The particular additional hardware and software depends upon whether it is of the same type of LAN or not. Where the LANs are of a similar type a bridge is used, whereas when the LANs are of a different type a gateway is used. Thus, a bridge would connect two ethernet LANs together, whereas a bridge would be used to connect a token ring and an ethernet together.

A LAN can also communicate with a WAN. It does this through the server to which it is attached. Similarly, a WAN can communicate with another WAN. This simply recognises that two servers can communicate with one another when connected through a WAN. Again, with different requirements, different technology is required.

It is not uncommon for a user to require access to several servers, be they on the same LAN or not. Users are becoming accustomed to open architecture, whereby connection can be made to wherever is necessary.

Irrespective of where the connection is being made to, the technology is now available to allow a user to use the same procedure to gain access. As an example, the user simply clicks on the appropriate icon under Windows and the connection is automatically established. This preferred method of connection is often referred to as *transparent connection* or *seamless connection*.

To satisfy the user requirements, the network manager needs to prepare script files in conjunction with the user. Obviously, this script file will only work while the parameters applicable to the network do not vary, so that for example if an application is shifted from one server to another, a corresponding change needs to be made to allow the connection to work.

With many applications changing from the traditional centralised approach to one involving the use of LANs and WANs, there is a need for security and privacy to be reviewed.

Very few sites now do not require some type of communications and the technology available can meet the most simple or most complex requirements. The pace of change in communications will not slacken. It is fast becoming a very important part (if not the most important part) of an information site.

Summary

With the vast array of technology available, it is necessary to ensure that a strategic approach is adopted. This is to make certain the information requirements are met, that compatibility is obtained and that investment in hardware and software is protected.

The health sector is moving very quickly to take advantage of the technology that is available and it will use LANs and WANs according to the different requirements. For these reasons it is imperative that a strategic approach is used to identify the most appropriate information and communication needs. In addition, network management is required to ensure that the network continues to serve the present and future requirements of the organisation.

REFERENCES

Ahituv N, Neumann S 1990 Principles of information systems for management, 3rd edn. Wm C Brown, Dubuque
Cooper J A 1989 Computer and communications security. McGraw-Hill, New York
Currid C C 1992 Planning, designing and staffing LANs. Network Management, March
Denning P J 1990 Computers under attack: intruders, worms and viruses. Addison Wesley, Reading, Massachusetts
Forgione D, Blankley A 1990 Micro security and control. Tutorial of Accountancy, June

Highland H J 1990 Communications checklist. Computers and Society 9(6) October

Highland H 1989 What if a computer virus strikes? EDPACS, July

Hovenga E J S 1994 Information systems and diagnostic imaging. Informatics in Healthcare Australia 3(20)

Kauffels F 1992 Network management: problems, standards and strategies. Addison-Wesley, Reading, Massachusetts

Mair A, Scott J 1994 High hopes for productivity and health gains from health communication network. Healthcover, April-May

Marcella A 1989 Telstramunications: a control strategy. EDPACS, May

Schweitzer J A 1987 Securing information on a network of computers. EDPACS, July

Scott J 1993 Health communication network: current status and future developments. Informatics in Healthcare Australia 2(4)

Stallings W 1993 Local and metropolitan area networks, 4th edn. Macmillan Publishing Company, New York

Stamper D A 1991 Business data communications, 3rd edn. Benjamin/Cummings, Redwood City, California

Stamper D A 1994 Business data communications, 4th edn. Benjamin/Cummings, Redwood City, California

Utter A 1989 The four essentials of computer and information security. Internal Auditor, December

Waters S 1989 15 questions to ask before you buy a LAN. PC World, 4 October

FURTHER READING

Brown N 1990 Internal controls and systems integrity. EDPACS, September

Parker C, Case T 1993 Management information systems, 2nd edn. Mitchell McGraw-Hill, New York

Reynolds G W 1992 Information systems for managers, 2nd edn. West, St Paul

11

Management support systems principles and concepts

GREGORY K WHYMARK

> Providing information to management is much more than an intellectual challenge: it is the art of organizing complexity, of mastering multitude and avoiding its bastard chaos as effectively as possible (adapted from Dijkstra 1982).

MSS is a category of software solutions that are intensely user oriented and it includes systems known as decision support systems (DSS), executive information systems (EIS), executive support systems (ESS), and expert systems (ES). The term MSS is used here to refer to any computer based system that aims to support a manager or professional in a decision making environment. It is an extension of the older concept of a DSS to include a wider range of computer based support systems. MSS has a wider meaning than just the quantitative models that have traditionally been referred to as DSS.

DSS, MIS and MSS

The term decision support system is used by many different groups in the computer industry, in management, and amongst workers in operations research. One of the traditional views of DSS is that it implies the use of mathematical or statistical models. Such systems focus on a single or recurring decision area and will usually support one decision maker or a small management team working on the one management problem. The problem must be at least semi-structured, but is more likely to be based on a well structured problem and the resulting DSS is model oriented. Standard operations research tools such as linear programming, queuing theory, inventory theory and simulation (Turban 1995) are well suited to such systems. This type of decision support system is problem oriented with a major contribution of the system being in the area of problem definition. A disadvantage is that being problem oriented the system must continue to be restructured, updated or expanded as the problem changes.

This definition of a DSS is too narrow. No matter how it is viewed, the process of management is fundamentally one of decision making, and the process of making decisions and acting on them is the business of management. Any decision support system must contribute something tangible to the decision making process. It must either enable the manager to make the decision more efficiently, or enable the manager to make a more effective decision. Hence the increasing use of the term MSS to include any computer based system that supports a decision making process.

Another type of MSS is the computer based system which transforms data into information which is useful in the support of decision making. It is commonly referred to as a management information system (MIS) (Thierauf 1988, Turban 1995). It is characterised by the use of internal data which is often stored, manipulated and reported on using relational data base technology. Management use is usually restricted to reports that may be printed or reviewed on screen although access to the MIS using a structured query language (SQL) may be given to management in some cases. However, unless the decision maker is a computer professional or occupies the lower levels of management it is unlikely that enough time will be invested in learning the query language for this to be useful. In fact the manager is unlikely to learn enough for the integrity of the MIS to be secure.

By their nature the development of an MIS tends to require a long lead time. They require a large investment in the analysis of the problem and of the data that will be processed to provide the information.

Considering automation and the state of computing technology today, it is common to see office automation and computing support for all levels of management in both private and government organisations. That technology cannot supply management support in isolation. The state of the technology is such that with the purpose that an MSS implies, it can bestow great benefits on the user in terms of productivity and effectiveness. Equally, without that purpose, an ill defined system will bestow confusion, lack of direction and worse of all it will distract the manager from the complex decision processes that it is supposed to support.

Management levels

Decisions are made by people and DSS are designed to support those people. That we now see an emphasis on the term *user oriented* (Thierauf 1988) implies that that component of decision support systems may not have received sufficient attention in the past. Some of the work in the field categorises decision makers according to their place in the hierarchy, and according to the types of decision making that they engage in (Jaques 1976, Khadem & Lorber 1986, Rockart & Delong 1988). This has been discussed elsewhere (Whymark 1989, 1991a), but a summary of some of the concepts is presented here to help establish the place that the function of management has in the development of MSS.

The information needed to support decision makers at opposite end of the management hierarchy is fundamentally different. Figure 11.1 divides it into *control information* and *planning information*. Lower management will spend almost all of their time using control information which tends to be centred on the internal environmental factors. On the other hand, the information required by top management will largely be planning information that centres on the external environmental factors. Government guidance on financial expenditure is a good example of the latter in public administration.

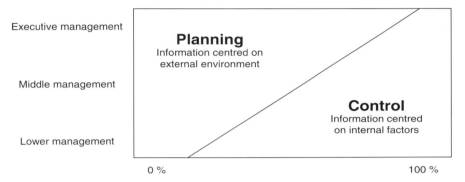

Fig. 11.1 Information requirements for control and planning processes
Source: Thierauf (1991)

Elsewhere, Thierauf (1988) categorises the decision maker according to the type of activity using a similar model to that first described by Jaques (1976). Figure 11.2 (Whymark 1991a) is a simplification of the model and is a useful guide in identifying the type of DSS required. Lower management is concerned with operational control. Therefore the type of information required is often detailed and accurate, and is sourced from within the organisation. The middle manager, according to this model, is concerned with organising programs into systems of work and ensures that goals are being met. The activity is referred to as managerial control and is tactical in nature. Reports that support this type of activity need to be comprehensive and may include some external information.

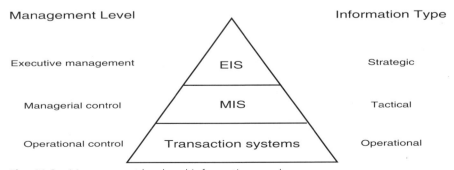

Fig. 11.2 Management level and information need
Source: Whymark (1991a)

As an example, the use of the characteristics of executive management to identify a system that supports executives (EIS) is described in Whymark (1991a), Watson (1992), and Turban (1995) among many others. Such managers are characterised by the strategic nature of their decision making, their long term goal seeking, and the higher level of abstraction in the mental models they use in managing their corporate affairs.

Components of information support systems

Another way of viewing and categorising an MSS is from the technology viewpoint. Figure 11.3 shows a convenient and often used description of four major components of a DSS. These are the database management system (DBMS), the model base management system (MBMS), the dialogue generation and management system (DGMS), and the most important, the user. Another component added by recent authors (Turban 1995) is the knowledge base management system (KBMS), in recognition of the role knowledge base sytems play in information support systems.

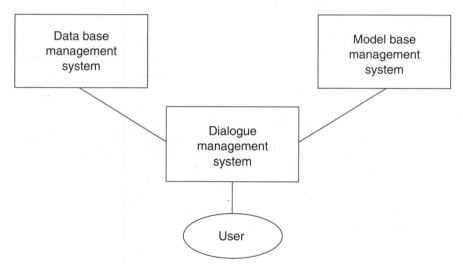

Fig. 11.3 Components of information support system
Adapted from Sprague & Watson (1993)

The model is used here to help describe the components of all management support systems. In doing so, the discussion has been kept as brief as possible as space precludes describing each modelling technique. Turban (1995) and many others provide further reading and references.

Modelling in MSS

There is much discussion about the relative merits of expert systems (ES), DSS, operations research and artificial neural networks. Often each is represented as an alternative to DSS. In reality each of these techniques is but one in a range of modelling techniques that can be used to form all or part of the model base for an MSS. The modelling techniques are described elsewhere (Turban 1995) and the discussion here concentrates on their relationship and their application in the decision making environment.

The use of models enables the analysis of large and complex scenarios. They can compress time for the decision maker, and allow the manipulation of variables to play *what-if* and *goal seeking* exercises as part of the decision making process (Turban 1995). They also enhance and reinforce learning, and providing they match the decision makers mental model of the decision environment, they can also greatly enhance the decision makers ability to reduce the complexity to simpler and easily handled decisions. The DBMS component also plays a part in this process.

To the non mathematically inclined, the concept of modelling can seem to be little more than a black art. However, the various modelling techniques can be treated as parts of a toolbox from which the appropriate tool for the job is selected.

The overlap of the different modelling techniques is illustrated by Figure 11.4. This figure is a simple Venn diagram drawn in the problem space of MSS. Each technique is suitable for use with certain problems, and for parts of the problem space more than one technique will perform. It depends on the skill on the MSS developer to choose the one that is most appropriate. Even without specific examples, it is now clear that a one method toolbox will no longer suffice.

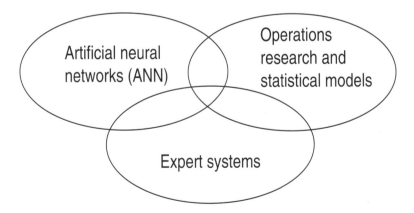

Fig. 11.4 Techniques used to model information and knowledge
Source: Smyrk (1992)

Data structures for MSS

Data models play an important role in MSS, far bigger than in most traditional DSS. The reason for this is twofold. First, the improvement in data base technology and distributed systems has made the access to data far easier for the MSS developer. Secondly, the role of data modelling plays a much bigger role than the model base in many modern MSS. This is particularly so for executive information systems and MIS that support middle managers in data intensive decision environments. The modelling of the data starts to play a crucial role in the enhancement of the user's mental model of the scenario and in the user's learning from the process.

Two data modelling technologies are useful here. The first, using the relational model and usually referred to as a relational data base management system (RDBMS) is described in another chapter. Most modern corporate systems are implemented using the relational model, and many large transactional systems uses RDBMS. There are now many proprietary systems that can provide an easy to access interface for managers at all levels to gain access to corporate relational systems.

The second approach to representing data in an MSS is called multi-dimensional modelling (MDM). The data is presented to the user as hypercube, with each dimension representing one way in which the decision maker breaks down the information for the problem at hand. An example might be a financial report that can be broken down first by organisational unit, secondly by service provided (administration, clinical, etc), thirdly by forecast, estimate and budget, and lastly by month and year. The data for this example could be presented to the user as a four dimensional hypercube which can then be interrogated by selecting components of different dimensions to gain the particular combination required. This is sometimes called *slicing the hypercube.*

MDM is an excellent way of presenting the data as it usually closely resembles the mental model used by the decision maker. This technique is further explained in Whymark (1991a), and is available in many MSS software packages such as EXPRESS[1] and EPIC[2]. SYSTEM/W[3] is a mainframe product that uses multi dimensional modelling for financial reporting systems as well as for MSS. A key property of these systems is that unlike a spreadsheet, the logic for calculations and consolidation is separated from the data and usually one logic file is used for many data files. This makes for much easier management of the underlying logic model than is the case with a spreadsheet approach. The technique also provides a powerful tool for financial reporting as the hierarchical structure of the dimensions makes for easy and efficient consolidation from cost control centres.

The interface

A typical MSS combines both the modelling and the data base systems to provide seamless support for a decision making professional or manager. The interface is the third component of the technology necessary for this seamless operation. Fortunately the technology has improved substantially to the point where serious MSS can be developed without a lot of technical expertise or help, especially when the support system relies mostly on the data modelling.

EIS are a good example of this type of system, but the idea is also extending down to other levels of management.

It is important that the interface matches the user's needs and skills. Executives need a system that is *executive friendly* (Whymark 1991a), but other MSS users may need training programs before using the system. The knowledge required by the user before using an MSS is an often overlooked aspect of system development.

The user

Thus we return to the fourth and most important component of any MSS, the user. The type of MSS ultimately depends on its purpose, and the purpose depends on the needs of the user. Understanding these needs can often be gained by considering the level of management practiced by the user, the information required, and the type of decision the user needs to make. This determines the model types and data base technology to be used, and also the type of interface required.

Development methods for MSS

The purpose of this section is to highlight the software development life cycles (SDLC) that are often most appropriate for the development of MSS. It is not intended to review basic software engineering theory in this paper, and the references used here (just a few of the many written on this topic) will provide further detail for the reader.

The classic life cycle of computer based information systems is described in Chapter 7 (Fig. 7.1), and should be the basis of the development of any transaction based operational system, especially those used by lower and middle management. MSS are different. In general, they have characteristics that will cause a project manager to adopt an approach that allows for greater flexibility in identifying the users needs, and that allows for flexibility throughout the life of the system. A caution is in order at this stage: a review as brief as this one attempts to provide general guidelines, and there will always be exceptions.

Common prescriptions for MSS development include the following.

- It must focus on the user, the decision process and the problem.
- It must involve the user in both development and change.
- It will induce change in the organisation, the MSS itself, in the user's work and in the decision making the MSS supports.
- The design process must be flexible.

This implies that one of two approaches to system development should be adopted: the iterative design approach or the adaptive design approach (Ahituv 1990). Both are similar to a general category of system development approaches called prototyping (Ahituv 1990, Pressman 1988) where the definition of the user requirements and final performance of the MSS is gradually refined during development. It is particularly useful in situations where both user and analyst have great difficulty in determining the functional characteristics before the system is built. It is almost essential in situations where the system is expected to change the way the user or the organisation will conduct work. MSS can be expected to perform in this way.

Iterative design

Iterative design (Ahituv 1990) is a series of rapid cycles or iterations through the full life cycle process. In each iteration the full life cycle is compressed into a very short period of time, and then repeated. It is a process where flexibility can be operationalised.

The steps in the iterative process are as follows:

1 User and designer jointly define the problem.
2 A small, useable system is developed.
3 The system is refined, expanded and modified.
4 The system is evaluated by the user, and the process continued.

The process of formal evaluation and modification of the problem definition is essential to the iterative design approach. The length of the cycle will depend on the size of the project.

Adaptive design

The adaptive design approach assumes that the final system must evolve through usage and learning. Whereas the iterative approach still relies on formal specifications, this approach relies on a prototype to define the system performance.

The basic principles are as follows:

- Find out quickly what is important to the user.
- Provide the user with something concrete.
- Define a clear architecture for the MSS so that it can be easily developed and modified.
- Pay careful attention to the user-MSS dialogue.
- Emphasise the importance of use learning in terms of using the system.
- Emphasise getting started rather than getting finished.

In some ways this approach reflects the philosophy of an old maxim for succeeding in any venture—*fail early*. The principles are in sharp contrast to those of the traditional SDLC. The designer's job goes well past the need for design in conventional systems as they become closely involved in the decision situation with the user. They also have to be responsive to the user and help to stimulate exploration and learning in all users.

The system continues to develop and evolve as the user develops further knowledge about how the system can be used, and most importantly, on what its impact on the decision making process will be. This was the approach used in developing EDIS, the EIS developed for the Royal Australian Navy. It is also the most appropriate development life cycle approach for most management support systems.

Application of MSS

EIS are one type of MSS that is easily identified by the users supported. They are highly focussed on the needs of the executive and the executive friendly software used for implementation of the system. The software used does not define an EIS, and it may be used to provide information support to other managers as well. The information content, style of delivery and the decision processes supported are unique to executive management, and it is these aspects that define the system as an EIS. Many examples of EIS will be found at the end of this chapter.

Managers in the health industry have the same needs and can be categorised in the same way as managers in other industry sectors. Executives are concerned with strategic planning, and so need external as well as internal information. Middle management also have similar needs in the administrative functions. These managers can be served by similar technology and development methods to managers in other industries.

The needs of clinical managers is the challenge of the 1990s. The technology is available, the development process is well understood, and the clinical processes are well understood. It is not clear however, just what impact the technology may have on process redesign and hence on the needs for information support by clinical management. Much of the software tools will be specific to professional practice.

Two commercial systems recently developed in Australia serve as examples. The first is a patient dependency system designed to be used by nursing staff at the ward level. Called TDS[4] (Total Dependency System), it is a cross between a transaction processing system and an MSS. It provides a means of capturing ward based activity and provides nursing management with information to support both operational and strategic decision making.

The Ca$eMax[5] system is a true MSS. The developers worked in close liaison with hospital managers to develop an application that supported their needs in a casemix environment. It is tailored to the needs of the Victorian hospital, but like all good MSS, these sorts of systems can easily be tailored to other environments. In this case the data are stored using multidimensional modelling techniques, and this allows the manager to easily compose a report that suits the needs of the moment. The interface is intuitive and is executive friendly. The system supports executive management with their internal data needs in the casemix decision making environment, and so will not provide all information needs for management.

This highlights another important point. It is rare that MSS or DSS are able to supply all the information a manager needs. The aim is to always provide as much of the routine requirements as possible, so freeing the professional or manager to concentrate on the non-routine.

MSS as a factor in organisational change

Information: the sixth resource

The five resources necessary to conduct any enterprise are people, machines, management, material and money (in past times referred to as the five Ms). Information is now an equally important commodity and can be considered to be the sixth resource. The information revolution has been likened to the industrial one of the eighteenth and nineteenth centuries, but has occurred in the space of about 20 years instead of over a period of a century or two.

Information is power in modern enterprises and is essential to decision. Not only is information power, but changes to the information flow can and will transform an organisation. Since many MSS deal directly with both the information and its flow within the organisation, they can act as change agents in a number of ways. This can happen by design or by accident. MSS can:

- change the lines of communication
- change the lines of power and control
- change the organisational structure, either directly or covertly
- support a corporate memory or knowledge base.

Impact at the personal level

Modern MSS (including interactive MIS) have the capacity to improve job satisfaction as well as job productivity, as decision making is pushed down to the lower levels of management. In addition, many professional workers will see the improved technology available in MSS removing the complexity imposed by multitudinous data inputs, therefore bringing them closer to the real problem and the real decision process required of them.

MSS are also increasing the flexibility of organisations and individuals. For example, expert systems have the capacity to bring expert knowledge to many others in the same profession. Many tasks that now require greater experience and knowledge will be carried out by *lesser experts* in the profession.

As our knowledge and skill at implementing computer human interaction (CHI) improve there will be less need for computer skills and more need for business and management skills. This is already evident with EIS, and is heading that way with ES. The trend is the same of MSS in general. It means a much closer relationship between the ultimate users and the development of the MSS, and this will further improve the job satisfaction of the professional and the middle manager. They will attain their proper position as directors of development instead of merely acting as receivers of inadequate technology.

Impact on training

The impact of new trends in MSS on training (more so than education) will be twofold. It will effect the type of training required, and secondly, it will effect the way that training is delivered.

As MSS provide more guidance to all levels of management and use modelling techniques more appropriate to the problem domain then the skills required to use the systems will change. The trend will be towards a requirement of greater skill in the decision making process, and less in the use of technology as such.

The way training will be delivered in the future will also be affected by the linking of MSS development and computer aided learning (CAL) systems. Research is very active in this area and results are starting to reach industry. This is another technology that gained a false start in the late 1960s and early 1970s, but is likely to deliver over the next decade. The ability of many MSS to provide a learning environment in addition to the primary purpose of decision support will support the integration of MSS and CAL.

Social impact

There are many aspects of our society that have been affected by MSS. Many problems solved using traditional DSS could not have been solved economically, if at all, with traditional computer based information systems (CBIS). Some of the positive implications can be far reaching and include furhter opportunities for the handicapped, working at home or telecommuting, and improvements in the quality of life for some workers (Turban 1995).

There are always negative affects. In the case of MSS they may include changes in employment availability and opportunity and changing gaps between socio-economic groups, a potential for new types of computer crime, problems with the centralisation of power via integrated computer systems and corporate data base systems, and an increasing 'blame the computer' attitude.

Conclusion

The potential of the role of MSS in organisational change is particularly important for project managers to understand as it has such a big impact on the success of the project. Senior management also need to be aware of the potential and to make a clear decision as to whether they wish to avoid or to take advantage of that potential.

To date, most MSS use has occurred at the lower levels of management, but the impact is increasingly being felt at all levels. Management support systems are taking over routine tasks and freeing decision makers to concentrate on the crucial decision making process. Is this an opportunity or a threat?

MSS support the decision making process. This gives the MSS developer the potential to change the process and even affect the decision making style of the manager. By shortening the intelligence phase of the decision making process MSS give the manager or professional the opportunity to concentrate on problem specification and problem finding, rather than just 'putting out bush fires'.

NOTES

[1] EXPRESS is a product of Information Resources.
[2] EPIC is a product of Planning Sciences UK and Australia.
[3] SYSTEM/W is a product of Comshare Inc.
[4] Total Dependency System (TDS) is a product developed by E J S Hovenga & Associates, and marketed by the CBIM (Centre for Information Management), a commercial arm of the Faculty of Business, CQU. Dr G K Whymark is the current director of CBIM.
[5] Ca$emax is a product developed by FHA Melbourne using EPIC as an MSS generator.

REFERENCES

Ahituv N, Neuman S 1990 Principles of information systems for management. Wm C Brown, Dubuque

Dijkstra E W 1982 Selected writings on computing: a personal perspective. Springer-Verlag, New York

Jaques E 1976 A general theory of bureaucracy. Gower, Hampshire

Khadem R, Lorber R 1986 One page management. Information Australia, Melbourne

Rockart J F, Delong D W 1988 Executive support systems. Dow Jones-Irwin, Homewood, Illinois

Pressman R S 1988 Software engineering: a beginner's guide, McGraw-Hill, New York

Smyrk J 1992 Artificial neural networks. 1992 ACS Lecturer of the Year.

Sprague R H 1980 A framework for the development of decision support systems. MIS Quarterly 4(4)

Sprague R H, Watson H J 1989 Decision support systems: putting theory into practice. Prentice-Hall, Sydney

Thierauf R J 1988 User oriented decision support systems. Merrill, Melbourne

Thierauf R J 1991 Executive information systems: a guide for senior management and MIS professionals. Quorum Books, New York

Turban E 1995 Decision support and expert systems: management support systems. Collier Macmillan, Sydney

Watson H J, Rainer R K, Houdeshell G. 1992 Executive information systems: emergence, development, impact. Wiley, New York

Whymark G K 1989 Systems that support decision makers. Asor Bulletin 8(2)

Whymark G K 1991 Development of the EIS concept and its implementation in the RAN. Australian Computer Journal 23(3)

3

Health informatics in clinical practice

12

Electronic medical records

TERRY J HANNAN

Historical overview

The importance of medical records in health care delivery has been recognised for a long time. Its relevance to patient care and health administration was documented by Florence Nightingale in 1873 a book entitled *Notes on a Hospital*. Health care is a continuous process in which data is progressively accumulated, therefore the record must function as a 'pre-birth to post-death system that meets the requirements for any clinical setting–whether intensive care or primary care' (Hammond 1993).

Ideally the medical record should be the primary repository of all information regarding patient care, provide decision support, and be a tool for supporting and maintaining ancillary health care activities such as administration, quality assurance, research and epidemiology.

Shortliffe & Perreault have defined medical (health) practice as medical decision making, (Shortliffe 1990) and it is recognised that there is an integral relationship between medical decision making, the accumulation of clinical data, health care costs, patient outcomes, and the quality of care (Johns & Blum 1973, James 1989). The delivery of quality, cost effective health care requires efficient decision support tools based on the medical record system if these end points are to be achieved.

Traditional medical record systems

Current medical record systems are predominantly hard copy paper based models with or without variable components of electronic data such as laboratory results and X-ray reports. The paper chart can be read by only one person at a time and they must have it physically in their possession. It is difficult to store and retrieve, requiring space, time and effort. It can be organised in one format at a time yet the demands of the users of the record require it to be in a multitude of formats to meet the individuals needs. To reorganise the record into a variety of formats requires major time commitments and the schematic format is easily corrupted. The paper record is not always legible, is often inaccurate, lacks clinical sensibility, and is not compatible with specified data standards or other information stored in the record (Tierney & Hannan 1992). Poor indexing of data makes the finding of information difficult or impossible (Brennan et al 1991, Leape et al 1991).

Reproduction of the manual record by transcription and photocopying adds to the costs of health care services without any corresponding proven benefit. It was recently calculated in the United States to cost an additional $15 billion per year to manually reproduce the medical record by transcription (Frawley 1993). Use of the paper chart as a medical record impedes efforts to monitor and improve health care by the inherent difficulty, time, and expense required to access individual charts (Payne et al 1990).

Technology and health care delivery

Since the 1960s there has been a rapid growth in the technology used to support medical care (Blum 1986, Orthner & Blum 1989, Shortliffe & Perreault 1990), and this has resulted in the creation of enormous volumes of *data and information* that is available to assess and manage the delivery of health care. Weed estimated that an individual patient can generate up to 50 000 data items during their life (Weed 1989), and to support good decision making individuals who provide health care require timely integration of this data. New and evolving technologies continue to produce and store large volumes of data and information for patient care (Blum 1986, McDonald 1989a, McDonald et al 1992a), but there only a few systems that provide *information processing tools* which support clinical decision making (Blum 1986, Orthner & Blum 1989, Shortliffe et al 1990).

It is recognised that the information processing capacity of the human brain is limited in its ability to accurately decipher this clinical data and information in a timely manner without errors (Miller 1956, Pryor & Clayton 1991, McDonald 1976). Errors in decision making are further increased when there is *random noise* data; for example, with unexpected data input in stressful situations, a common occurrence in health care.

Consequences of using manual-based record systems

The use of predominantly manual, non-integrated medical records systems has led to increasing costs in patient care (Johns & Blum 1973, Blum 1986) and administration (Woolhandler & Himmelstein 1991), decreased compliance with health care standards (McDonald 1976, Gardner & Schaffner 1993), inappropriate variation in health care delivery (Wennberg & Gittelsohn 1973), and possible negligent behaviour by health care providers (Brennan et al 1991, Leape et al 1991). A Harvard study into the incidence of adverse events during hospitalisation led the authors to conclude that, 'Lawyers generally believe that investigation of substandard care only begins with the medical record; that in many instances the medical record even conceals substandard care; and that substandard care is not reflected in, or "discoverable" in the medical record' (Brennan et al 1991, Leape et al 1991).

Concept of Electronic Medical Record (EMR)

What is the Electronic Medical Record (EMR)? It is the storage of all health care data and information in electronic formats with the associated information processing and knowledge support tools necessary for the managing the health enterprise system.

In the early 1970s several institutions investigated the concept of creating an EMR to improve patient care. An important feature each of these projects was the concept that the medical record should be the cornerstone for all information systems within the health care environment (Blum 1986, McDonald et al 1992a, Safran et al 1990, Enterline et al 1989, Kuperman et al 1991) and that the data supporting ancillary patient care activities such as administration, pharmacy and laboratories could and should be generated as a by-product of the patient care process (Blum 1986, Slack 1990, Bleich et al 1985).

One of the earliest successful implementations of EMR functions was at the Regenstrief Institute, Indianapolis. Using the Regenstrief Medical Record System (RMRS) McDonald demonstrated that the use of computer generated reminders based on patient specific laboratory data resulted in a reduction of physicians errors in the detection of life-threatening events, and also confirmed that busy physicians were often unable to detect many of the critical abnormalities occurring in the patient record. He concluded that, 'the amount of data presented to the physician per unit time is more than he can process without error. The computer *augments* the physician's capabilities and thereby reduces his error rate... It is very likely that the physicians in these studies were simply unable to detect all the multitudinous conditions specified by the standards' (McDonald 1976). Computer generated reminders are now used as standard tools for patient care in the RMRS and other EMR systems used in hospitals and ambulatory care environments (Tierney et al 1986, Tierney et al 1987, McDonald et al 1992a, Safran et al 1990, Safran et al 1991, Enterline et al 1989, Kuperman et al 1991).

The Institute of Medicine study into electronification of the patient care record

In 1992 the Institute of Medicine (Dick & Steen 1991) of the American National Academy of Sciences, published the results of its study into computerised medical records, their functionality, and how technology could bring the benefits of these records within the reach of all those within the health care system. The recommendations from this study are summarised in the following list:

1 Health care professionals and organisations should adopt the computer based patient record (CPR) as the standard for medical and all other records related to patient care.

2 To accomplish Recommendation 1, the public and private sectors should join in establishing a Computer based Patient Record Institute (CPRI) to promote and facilitate development, implementation, and dissemination of the CPR.

3 Both the public and private sectors should expand support for the CPR and CPR system implementation through research, development, and demonstration projects. Specifically, the committee recommends that Congress authorise and appropriate funds to implement the research and development agenda outlined herein. The committee further recommends that private foundations and vendors fund programs that support and facilitate this research and development agenda.

4 The CPRI should promulgate uniform national standards for data and security to facilitate implementation of the CPR and its secondary databases.

5 The CPRI should review federal and state laws and regulations for the purpose of proposing and promulgating model legislation and regulations to facilitate the implementation and dissemination of the CPR and its secondary databases and to streamline the CPR and CPR systems.

6 The costs of CPR systems should be shared by those who benefit from the value of the CPR. Specifically, the full costs of implementing and operating CPRs and CPR systems should be factored into reimbursement levels or payment schedules of both public and private sector third-party payers. In addition, users of secondary databases should support the costs of creating such databases.

7 Health care professional schools and organisations should enhance educational programs for students and practitioners in the use of cmputers, CPRs, and CPR systems for patient care, education, and research.

Publication of this report has resulted in a wide range of activities directed towards standardised EMR developments. In the US, the Department of Health and Human Services has implemented a national policy on a health information communication infrastructure based on automation of the patient record (US Department of Health and Human Services 1993). This group sees a national interconnected communication network linking all participants in the health care system via their own *computer based patient record system*—an information system that would have the ability to create, store, retrieve, transmit and manipulate patients 'health data in ways that best support decision making about their care.' These record systems would be linked to reference bases of aggregated patient data and computerised knowledge based systems which use decision support logic and practice guidelines to help caregivers make better decisions about diagnosis and treatment options (Safran et al 1990, Kuperman et al 1991).

Software applications providing decision support in EMRs

No complete EMRs currently exist; however standards for software function and decision support have been defined and are seen as core elements for future EMR developments (Dick & Steen 1991). The basic software components necessary for future EMRs as defined by McDonald (1988) are as follows:

- maintain a data dictionary
- orientation
- introspection
- selectivity of data input
- query languages

In systems which maintain a *data dictionary* all data and observations are stored in records, which include fields that link or point to the dictionary files. This means that the data is stored in coded formats providing for more consistent recording and ease of data entry. They also provide facilities for declaring the data entry fields prior to the recording and storage of data, without the need to define in advance the space to be occupied by the recorded data, thus allowing a much more economical use of computer storage space, and more rapid access to the data.

Orientation provides the facility to produce an array of time-oriented flow sheets from the stored data. Figure 12.1 shows summary flow chart of clinical data taken from a patient on chemotherapy for leukaemia. The capacity for displaying clinical data in user defined, time oriented formats, is a decision support tool fundamental to good clinical practice (Blum 1986, Orthner & Blum 1989, Hannan 1991).

Introspection is a decision support tool where the computer is able to examine data and information stored within the EMR database using pre-defined clinical rules, and to identify certain conditions that require attention (McDonald et al 1992a, Kuperman et al 1991, Safran et al 1990). These record systems automatically produce drug alerts, warnings, protocol generated reminders and are able to detect significant alterations in data elements which complement the medical decision making process (McDonald 1976, Tate 1990, Kuperman et al 1991).

The users of EMR systems must decide on the *selectivity of data input* and how it will be entered into the medical record, manually, electronically, or by other processes (McDonald 1990a). Quality data input can be expensive to maintain because it requires disciplined, well-trained staff (Orthner & Blum

CCCIS CLINICAL INFORMATION SYSTEM

HISTORY NO: 808080
NAME: MARROW,BONE
DATE: 30/10/88

FULL FLOW

CURRENT		04SEP87	05SEP87	07SEP87	08SEP87	09SEP87	10SEP87	11SEP87
PROTOCOL/CYCLE								
525					DAY 1	DAY 2	DAY 3	DAY 4
CYCLE					C2D1	C2D2	C2D3	C2D4
737		DAY 24	DAY 25	DAY 27	DAY 28			
CYCLE		C1D24	C1D25	C1D27	C1D28			
CHEMO								
ARAC	MG					220	220	220	220
DAUNORUB	MG					110	110		
VP-16 IV	MG					165	165	165	165
HAEM.								
WBC	10^9/L	4.1	5.1	7.8	8.4		5.7	
RBC	10^12/L	3.88	4.15	4.23	4.13		4.74	
HGB	g/dl	11.7	12.2	12.8	12.7		14.6	
HCT	%	33.3*	36.5*	37.8	37.1		42.7	
MCV	fL	86.0	88.0	89.0	90.0		90.0	
MCH	pg	30.2	29.4	30.3	30.8		30.8	
MCHC	g/dl	35.1*	33.4	33.9	34.2		34.2	
BAND FMS	%				2			
NEUTROPH	%		30*	36*	44	45		68	
PLATELET	10^9/L	67*	103*	214	247		200	
BLASTS	%			7				
MYEL	%		3					
METAMY	%		2					
EOS	%			1		5		
TOX.GRAN		SL		SL	SL			
LYMPH	%	43.0	46.0	42.0	36.0		23.0*	
MONO	%	22.0*	10.0	12.0*	14.0*		9.0	
ANISOCYT					MO			
OV.POIK					MO			
POLYCHRO					SL			
RNDMACRO					SL			
CHEMSTRY								
SODIUM	MMOL/L	144		139			138	
POTASS	MMOL/L	3.5		4.3			3.5	
CHLOR	MMOL/L	105		103			108	
CO2	MMOL/L	26		25			26	
UREA	MMOL/L	6.3		5.5			6.3	
CREAT	MMOL/L	0.08		0.09			0.08	
GLUCOSE	MMOL/L	5.6*						
BILI.T	UMOL/L				18*		14	
AST	U/L				53		34	
ALT	U/L				131*		86*	
GGT	U/L				114*		83*	
ALK.PHOS	U/L				198*		143*	
TOT.CALC	MMOL/L				2.26		2.16	
PHOS	MMOL/L				1.3		1.2	
T.PROT	G/L				74		66	
ALBUMIN	G/L				39		34*	

(C)ONTINUE OR (Q)UIT

(C)URRENT   (E)ARLIEST   (D)ATE   (B)ACKWARD   (F)ORWARD   (P)RINT   (Q)UIT

Fig. 12.1 User defined flow chart of clinical data

1989, Enterline et al 1989). However, once data are stored the users have access to the computer's powerful report generator functions that provide useful data and information displays and reports that support all components of health care delivery (Enterline et al 1989, Safran et al 1990).

It is now possible to access these large volumes of clinical data stored in electronic formats using *medical query languages* for the purposes of research, epidemiology, health care planning, and for producing reports based on data analysis. The collection of information on large numbers of patients to answer specific problems is expensive, time consuming and personnel intensive and is often restricted to small numbers of patients for a limited range of conditions (Tierney & Hannan 1992). For example, to answer the question whether the post menopausal oestrogen use protected women against cardiovascular morbidity and mortality, Stampfer and others had to receive regular mailed reports on specific clinical events from more than 48 000 women for 10 years (Stampfer et al 1991). These tasks could have been performed more easily and cheaply if the data were available in a single EMR database or accessible over a range of standardised EMR systems.

Computerised clinical decision support tools

Specific decision support tools for use within EMRs which provide benefits to health care have been defined (Pryor & Clayton 1991), and these are as follows:

- alerting
- intepretation
- assisting
- critiquing
- diagnosing
- management

Alerting automatically provides decision makers with data and information in situations where rapid, sometimes life threatening, decisions are required. Examples are abnormal laboratory values, vital sign trends, failure to perform nursing procedures and medication contraindications. These clinical situations often have episodes of unpredictable *random noise* data which impair the decision making process leading to errors in patient care.

A system of alerts is used routinely in HELP (Health Evaluation through Logical Processing) (Bradshaw et al 1989) and Regenstrief Medical Record Systems (RMRS) (McDonald et al 1992a). Established benefits from the use of alerts are a reduction in physician and nursing errors in patient management, increased compliance with predefined standards of care, (McDonald et al 1984) decreased length of stay in hospital and time spent in life-threatening situations (Kuperman et al 1991, Sittig et al 1989).

Using automated alerts in the HELP system during surgery for non-indicated and non-ordered antibiotics Classen demonstrated a fall in the post-operative infection rate from 13% patients per day to 5.5%, and a fall from 35% to 18% in the percentage of patients receiving antibiotics late for surgery. As a consequence there was a reduction in the number of patients receiving antibiotics for an excessive time post-operatively which produced overall savings of $59 000 in 6 months (Classen et al 1992). This system for recommending antibiotics has now been extended to primary and ambulatory care (Evans 1991, Evans et al 1993).

Interpretation is the assimilitation of stored clinical data leading to an improved understanding of what the data means. Examples are ECG interpretation, blood gas data analysis and the interpretation of X-ray findings (Blum 1986, Orthner & Blum 1989, McDonald 1989, 1990b, 1991).

Assisting is the use of decision support tools to speed up or simplify some clinical action. This technique is used in the production of clinical orders, nursing assessment of patients, and history and physical examination. Patient pre-printed encounter forms improve history taking and standardise data recording. Assisting also facilitates direct data entry on to computer terminals making the data immediately available to authorised users of the EMR (McDonald et al 1992b).

Where assisting is used in the ordering of blood samples the specimen is ordered 'on-line' and the EMR system indicates the tube type, laboratory to which the specimens are to be sent and when the last specimen was ordered. In this situation the system may also recommend how many times and on what dates a given sample is to be collected within a specified time interval (Enterline et al 1989, McDonald et al 1992b). At the Johns Hopkins Oncology Center (JHOC), computerised protocol directed care plans were used to manage blood-product facilities by recommending specific numbers of platelet units for thrombocytopenic patients who were at risk of bleeding. This produced cost savings of $250 000 per year, decreased the use of a limited resource (platelets), and improved patient outcomes (no increase in bleeding) (Enterline et al 1989).

Critiquing is the analysis of decisions within the EMR using defined knowledge rules to verify the appropriateness of those decisions. The system is able to recommend to the physician, nurse, etc. the most appropriate decision to make (McDonald 1976). Examples of critiquing include clinical orders, protocol-directed care plans, diagnosis making and management plans (Blum 1986, Orthner & Blum 1989).

Diagnosing is the application of a specific clinical model for the purpose of understanding a complex clinical situation. In these situations the computer may provide a probability list for a range of differential clinical diagnoses based on the data has stored within it (Miller et al 1982, Safran et al 1991). Currently these systems are limited to small clinical domains, such as intensive care, and are expensive because of the expertise needed to maintain the knowledge rules within them (Blum 1986, Orthner & Blum 1989).

Management is the generation of action oriented decisions designed to improve the function of the current system state. Examples include hospital operations, resource allocation (including personnel) and the current status of changing clinical disease patterns, either acute or chronic. In HELP the decision support system will recommend changes in FI02 (Fraction of Inspired Oxygen) with patients on respiratory support and suggest when to draw the next blood gases based on existing laboratory and clinical data (Kuperman et al 1991). Pooled data from HELP made available to surgeons performing uncomplicated prostatic resections resulted in reduced length of stay and costs of the procedure over a range of hospitals in the region (James 1989, Grandia 1994).

The Oncology Center Information System (OCIS) uses nurse generated patient dependency ratings to allocate staff during hospital admissions, and patients are scheduled in outpatient clinics according to the procedures performed so that the doctor-patient encounters coincide with the availability of the clinical data.

Many decision support applications coexist within EMR systems and they must be integrated to the continuously expanding database of individual patients and groups of patients. Data required for patient care must be available in a timely, reliable and complete manner with the user being able to extract data they require in the format that best suits their decision making (Blum 1986, Kuperman et al 1991). Timeliness of data retrieval is critical in patient care and it has been recommended that data recall times of less than two seconds should be achieved irrespective of the complexity of the decision support function (Pryor & Clayton 1991). An example of how access, storage, and manipulation of clinical data is able to assist all levels of health care is illustrated in Figure 12.2 (a plot of white blood cells and platelets on a patient undergoing chemotherapy).

The display shows user-defined levels (horizontal dashed lines) at which decisions relating to platelet or white cell transfusion, or prophylactic antibiotic therapy may be made. Using accumulated data from groups of patients based on the time interval in which they have a low cell counts, the length of stay in hospital can be predicted by treatment and diagnosis, thus aiding bed allocation and rostering of nursing staff based on patient dependency status. Resource utilisation such as the number of tests ordered, medications utilised and bed occupancy can be evaluated from the data accumulated during the patient care process, thus demonstrating how administrative and health planning data can be generated from the patient care record. The data displayed is linked to the complete medical record so complex interrelationships of data within the EMR can also be evaluated (Bleich et al 1985, Slack 1990 Safran et al 1990, and 1991, Grandia 1994).

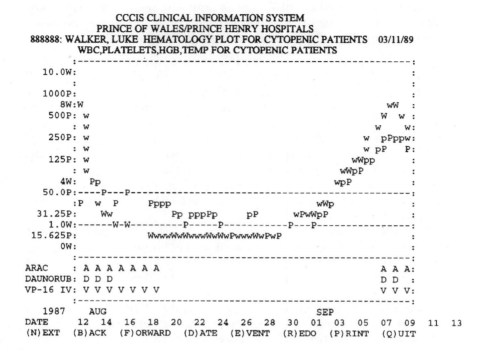

Fig. 12.2 Daily plot of white blood cells and platelets with chemotherapy

Existing EMR models and confirmed benefits of EMRs

Complete automation of the medical record system has not yet occurred; however there are a range of EMR systems which provide information demonstrating the real and potential benefits of electronically stored medical information. Recent advances in technology relating to data and information storage, such as Compact Disks—Read Only Memory (CD-ROM), provide facilities for lifelong repositories of medical data. There are functioning EMR systems storing in excess of one million patients on line, representing billions of data points accessible within seconds (Safran et al 1990, McDonald 1989a), and the ability to manage these large volumes of data is another area where the benefits of computerisation can be seen. For example:

- Fries and his co-workers, using the American Rheumatological Association Medical Information System (ARAMIS), showed that physicians using a computerised data flow sheet were able to find specified information twice as fast as physicians using the traditional paper record (Fries 1974). The physicians in this study were able to find the relevant information virtually all the time with the computer record but failed to find 10% of the information in the paper chart.

- Whiting-O'Keefe and his colleagues used the Summary Time-Orientated Record (STOR) to show that physicians were better able to predict their patients laboratory results when using the computerised record (Whiting-O'Keefe 1980).
- Computer generated reminders used in the RMRS have improved compliance with practice standards particularly in the area of preventive care (McDonald et al 1984, 1989b, Litzelman et al 1990).
- HELP has an extensive alerting system based on data generated from laboratory auto-analysers which has resulted in shorter length of stay in hospital, reduced costs and time spent in life-threatening situations (Kuperman et al 1991).
- Research using OCIS has confirmed the benefits of protocol-directed care plans by reducing resource utilisation and costs without reducing the quality of care (Enterline et al 1989).
- Use of the Beth Israel Hospital (BIH) system has improved access to medical records, provided decision support through rapid access to bibliographic databases and to cumulative patient data subsets via its medical query language (Safran et al 1990 and 1991).

The benefits from effective automation of health care delivery using EMR systems based on the IOM criteria can be viewed from different domains, namely patient care, quality assurance, costs, epidemiology, research, and administration.

Patient care

Preventive care is recognised as one area for providing major cost savings in health care delivery. The use of an electronic reminder system based on the patient record has resulted in the more effective implementation of preventive care protocols, immunisation procedures, better use of vaccines, and a reduction in morbidity and mortality from infectious diseases (Fries et al 1993, Gardner & Schaffner 1993).

Quality assurance

Effective quality assurance in health care requires a *reduction of inappropriate variation in health care delivery and adequate documentation of procedures* to improve the processes involved in health care delivery (Wennberg & Gittelsohn 1973, James 1989). At the Regenstrief Institute rheumatologists use the RMRS to identify patients with rheumatoid arthritis and other connective tissue disorders who are being treated with 'second line' drugs such as gold, methotrexate, azathioprine, and penicillamine. The monitoring program detects whether the appropriate pre-treatment haematology and urine tests have been performed, if the results are abnormal and whether the drugs were held or given in reduced dosages. Patients whose records do not meet these standards have their outpatient charts reviewed and, if substandard care has been delivered, the providers are contacted (McDonald 1990b). The same system using data accumulated within the first 24 hours following admission has been used to identify patients who are likely to have high hospital costs (McDonald et al 1990b). Tierney and others (Wilson et al 1982, Tierney et al 1993) demonstrated how the use of an electronic medical record system to control orders for inpatients significantly lowered patient charges and hospital costs. In this situation the ordering of blood tests, medications, etc, was performed at the computer terminal by the medical officers and the justification for requesting each test was prompted by reminders from the EMR.

Research

Research costs represent a significant component of the health care budget as the acquisition of accurate data is difficult and costly in both time and dollars (Tierney & McDonald 1991). Payne et al (1990) demonstrated the cost and time savings benefits of the electronic medical record system Computer Stored Ambulatory Record (COSTAR) over the paper record when evaluating the effects of anti-arthritic medications in hypertensive patients. The costs saving were in the tens of thousands of dollars and the time savings were measured in hundreds of person hours.

Epidemiology

As chronic diseases become more prominent in modern health care, larger patient populations will need to be studied to detect variations in diseases and changes in health outcomes resulting from therapeutic interventions, and the size of these populations make it impractical to undertake studies using existing paper based medical record systems (Tierney et al 1985). Effective studies of these large patient populations will require new analytical methodologies to be created so we can harness all the information they contain (McDonald 1989b).

EMR systems have been used to identify those patients with hypertension prescribed non-steroidal anti-inflammatory drugs who are likely to develop renal insufficiency (Tierney et al 1989, Murray et al 1990), and identify clinical factors that predict which patients taking diuretics are likely to develop hypokalemia (Tierney et al 1985a) and ventricular ectopy (Tierney et al 1985b).

Administration

Data stored within the HELP clinical system has been used in the Utah Intermountain Health Centre to evaluate the costs and quality of care for a variety of medical and surgical procedures. The EMR provided information on variations in length of stay, surgical procedure time and costs for uncomplicated surgical resections of the prostate. This information was relayed to the medical practitioners who performed the operations in a range of institutions and they co-operated in altering their surgical techniques and procedures to reduce the mean length of stay and costs of routine Transurethral Resections of the Prostate (TURP) (James 1989). In the evaluation process it was found that certain preoperative procedures such as chest X-rays, were unnecessary if a patient had an uncomplicated medical history. The same clinical data generated from the patient care process is being used to measure and evaluate the effectiveness of Diagnostic Related Group (DRG) studies, and has led to a reduction in DRG costings. Similar hospitals not using a patient-based EMR system have expanding DRG and other health costs (Gardia 1994). This confirms Howard Bleich's observation that 90% of administrative cost data can be generated as a by-product of the patient care process (Bleich et al 1985).

To achieve these results EMR systems must provide standardisation of data recording so that data and information can be shared across institutions and internationally. Achieving the end points of EMR integration is not easy; however successful implementations have been completed and they provide answers to many of the difficulties faced and how they can be overcome (Martin 1992, Hannan 1994).

Conclusions

With the knowledge that established models of EMRs have been shown to improve the health care process, what is the recommended course for future EMR projects?

Developers, project directors and users of clinical information systems must begin to share the experiences, and use existing and evolving software tools to reduce implementation costs. This will result in the most effective delivery of quality health care.

REFERENCES

Bleich H L, Beckley R F, Horowitz G L, et al 1985 Clinical computing in a teaching hospital. New England Journal of Medicine 312:756-764

Blum B I 1986 Clinical information systems. Johns Hopkins Oncology Center. Springer-Verlag, New York

Brennan T A, Leape L L, Laird N M, et al 1991 Incidence of adverse events and negligence in hospitalized patients. Results of the Harvard Medical Practice Study I. New England Journal of Medicine 325(3):210

Bradshaw K E, Gardner R M, Pryor T A 1989 Development of a computerised laboratory alerting system. Computers and Biomedical Research 22:575-587

Classen D C, Evans S, Pestotnik S L, Horn S D, Menlove R L, Burke J P 1992 The timing of prophylactic administration of antibiotics and the risk of surgical wound infection. New England Journal of Medicine 326:281-286

Dick R S, Steen E B 1991 The computer-based patient record. An essential technology for health care. National Academy Press, Washington DC

Enterline J P, Lenhard R E Jr, Blum B I A 1989 Clinical information system for oncology. Springer-Verlag, New York

Evans R S 1991 The HELP system: a review of clinical applications in infectious diseases and antibiotic use. MD Computing 8:282-288

Evans R S, Pestotnik S l, Classen D C, et al 1993 Development of an automated antibiotic consultant. MD Computing 10:17-22

Frawley K A 1993 Health information: overview of privacy and confidentiality issues. Tutorial 3 AMIA Spring Congress St Louis, Missouri, May 9-12

Fries J F 1974 Alternatives in medical record formats. Medical Care 12:871-881

Fries J F, Koop C E, Beadle C E et al 1993 Reducing health care costs by reducing the need and demand for medical services. New England Journal of Medicine 329:321-325

Gardner P, Schaffner W 1993 Immunisation in adults. New England Journal of Medicine 328:1252-1258

Gardner R M, Golubjatnikov O K, Laib R M, et al 1990 Computer-critiqued blood ordering using the HELP system. Computers and Biomedical Research 23(6):514-528

Grandia L D 1994 Intermountain health care's medical informatics strategy. Plenary Session AMIA Spring Congress, San Francisco May 5

Hannan T 1991 Quality assurance. Australian Clinical Review 11:22-27

Hannan T 1994 International transfer of the Johns Hopkins Oncology Center Information System. MD Computing 11(2):92-99

Hammond W (ed) 1993 An in depth look at the data structure of a computer-based patient record—TMR. AMIA Spring Congress, St Louis, Missouri. May 9-12, p 43

James B C 1989 Quality management for health care delivery. The Hospital Research and Educational Trust. Chicago, Illinois

Johns R J, Blum B I 1973 The use of clinical information systems to control costs as well as improve patient care. Trans American Clinical Climatological Association 90:140-152

Kuperman G J, Gardner R M, Pryor T A 1991 HELP: a dynamic hospital information system. Springer-Verlag, New York

Leape L L, Brennan T A, Laird N, et al 1991 The nature of adverse events in hospitalized patients. Results of the Harvard Medical Practice Study II. New England Journal of Medicine 324:377-384

Litzelman D K, Dittus R S, Miller M E, Tierney W M 1990 Improving compliance by 'forced choice' preventive care reminders. Clinical Research 38

Martin D K 1992 Making the connection: the VA-Regenstrief project. MD Computing 9:91-96

McDonald C J 1976 Protocol-based computer reminders, the quality of care and the non-perfectibility of man. New England Journal of Medicine 319(18):1351-1355

McDonald C J 1988 Computer-stored medical record systems. MD Computing 5(5):4-5

McDonald C J 1989a Risk versus benefits of tests and treatments. MD Computing 6(2):63-64

McDonald C J 1989b Medical information systems of the future. MD Computing 6(2):82-87

McDonald C J 1990a Interchange standards revisited. MD Computing 7(2):72-74

McDonald C J 1990b Input technology. MD Computing 7(4):201-204

McDonald C J 1991 Analysis of complex data, image reconstruction, and Joshua Willard Gibbs. MD Computing 8:272-274

McDonald C J 1992 Delivering X-ray images on hospital computer networks. MD Computing 9:348-350

McDonald C J, Hui S L, Smith D M, et al 1984 Reminders to physicians from an introspective computer medical record: a two year randomized trial. Annals of Internal Medicine 100:130-38

McDonald C J, Hui S L, Tierney W M 1986 Diuretic-induced laboratory abnormalities that predict ventricular ectopy. Journal of Chronic Disease 39:127-135

McDonald C J, Hui S L, Tierney W M 1992 Effects of computer reminders for influenza vaccination on morbidity during influenza epidemics. MD Computing 9:304-12

McDonald C J, Tierney W M, Miller M E, et al 1990 Toward qualification of small area variations. Clinical Research 38:914

McDonald C J, Tierney W M, Overhage M, et al 1992 The Regenstrief medical record system: 20 years experience in hospitals, clinics, and neighbourhood health centers. MD Computing 9(4):206-217

Miller G A 1956 The magical number seven plus or minus two: some limits on our capacity for processing information. Psychology Review 63:81-97

Miller R A, Pople H E Jr, Myers J D 1982 INTERNIST-1: an experienced computer-based diagnostic consultant for general internal medicine. New England Journal of Medicine 307:468

Murray M D, Brater D C, Tierney W M, McDonald C J 1990 Ibobrufen-associated renal dysfunction in a large general internal medicine practice. American Journal of Medical Science 299:222-229

Orthner H O, Blum B I 1989 Implementing health care information systems. Springer-Verlag, New York

Payne T H, Goroll A H, Morgan M, et al 1990 Conducting a matched-pairs historical cohort study with a computer-based ambulatory medical record system. Computers and Biomedical Research 23(5):455-472

Pryor T A, Clayton P D 1991 Decision support systems for clinical medicine. Tutorial II 15th Annual Symposium on Computer Applications in Medical Care, Washington DC, November 17

Safran C, Porter D, Rury C D, et al 1990 Clinquery: searching a large clinical database. MD Computing 7(3):144-153

Safran C, Rury C, Rind D M, et al 1991 A computer-based outpatient medical record for a teaching hospital. MD Computing 8:291-299

Shortliffe E H, Perreault L E 1990 Medical informatics. Addison-Wesley, Massachusetts

Sittig D F, Nathan L P, Gardner R M, et al 1989 Implementation of a computerised patient advice system using the HELP clinical information system. Computers Biomedical Research 22:474-487

Slack W V 1990 Type 1 and Type 2 administrators. MD Computing 7(2):69-70

Stampfer M J, Colditz G A, Willett W C, et al 1991 Postmenopausal oestrogen therapy and cardiovascular disease. New England Journal of Medicine 325:756-762

Tate K E, Gardner R M, Weaver L K 1990 A computerised laboratory alerting reminder system. MD Computing 7(5):296-301

Tierney W M, McDonald C J, McCabe G P 1985a Serum potassium testing in diuretic-treated outpatients: a multivariate approach. Medical Decision Making 5:89-104

Tierney W M, Roth B J, Psaty B, et al 1985b Predictors of myocardial infarction in emergency room patients. Critical Care Medicine 13:526-531

Tierney W M, Hui S L, McDonald C J 1986 Delayed feedback of physician performance versus immediate reminders to perform preventive care-effects on physician compliance. Medical Care 24:659-666

Tierney W M, McDonald C J, Martin D K, et al 1987 Computerised display of past test results: effects on outpatient testing. Annals of Internal Medicine 107:569-74

Tierney W M, McDonald C J 1991 Research using practice databases. Statistical Medicine 10:541-557

Tierney W M, Hannan T J 1992 The medical record, clinical care, and the information revolution. Royal Australasian College of Physicians, Fellowship Affairs 11(1):17-18

Tierney W M, Miller M E, Overhage J M, McDonald C J 1993 Physician inpatient order writing on microcomputer workstations: effects on resource utilisation. Journal of the American Medical Association 269:379-383

US Department of Health and Human Services 1993 Toward a national health information infrastructure. Report of the work group on computerisation of patient records.

Weed L 1989 New premises and tools for medical care and medical education. Proceedings international symposium of medical informatics and education. University of Victoria, British Columbia, Canada, p19

Wennberg J, Gittelsohn A 1973 Small variations in health care delivery. Science 182:1102-1108

Whiting-O'Keefe Q E, Simborg D W, Epstein W V 1980 A controlled experiment to evaluate the use of a time-oriented summary medical record. Medical Care 18(8):842–52

Wilson G A, McDonald C J, McCabe G P 1982 The effect of immediate access to a computerised medical record on physician test ordering: a controlled clinical trial in an emergency room. American Journal of Public Health 72:698-702

Woolhandler S, Himmelstein D U 1991 The deteriorating administrative efficiency of the US health care system. New England Journal of Medicine 324(18):1253-8

13

Expert systems

SHIRLEY GREGOR

Expert systems were one of the first areas to be commercially fruitful within the field known as *artificial intelligence* (AI). These systems are now operational in many areas, including medicine and health care. Expert systems are related to *decision support systems*, which are discussed in Chapter 14. Both expert systems and decision support systems assist humans carrying out difficult tasks, but decision support systems traditionally provide assistance with complex calculations and modelling, while expert systems provide assistance with qualitative knowledge and reasoning, assisting the human memory with complex rules or regulations, and providing expert strategies for attacking a problem. There are also differences with respect to the amount of responsibility the human user takes for problem-solving methods and the final decision. With a decision support system the user is required to contribute more in choosing problem-solving methods. With an expert system the choice of methods and even the final decision may be completely, or almost completely, automated.

Artificial intelligence is a broad disciplinary field which encompasses work in robotics, computer vision and natural language processing, as well as expert systems. Definitions of artificial intelligence (Charniak & McDermott 1987) vary from 'the study of mental facilities through the use of computational models' to 'the science of making machines do things that would require intelligence if done by men' (accredited to Minsky). The beginning of the modern field of artificial intelligence is often traced to the so-called Dartmouth conference in 1956, organised by John McCarthy and Marvin Minsky. McCarthy at Stanford University, and Minsky at the Massachusetts Institute of Technology, have continued as leaders in the field of artificial intelligence, together with Allen Newell and Herbert Simon of Carnegie-Mellon University.

Expert system development began in the late 1960s. Earlier work in artificial intelligence had focused on developing systems for general purpose problem-solving. An example was the GPS (General Problem Solver), developed by

Newell, Simon and J.C. Shaw. Though work on such systems has had enormous influence, the systems themselves were not suitable for practical application. It was not until work began on building systems for more limited areas of knowledge, where the use of specific rules and heuristics (rules-of-thumb) enabled more efficient processing, that systems could be applied successfully to practical problems. It is these narrower systems that are known as expert systems.

Perhaps the earliest expert system was DENDRAL, a system originally intended to do chemical analysis of the soil on Mars. Eventually, the program (and the computer it ran on) were too large to travel on the NASA vehicle to Mars, but the value of encoding the expertise of a human expert in a computer program was demonstrated. DENDRAL has outperformed human experts in carrying out mass-spectogram analysis of chemical structures, and has discovered errors in published literature (Parsaye & Chignell 1988). Another early and influential system was MYCIN, also developed at Stanford University (Buchanan & Shortliffe 1984). MYCIN diagnoses bacterial infections and prescribes treatment.

An expert system can be defined (Firebaugh 1988) as possessing the following characteristics:

- Performance is at a level generally recognised as equivalent to that of a human expert or specialist in a particular field.
- Knowledge is highly domain specific; that is, the system has a narrow range of knowledge relevant to one problem area.
- The system can explain its reasoning, being able to justify its advice, analysis, and conclusions (though not all systems can do this).
- Systems can be built where some knowledge is uncertain, probabilistic or fuzzy, and give a range of alternative solutions with associated likelihoods.

The term *knowledge-based system* (KBS) is now used almost synonymously with the term expert system. The former term, however, has a more general meaning, to reflect the ideas that these systems can include knowledge drawn from sources other than human experts, and that systems may be useful although they are not, strictly speaking, equivalent in performance to a human expert.

Systems with some similarities to expert systems are *neural net* systems. These systems also focus on qualitative rather than quantitative reasoning, but were originally inspired by attempts to model the reasoning processes of the human brain. In the human brain, activity consists of impulses passed from one neurone to another in a complex network. Neural networks employ a *black box* approach, where the system is given sets of inputs and outputs, and *learns* the relationships between the inputs and outputs in a number of training sessions. These learned relationships are then used to evaluate future cases. The system is a black box because it is usually not obvious to the outside observer what the learned relationships are. Thus, it is not usual for these systems to be able to explain how they reach conclusions. Neural nets are particularly good for identifying patterns. For example, a hospital system developed in South Carolina predicts length of stay and type of hospital discharge from a given diagnosis (Kestelyn 1991). It is claimed that this system has saved millions of dollars by allowing the hospital to administer resources more effectively.

Architecture and functioning of expert systems

A knowledge-based system includes a *knowledge base*, an *inference engine* (which may include routines for providing explanations), and a *user interface*. Figure 13.1 shows the main components of a knowledge-based system.

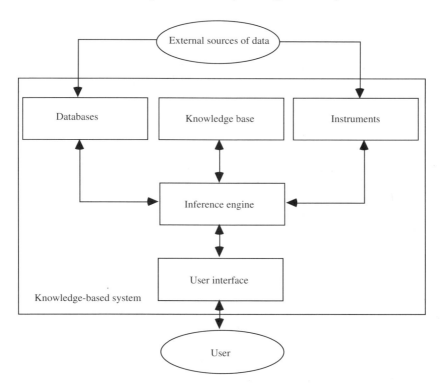

Fig. 13.1 Components of an expert, or knowledge-based, system

The inference engine is the main driving component for the expert system and controls the operation and accessing of the other components. The inference engine acquires necessary information from the expert-system user through the user interface, controls the way the knowledge in the knowledge base is accessed and communicates results to the user, again through the user interface. The inference engine may have access to internal or external databases, and instruments such as sensors in process control, or devices for monitoring patients. It is possible to use the same inference engine with different knowledge bases, and in effect, this is what is done when we use an *expert-*

151

system shell, a software tool that can be used to build an expert system for a particular problem area.

The user interface can be thought of as simulating the interaction which would occur when there is a consultation between a human expert and a seeker after advice. This simulation is virtual rather than substantive; though some systems provide forms of natural language processing, most systems use interface methods similar to those in other programs: menu, question-and-answer, form fill-in and graphical interfaces. These methods appear to work well in practice. It is not clear that users wish to have interactions with computers that are imitations of human-to-human interactions.

The knowledge in the knowledge base may include implicit (tacit) or explicit knowledge from an expert; formal knowledge such as that found in texts or legislation; heuristic knowledge; procedural (problem-solving) knowledge and declarative (factual) knowledge. There are many different ways of representing this knowledge including logic, production rules, semantic nets, and frames. These methods are covered in greater detail in Chapter 14. Many systems are rule-based and are relatively simple, easy to understand, and efficient in diagnostic situations. An example of a simplified rule from MYCIN is:

Rule 543

If 1 the infection which requires therapy is meningitis
   2 only circumstantial evidence is available for this case
   3 the type of the infection is bacterial
   4 the patient is receiving corticosteroids

then there is evidence that the organisms which might be causing the infection are e.coli (.4), klebsiella-pneumoniae (.2), or pseudomonas-aeruginosa (.1) (Clancey 1983).

When an expert system is consulted about a particular problem it gathers facts specifically to do with the problem addressed. Some systems also allow for *machine-learning,* where new knowledge updates the existing knowledge in the knowledge base. For example, a new set of facts may lie outside of the existing knowledge, so a new rule is added to cover them. Knowledge representation systems also often allow for uncertainty, or less than perfect confidence in aspects of the knowledge held, as shown in the example from MYCIN above, where the numbers in brackets represent certainty factors.

Blackboard systems are a newer development in which the knowledge base is divided into independent knowledge sources, and each independent source communicates via a blackboard, which is organised in a hierarchical structure representing the problem to be solved.

The emphasis on the separation of knowledge from processing is the main distinguishing feature of expert systems when compared with more conventional programs. More traditional programs may have knowledge incorporated into their procedures, but it may not be explicitly recognised that this is so. For example, in a billing system, the rules for charging patients may be buried in the depths of a large program amongst the procedures for printing accounts and updating files. Recognising that the knowledge base is a separate component is important as it allows us to think more clearly about problem areas which are specifically to do with the knowledge base: acquiring the knowledge in the first place, finding an appropriate representation method, and keeping the knowledge up to date.

When is an expert system feasible?

A survey of reports of expert system use in Australia (Parakala & Gregor 1992) identified over 60 systems in use in government, health and industrial organisations. The largest number of systems were in engineering, science, industry, business and agriculture. Progression from research to successful commercial systems has been slow. Analysis suggests that successful deployment involves considerable effort, integration of knowledge based systems with mainstream technology, emphasis on ease of use, systems which assist experts rather than replacing them, and the use of special purpose shells for developing the systems. Many successful systems, especially in business, have an automated, intelligent checklist approach.

In general, expert systems can be developed where:

- the task requires symbolic reasoning more than numeric calculations
- heuristic search is required more than algorithmic procedures
- domain-specific knowledge is more dominant than common sense
- the task has well defined solutions that can be specified in advance
- the inference logic is predetermined
- the task is of manageable size, but complex enough to benefit from an expert system (Klein & Methlie 1990).

Advantages of expert systems include:

- increased output and productivity
- increased quality
- capture of scarce expertise
- flexibility in services offered
- reliability
- shorter response time
- integration of several experts' opinions
- educational benefits: training of novices may occur as a side-effect of expert-system use
- enhancement of problem solving
- use in remote locations where experts are unavailable.

Disadvantages of experts systems include:

- updating the knowledge base may be laborious and error prone
- the systems have no common sense

- brittleness: performance does not degrade gracefully at the limits of the expert system's knowledge, and a novice user may not be aware of the limitations of the system
- legal responsibility for the advice offered is an ill-defined area.

Examples of expert systems in use

The first expert system to be used daily in Australia was a medical system (Catlett 1990). Garvan-ES1 was introduced in 1984 at the Garvan Institute of Medical Research at St Vincent's Hospital in Sydney to assist with the interpretation of laboratory tests on patients' thyroid levels. The program was written in the C language, and is said to produce reports that are 99% correct, with a higher quality product at a lower cost.

Miller (1994) gives a full review and bibliography for medical diagnosis decision support systems from 1954 to 1993. Miller states that medical diagnosis systems, many simple, and some complex, are now ubiquitous and such systems have become an established component of medical technology. In particular, he notes many highly successful systems are specialised and focused. For example, commercial systems for EEG analysis are now in widespread use. Systems for cytologic recognition and classification have also found successful application in devices such as automated differential blood count analysers.

Further examples of expert and decision support systems used in nursing can be found in Ozbolt et al (1990).

Developing expert systems

Guidelines for the development of expert systems exist, although a variety of approaches is available. Prerau (1990) gives useful guidance. One point of reasonable general agreement is that prototyping and some form of evolutionary or iterative design is needed. A *prototype* is a rough, small-scale system which is developed quickly. The prototype helps the users to see what they really want and express what needs to be done to achieve this. Using a prototype must be an iterative process, as a number of cycles through the adaptation of the prototype and retesting on users is necessary.

Weitzel and Kerschberg (1989) argue that knowledge engineering can be done by average people (ordinary systems analysts) rather than high priced *knowledge engineers,* who are specialised staff with knowledge of the technical side of expert system development. These authors feel that new software and new development methods are needed. Shells and programming environments facilitate prototyping by allowing knowledge engineers to focus on the problem instead of coding. Definition of the problem and feasibility assessments are more difficult and are done tentatively at first, becoming firmer in subsequent passes. Identifying the conceptual structure that underlies the expert's thinking is important and differs from the basic systems analysis tasks in transaction processing systems. Objects about which data are to be gathered for a transaction system may be peripheral details in a knowledge based system. What is more important is how the experts make decisions; for example, what concepts require value judgements from the expert. Multiple points of view during conceptual design are important, to allow different knowledge representations. It is important to have validation carried out by people outside the development process so that assumptions peculiar to individuals are uncovered.

It is still important to use methods from conventional system development that are considered good practice when developing and testing expert systems. These methods include the use of structured programming techniques when appropriate, the reduction of the complexity of programs by the use of relatively self contained modules, documentation of coding and use of meaningful data names, an emphasis on program readability and maintainability rather than efficiency, and the use of configuration management and control procedures. The validation of knowledge and the assessment of expert system performance can be extremely difficult. It should also be recognised that validation of knowledge should be an ongoing process; a system cannot be specified as correct at just one point in time.

Knowledge acquisition

Knowledge acquisition refers to the extraction and formulation of knowledge from various sources, especially from human experts. Knowledge acquisition is recognised as one of the particularly difficult and time consuming aspects of expert system development, which leads to the concept of a *knowledge engineering bottle-neck*.

Approaches to knowledge acquisition include:

* interviewing, where the knowledge engineer obtains knowledge from the human expert through a series of interviews and encodes it in the expert system. These interviews may be structured or unstructured and questionnaires may be used.
* learning by interaction, where experts directly interact with a computer program that helps to capture their knowledge. A technique can be used called *repertory-grid analysis*, where relationships between actions and results can be developed and tested.
* *verbal protocol analysis*, a *process tracing* method, where individuals are asked to think aloud while they solve a problem (Ericsson & Simon 1980).
* learning by *induction* or machine learning, where a computer program distils knowledge by examining data and examples.

Interviewing is very common. Learning by induction is not uncommon, and can be done with even moderately priced shells, for example, VP-Expert. In Australia, Ross Quinlan, of the University of Sydney, has made significant contributions in the area of machine learning, having developed Interactive Dichotomizer 3 (ID3), which uses classification to learn the essential features of a set of examples. ID3 has provided the basic inference algorithm for a number of commercial systems.

Also, a considerable number of systems rely heavily on the systemised knowledge codified in manuals, regulations and books rather than on knowledge extracted directly from experts. A survey of reported systems in the legal domain (Gregor & Watts 1991) showed that systems which were legislation based had reached more advanced stages of development than other types.

Keeping knowledge in systems current is a major undertaking. A novel approach is reported by Edwards et al (1993), who, in work following from Garvan-ES1, have introduced the notion of ripple down rules. Newer rules are patched on to the old rules at an appropriate point. The authors report that this approach allows the knowledge base to be easily maintained and updated by the pathologists using the system.

There are a number of problems in knowledge acquisition, including:

- insufficient availability of the expert
- lack of enthusiasm by the expert
- communication difficulties between the expert and the knowledge engineer
- lack of domain knowledge by the knowledge engineer
- inarticulateness of the expert
- implicit or tacit knowledge held by the expert, which is not accessible to awareness
- knowledge is only collected from the first available or most convenient source. For example, the knowledge engineer may rely on books or manuals when these contain parts that are not used by experts in practice, or have exceptions that the expert has discovered and learned to work around.
- irrelevant knowledge is collected from the expert. One way of identifying which knowledge is relevant is by comparing the knowledge of people with different levels of expertise on the task. Critical knowledge will be indicated when it is known by experts but not by those with less expertise.
- the range and flexibility of the expert's knowledge is not sufficiently explored. A working system can be expected to encounter many different situations in the field. Thus it is essential that its knowledge base contain as many exceptions and unusual cases as possible.
- difficulties in observing behaviour. Experimenter effects, where people's behaviour changes when they know they are being observed, are well known.

Johnson's (1983) article on the development of expertise is interesting for its insights into the problem of implicit knowledge. Johnson observed that a colleague's teaching of medical diagnosis differed from how he carried out the diagnosis in practice. He did not teach what he seemed to do. When asked about this, the colleague said: 'Oh, I know that. But you see I don't know how I do diagnosis, and yet I need things to teach students. I create what I think of as plausible means for doing tasks, and hope students will be able to convert them into effective ones.' This anecdote illustrates both the problem of reconstructed methods of reasoning, and implicit or tacit knowledge. Implicit knowledge is knowledge acquired as expertise develops,which is no longer available to the expert's own awareness. The protocol method of knowledge acquisition is one means of uncovering implicit knowledge. For a more detailed discussion of knowledge acquisition see Turban (1992).

Tools used in development

When building expert systems, the choice of tools to assist in the task includes:

- conventional programming languages; for example LISP, Prolog, C
- special purpose programming languages; for example, OPS5
- expert system shells that are special purpose environments with most of the mechanisms needed in an expert system already present. Just the knowledge base needs to be added.

Brody (1989) gives a good discussion of the relative merits of various expert system shells, as well as a checklist of features which can be used when comparing different products. Stylianou et al (1992) give a comparison of the perceived importance of selection criteria for expert system shells.

Following are some of the important questions to ask before purchasing a shell:

- How much does it cost?
- Can run-time (executable) versions of the program be produced, to execute separately from the shell? This is important if you wish to have the program used by many users. Otherwise, each user who uses the program must pay for the licence to run the shell.
- Is the final program as efficient as needed? Does it operate quickly enough? In some cases, especially where a separate run-time version of the program cannot be obtained, the program plus the shell will need a large amount of disk space and will be slow once the system reaches any appreciable size.
- What does the user interface of the final system look like? Is it easy to use? Can a graphical user interface, like Windows, be produced?
- Can explanations of the system's reasoning be produced?
- Is the shell easy to use and well-documented?
- Is local support available in case of difficulties?
- Is the system compatible with other languages? For example, it may be necessary to link to routines written in some other language such as C.
- Is the system compatible with external files and databases? For example, it may be necessary to access data held in Lotus 1-2-3 or dBase format.
- Is there a subroutine library to carry out commonly required statistical routines, date manipulations and other calculations?
- What forms of knowledge representation are available? Opinions include rules, objects, and frames. Many systems now offer more than one form of knowledge representation, and are known as *hybrid* systems.
- What methods are used to control reasoning? Options include forward and backward chaining.

- Is it possible for the system to learn by induction from examples or from updated knowledge bases?

Legal issues

Legal issues surrounding experts system development and use are still somewhat ill-defined. There have been insufficient cases to establish precedents, though Mykytyn and Mykytyn (1991) discuss eight legal cases in the US pertaining to expert systems.

Organisations, however, should be aware of potential liabilities that necessitate careful planning in the testing, evaluation and documentation of systems. Potential liabilities arising from the use of expert systems include the following (Mykytyn et al 1990):

- The erroneous, incomplete, or conflicting opinions of experts could lead to the development of a faulty system. In this case, the experts may be held liable. Developers should chose experts carefully and carry out thorough reliability testing.
- The knowledge engineer might be held liable for errors or incompleteness in the knowledge base if these were thought to result from incompetence, bias or negligence. The knowledge engineer should document the development process carefully to guard against such charges.
- An organisation selling an expert system might be held liable for defective advice, especially if the system is regarded as a service, rather than a product, which could be covered under a warranty.

Consideration can also be given as to whether there are legal consequences from the non-use of an expert system. For example, in the absence of a doctor, a nurse may choose not to use an available expert system which could, potentially, give critical advice.

The provision of explanations by a system may be relevant to the question of liability. If a system has the capability of explaining how it reaches conclusions, the users do have some opportunity to verify for themselves the accuracy of the conclusions and to use their own judgement in qualifying the system's advice. It is interesting to note, however, that users often express little interest in explanations. Botsman and Smith (1992) report on the development of a drug advisory system at Mackay Base Hospital where there is a narrow margin between therapeutic and toxic levels of a drug and, in the worse case, inadequate prescription could result in death. The authors comment that 'There was very little curiosity—even after some gentle prodding—about the mechanics (how and why) of the system'.

Conclusions

Expert systems are already being used to advantage in many fields. It seems probable that use will continue and increase. One prediction (Turban 1992) is that expert systems, as well as other applications of artificial intelligence, will tend increasingly to be embedded in traditional software. A recommendation to readers is that they obtain one of the lower priced, or public-domain, expert system shells and experiment with building a simple system themselves. This experience will help with the appreciation of the material covered in this chapter, and could lead to some useful systems!

REFERENCES

Botsman K, Smith J D 1992 A drug dosage advisory system for use by physicians and others: experience with the implementation of an exemplary system. In: Adams A, Sterling L (eds) Proceedings of the 5th Australian Joint Conference on Artificial Intelligence. AI'92, Hobart

Brody A 1989 The experts. Infoworld 11(25)

Buchanan B G, Shortliffe E H (eds) 1984 Rule-based expert systems the MYCIN experiments of the Stanford heuristic programming project. Addison-Wesley, Reading

Catlett J 1990 Expert systems: the risks and rewards. Hub Information Technology 2(7)

Charniak E M, McDermott D 1987 Introduction to artificial intelligence. Addison-Wesley, Reading

Clancey W J 1983 The epistemology of a rule-based expert system—a framework for explanation. Artificial Intelligence 20

Edwards G, Compton P, Malor R, Srinivasan A, Lazarus L 1993 Piers: a pathologist-maintained expert system for the interpretation of chemical pathology reports. Pathology 25

Ericsson K A, Simon H A 1980 Verbal reports as data. Psychological Review 87

Firebaugh M W 1988 Artificial intelligence a knowledge-based approach. PWS-Kent, Boston

Gregor S D, Watts J 1991 The use of intelligent systems in taxation practice. In: Proceedings of the Annual Conference of the Accounting Association of Australia and New Zealand, Brisbane

Johnson P E 1983 What kind of expert should a system be? Journal of Medicine and Psychology 8

Kestelyn J 1991 Application watch. AI Expert February

Klein M, Methlie L B 1990 Expert systems a decision support approach with applications in management and finance. Addison-Wesley, Wokingham

Miller, R A 1994 Medical diagnostic decision support systems: past, present, and future. Journal of American Medical Informatics Association 1

Mykytyn K, Mykytyn P P, Slinkman C W 1990 Expert systems: a question of liability. MIS Quarterly March

Mykytyn P P, Mykytyn K 1991 Legal perspectives on expert systems. AI Expert December

Ozbolt J G, Vandewal D, Hannah K J (eds) 1990 Decision support systems in nursing. Mosby, St.Louis

Parakala S R K, Gregor S D 1992 Critical factors in the successful implementation of knowledge-based system technology in Australia: a recent survey. In: Proceedings of the Australian Computer Society Queensland branch conference, Bond University

Parsaye K, Chignell M 1988 Expert systems for experts. John Wiley, New York

Prerau D S 1990 Developing and managing expert systems proven techniques for business and industry. Addison-Wesley, Reading

Stylaniou A C, Madey G R, Smith R D 1992 Selection criteria for expert system shells: a socio-technical framework, Communications of the ACM 35(10)

Turban E 1992 Expert systems and applied artificial intelligence. Macmillan, New York

Weitzel J R, Kerschberg L 1989 Developing knowledge-based systems: reorganizing the system development life cycle. Communications of the ACM 32(4)

FURTHER READING

Jackson P 1990 Introduction to expert systems. Addison-Wesley, Wokingham

Lucas P, Van der Gaag, L 1991 Principles of expert systems. Addison-Wesley, Wokingham

Olson D L, Courtney J F 1992 Decision support models and expert systems. Macmillan, New York

Zahedi F 1993 Intelligent systems for business expert systems with neural networks. Wadsworth, Belmont

14

Decision support in clinical practice

TENG LIAW

What is decision support?

Decision support is aimed at assisting professional activity. Clinical decision support is focused on the information required for and generated by the clinical decision making process to make a diagnosis, manage the patient and solve problems during or outside the clinical encounter. The aim is to support and augment the skills of the professional rather than to substitute them as had been the trend with many of the early stand-alone paternalistic 'Greek Oracle' diagnostic decision-making 'expert' systems like MYCIN (Shortliffe 1976). It is now recognised that a decision-support system developed as part of a larger patient and institutional information system may facilitate a more meaningful dialogue between the clinician and computer. The clinician, who has broad skills, common sense and detailed knowledge of the patient, remains integral to the decision making and decision support process.

Shortliffe (1989) identified three overlapping types of decision support function based on tools for information management, focusing attention, and patient specific consultation. Decision support covers the whole range of clinical activities and include:

1 Information management tools:
   - A knowledge base which may be on-line or off-line e.g. Oxford Textbook of Medicine on CD-ROM.
   - A patient health summary generator (Liaw & Chan 1993).
2 Tools to focus attention:
   - A patient recall system e.g. for PAP smears (Hogg 1990).
   - A patient and/or doctor reminder or alert system e.g. flu vaccination (McDonald et al 1980).
   - Structured and/or prompted data entry e.g. problem-knowledge coupler (Weed & Zimny 1989).

- Structured and/or prompted management protocols e.g. health maintenance activities (Hanh & Berger 1990) or geriatric assessment (Devore 1991).
3 Tools for patient specific consultation:
  - A background 'watch-dog' and/or critic of decisions made e.g. abdominal pain (de Dombal et al 1991).
  - A post-hoc evaluator of diagnostic and management decisions and/or tasks e.g. hypertension management (HYPERCRITIC) (van der Lei 1991)
  - A decision maker or expert system e.g. the Quick Medical Reference (QMR) (Miller et al 1992).

To facilitate meaningful and useful dialogue between the clinician and the decision support system, both must be capable of 'learning' together. Like its human counterpart, a decision-support system can learn by instruction, experience or both. Learning by instruction is relatively much easier to understand, design, and write code for than experiential learning. For instance, the McGill University Family Folder Information Network (MUFFIN) (Liaw & Chan 1993) allows new evidence based information such as drug interactions or effective health promotion protocols to be taught to the decision support system. Experiential learning is usually associated with artificial neural networks, which use serial and parallel processing, connectivity and non-linear programming to model the multisynaptic, excitatory and inhibitory neuronal structure of the brain. The pattern recognition property of neural networks used to model experiential learning is still limited to very narrow decision support application areas such as mammography (Patrick et al 1991). An appreciation of learning capability is important in understanding decision support, although a detailed understanding of cognitive science, belief networks, neural networks and knowledge representation is not essential.

Components of a decision support system

The fundamental components of a decision support system are:

1 A comprehensive and current knowledge base containing information based on high quality evidence.
2 A decision support (or inference) engine to implement the decision rules. It may include experiential learning techniques.
3 A well-structured patient database upon which the decision support rules are applied.
4 Interfaces to allow ongoing mutual teaching, learning and feedback by instruction between clinician and computer as well as the updating of the various information databases.

Techniques for decision support

The techniques have traditionally been one or more of the following:

1 Knowledge bases with data elements linked by relational algebra (*categorical reasoning*).
2 Quantitative handling of uncertainty and probability based on Bayes theorem (*probabilistic reasoning*).
3 Symbolic inference techniques as used in artificial intelligence research (*symbolic reasoning*).

Higher level techniques have been developed to address the fact that health data and health knowledge are often incomplete, inaccurate and inconsistent. They include:

- Heuristic systems, which combine categorical and/or symbolic reasoning with probabilistic reasoning e.g diagnostic systems such as RECONSIDER (Blois et al 1981), QMR (Miller & Masarie 1992) and ILIAD (Lau & Warner 1992). Bayesian belief networks are more mathematically complex systems which include probabilistic dependencies of symptoms and signs (Herskovits & Copper 1991). For example, the breathless patient with a family history of asthma, wheeze and productive cough is more likely to have asthma than cardiac failure.
- Diagnostic systems based on fuzzy set theory (Adlassnig 1980).

All these techniques have limited applicability to real life and clinical practice. Acceptance depends on the users' personal beliefs in computer-based modelling techniques. Most of the decision support systems that have a broad application domain tend to be rule based with mostly categorical and probabilistic reasoning. Symbolic reasoning and applications capable of experiential learning are still limited in their scope.

The definition and organisation of the critical data elements

The traditional preference by clinicians to record text rather than data elements makes knowledge representation difficult although some effort, e.g. the Linguistic String Project, has been devoted to natural language processing (Sager et al 1994). Knowledge representation and logic engineering techniques prefer the data elements to be structured and defined at the most basic (*atomic*) conceptual level, allowing greater flexibility and combinations to build more complex concepts (*molecules*) from these simple ones (*atoms*). A nomenclature, or a list of terms/codes to describe the atoms, is essential. A taxonomy, or classification, is important to guide the construction of the molecules and give meaning to the knowledge accumulated.

The issue of which conceptual level is the most clinician friendly and relevant to health care is being addressed with increasing discourse and research into coding, classification and knowledge representation. The most widely used coding and classification systems are the International Classification of Diseases (ICD), Systematised Nomenclature of Medicine (SNOMED) (Cote & Robboy 1980), Read Codes (Read 1990), and International Classification of Primary Care (ICPC) (Lamberts & Wood 1987). The ICPC is a classification system with a low level of specificity, while the ICD and SNOMED have very detailed and specific nomenclatures. For further discussion of this topic refer to Chapter 4.

Knowledge bases

A decision support system is only as good as the quality of its knowledge base, decision rules and patient database—the information must be current, valid and reliable. The design of the decision support system must allow easy and specific updating of the decision support logic (rules and probability) when new high quality evidence becomes available. Electronic knowledge must be easily shared and re-usable. Maintenance of the quality of the knowledge base over time is a problem in terms of the continued availability of skilled personnel, time and other resources, a general lack of high quality evidence and the lack of connectivity to allow the easy sharing of knowledge and logic modules between different decision support systems.

Structured collection of patient data

Structured data entry is an attempt to reduce the uncertainty, indecision and noise that contribute to the large variations in estimates of prevalence of health problems and use of services by patients and clinicians in various health care settings and regions. At the least specific conceptual level, data collected in an encounter can be categorised into the reason for encounter (RFE), diagnosis (Dx) and process of care. RFE is the outcome of a consensus between the patient's demand for care and the clinician's assessment of that demand. The decisions made can and should be qualified by the degree of certainty based on objective criteria e.g. diagnostic criteria. By making explicit the three main components of the encounter as sources of uncertainty, variance and error, the structured *RFE-Dx-Process* approach to data entry can limit the number of possibilities and reduce the potential for errors, leading to enhanced accuracy of data collection.

The structure of the patient database need to facilitate longitudinal, temporal and lateral linkages among the data elements. Lateral linkages concern information like blood or family relationships which must be 'taught' to the computerised patient database. Automated longitudinal and temporal linkages will allow the creation and maintenance of a longitudinal record and patient summary organised into problem contacts, encounters and episodes of disease/ ill-health and care. This structured patient database will enable easier, more flexible and more efficient design of the decision support engine which will allow a more varied examination of the database e.g. relating process to outcome of care, family based or genetic analysis of the data, or predicting natural history of symptoms during an episode of a health problem.

Computer assisted data collection to enhance data quality

Computer assisted data collection based on 'problem-knowledge coupling' (Weed & Zimny 1989) can improve the quality of the data. The clinician must be critically aware of the nature and quality of the evidence for his/her diagnostic and management decisions and the conceptual and practical limitations of the decision support system involved. These broad critical skills are essential 'core behaviour' to allow the best use of decision support to make diagnostic decisions, facilitate best practice in the management of health problems, and record the encounter accurately and comprehensively. This broadly skilled clinician is the best guarantee of optimum data quality in the patient database.

A clinical framework to establish the information requirements for decision making

Coexisting physical and mental health problems, compounded with family, social or work problems present considerable diagnostic and management difficulties and uncertainty in clinical practice. The need to establish the information requirements at each clinical encounter is most acute in general/family practice which is mainly concerned with ill-defined and undifferentiated problems in an environment of many short encounters with many patients over time. The context and the degree of uncertainty may vary, but the primary focus of all clinicians is the patient and his/her reason for encounter. Loosely based on a list of consultation tasks (Pendleton et al 1984), Fig. 14.1 summarises a patient centred clinical framework which shows the information needed for and generated by each step of the encounter and decision making process and highlights the relevance of information and responsibility sharing. The various points in the model are amenable to decision support. The choice of a particular type of clinical decision support depends on:

• the nature of the problem and degree of uncertainty
• the nature of the decision and degree of indecision
• the environment in which the decision is made
• the character and preferences of the individual clinician.

Thus less experienced clinicians may value a diagnostic decision support more than experienced ones particularly if the medico-legal environment is highly charged as in situations of rape and criminal injury.

165

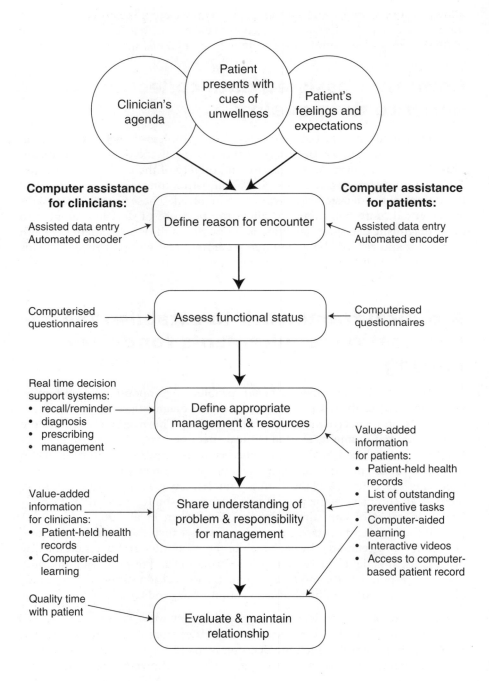

Fig. 14.1 Clinical information needs and areas for decision support

Decision support systems available within this clinical framework

Defining and coding the reason(s) for encounter

Structured and computer assisted data entry by patient and/or doctor is the main form of decision support available for these clinical tasks. These may be stand alone packages or are part of an integrated computer based patient record system. The problem-knowledge coupler (Weed & Zimny 1989) prompts the clinician to ask relevant questions associated with the presenting complaint. However, the choice of a particular problem-knowledge coupler, e.g. cardiovascular or psychiatric coupler, remains with the clinician.

Assessment of functional status and lifestyle factors

There are numerous automated questionnaires to assess health, functional status, diet, lifestyle factors and problems like anxiety and depression. Using data entered by the patient and/or the clinician, these systems use a simple scoring and ranking capability to generate either raw or interpreted scores which may help decision making. While these are usually stand-alone applications used in specialty areas, they can also be incorporated into a patient database as on-line decision support for patients and clinicians.

Defining the diagnosis and/or labelling the problem

Diagnostic decision support systems may take the form of:

- an on-line prompt (Weed & Zimny 1989).
- an on-line information/knowledge base e.g. a hypermedia document collection (Timpka et al 1982).
- a 'watchdog' to warn of mistakes (de Dombal et al 1991).
- a 'decision-maker' e.g. QMR (Miller et al 1986).

The problem-knowledge coupler (Weed & Zimny 1989) provides a list of associated symptoms and differential diagnoses as part of on-line decision support. The use of a 'watchdog' computer-aided diagnosis of abdominal pain has been shown to improve the management of patients who present to emergency departments with abdominal pain (de Dombal et al 1991). The pattern recognition capabilities of artificial neural networks have been used to analyse pain drawings by patients with low back pain to recognise and classify the pain with some success (Mann & Brown 1991). 'Decision-makers' are popular in the various specialty areas, where the breadth of knowledge is small but the depth of knowledge is great e.g. the diagnosis of colonic lesions has been shown to be 98% accurate (Graham et al 1990); MAGIC (*Melanoma Analysis and Graphic Imaging by Computer*) (White et al 1991) which uses a set of rules to decide if a video image of a lesion was a melanoma or not; or the Outcome Advisor, a diagnostic decision support for mammography which also uses neural network concepts to learn (Patrick et al 1991). QMR attempts to give an answer to the symptoms and signs presented by the patient.

Defining appropriate management and use of resources

On-line reminders which prompt important health information e.g. drug allergies or outstanding preventive activities when the patient file is opened are simple management decision support systems (McDonald et al 1980). This information may be picked up automatically from the patient files or entered manually by the patient, clinician or office staff. Recall lists e.g. influenza vaccinations or PAP smears and patient registers e.g. diabetes are other simple forms of management decision support based on time and disease (Hogg 1990).

More sophisticated decision support systems involves automated knowledge based decision support protocols which examine the patient database and make a series of decisions on the completeness of the information. For instance, MUFFIN uses health maintenance protocols to generate a list of outstanding health promotion and disease management tasks for each patient to facilitate opportunistic health promotion and chronic disease management during the encounter. A prototype prescribing decision support system searches the patient database, highlights drug allergies and potentially adverse drug combinations, and recommends a medication for diagnoses made during the encounter. The adverse reactions probability scale (APS) (Naranjo et al 1991), Yale algorithms (Kramer et al 1979) and other medication databases have been added to the QMR to provide decision support for good quality prescribing. Use of structured hypertension management protocols has been shown to improve understanding and management of compliance (ARTEMIS) (Degoulet et al 1982). HYPERCRITIC, which allows a clinician to reflect on his/her decisions after the encounter, has also been shown to improve the management of hypertension (van der Lei 1991). DIACON, a microcomputer based decision support system for diabetes, provides (i) information management including statistical analysis of patient and laboratory data, diagnosis of diabetic keto-acidosis, advice to patients on insulin dose based on glucose readings, therapeutic education programs and computer assisted implanted pump devices; (ii) computer aids including memory glucose reflectance meters and an insulin dosage computer, and (iii) educational programs on computer (Laron et al 1989).

Information and responsibility sharing

A shared understanding and the involvement of patients in the management of their health problems is an axiom of clinical care. A computer generated patient summary, which contains personal health information, outstanding health promotion tasks and general health education information, given to patients to keep and use can act as a patient and clinician reminder, achieve this shared understanding, and increase patients' responsibility for their own health care (Liaw 1995). A dilemma in information sharing is that while information theory reassures us that messages can be transmitted reliably, physical laws and probability tell us that these messages tend to become garbled easily. Ley et al (1976) emphasised that patient satisfaction and compliance depend on accurate, unambiguous, relevant and simple messages and measures to improve comprehension and recall. Computer generated patient-held health records (PHR) summarise and present patient information consistently and legibly to facilitate information and responsibility sharing. Patient access to on-line personal health information via a modem has also been shown to be practical and feasible (Jones et al 1992)

Evaluating and maintaining the relationship

Computer assistance in diagnostic and management decisions, which also facilitate the sharing of information and responsibility, can improve the quality and efficiency of the clinical encounter and promote a comprehensive approach to health care by patients and clinicians. More time is made available to establish, evaluate and maintain an effective long term patient-clinician relationship.

Some issues with decision support

A recent overview of trials of clinical decision support systems suggests that they can improve clinician performance (Johnston et al 1994). However, there are also problematic issues such as unproven effectiveness, high costs, potential adverse effect on the patient-doctor relationship, legal accountability for mishaps, implementation problems including lack of use of computer based patient records, lack of inter-operability between different operating systems, and indifferent or antagonistic attitudes of clinicians. The legal aspect of decision support depends on whether the courts view decision support under negligence (medical malpractice) law or product liability law or both. Consider DIACON: the information management module may raise issues relevant to negligence law while the computer assisted implanted pump device module will be viewed as a medical device. On the other side of the coin, are clinicians liable for malpractice if they chose not to consult a decision support system?

The philosophical question of control of knowledge and behaviour must also be appreciated. Opinions differ on how computer assistance in clinical practice should be taught and used. At one end of the spectrum, Weed (1990) advocates a paradigm change from teaching a 'core of knowledge' to teaching a 'core of computer based behaviour'. Others, more wary of the enormity of the task in effecting behaviour change, advocate the use of computers to facilitate the teaching and maintenance of this 'core of knowledge'. This less radical approach appear to be the majority view as reflected by the relative abundance of applications employing techniques such as natural language processing, temporal and spatial reasoning to try to make sense of data collected by clinicians trained under this 'core of knowledge' paradigm. The differences in opinion remain although the literature and recent developments in the American Medical Informatics scene suggest that these views are becoming less polarised.

The next steps

Because only a minority of clinicians use computer based patient records to any extent, the strategy to define and facilitate the use of decision support systems must include:

- appreciation of the decision support needs of clinicians
- consensus on the appropriate technique(s) of decision support to improve quality of care
- the development of practical systems that can learn from and teach clinicians
- modular approaches to design to encourage clinicians with varying levels of computer literacy to use decision support
- rigorous evaluation of the accuracy, consistency, adaptability, learning capability and usefulness of such systems.

Evaluation must examine if a decision support system models an expert's activity and knowledge adequately and appropriately i.e. *is it practical, useful, open to ideas (i.e. can learn), and able to teach*? The main problem with evaluation is a lack of acceptable and valid 'gold standards' in clinical decision-making or, often, the decision itself. Some of the standards used have been a clinical expert or a cluster analysis of the decisions of a panel of clinical experts. The extent of utilisation of a system is an indicator of its usefulness: clinicians will only use decision support if it is useful. Other evaluation questions must address the impact of decision support on health care, health costs and health.

Conclusion

The potential for decision support systems in clinical practice remains great. Computer based modelling must be used in conjunction with well established knowledge bases and decision rules within the context of well-structured patient information. The broadly skilled clinician with intimate knowledge of the patient is central to the decision support and decision making process. The evolution *from* the paternalistic 'Greek Oracle' model, which substitute professional decisions, *to* the collaborative model of decision support, which facilitate professional and clinical decision making, suggests that we are heading in the right direction.

REFERENCES

Adlassnig K P 1980 A fuzzy logical model of computer-assisted medical diagnosis. Methods of Information in Medicine 19

Blois M S, Tuttle M S, Sheretz DD 1981 RECONSIDER: a program for generating differential diagnoses. In: Hefferman H G (ed) Proceedings of the Fifth Annual Symposium on Clinical Applications in Health Care. IEEE Computer Society Press, Washington

Cote R A, Robboy S 1980 Progress in medical information management. Systematised nomenclature of medicine (SNOMED). Journal of the American Medical Association 243(8)

de Dombal F T, Dallos V, McAdam W A F 1991 Can computer aided teaching packages improve clinical care in patients with acute abdominal pain? British Medical Journal 302

Degoulet P, Vu H A, Chatelier G et al 1982 Hypertension management: the role of the computer in improving patient compliance. Medical Informatics 7(1)

Devore P A 1991 Computer-assisted comprehensive geriatric assessment in a family physician's office. Southern Medical Journal 84(8)

Graham A, Paplanus S, Bartels P 1990 A diagnostic expert system for colonic disease. American Journal of Clinical Pathology 94 (Suppl 1):S15-S18

Hahn D L, Berger M G 1990 Implementation of a systematic health maintenance protocol in a private practice. Journal of Family Practice 31(5)

Herskovits E H, Copper G F 1991 Algorithm for Bayesian belief-network precomputation. Methods of Information in Medicine 30:81-89

Hogg W 1990 The role of computers in preventive medicine in a rural family practice. Canadian Medical Association Journal 143(1)

Johnston M E, Langton K B, Haynes B, Mathieu A 1994 Effects of computer-based clinical decision support systems on clinician performance and patient outcome. A critical appraisal of research. Annals of Internal Medicine 120

Jones R B, McGhee S M, McGhee D 1992 Patient online access to medical records in general practice. Health Bulletin 50(2)

Lamberts H, Wood M (eds) 1987 ICPC: the International Classification of Primary Care. Oxford University Press, Oxford

Laron Z, Flexer Z, Albag Y, Ofan R 1989 The use of computers in the control of diabetes in children and adolescents. Journal of Endocrinological Investigation 12(8 Suppl 3)

Lau L M, Warner H R 1992 Performance of a diagnostic system (ILIAD) as a tool for quality assurance. Computing and Biomedical Research 25

Ley P, Whitworth M A, Skilbeck C E, Woodward R, Pinsent R J H F, Pike L A, Clarkson M E, Clark P B 1976. Improving doctor-patient communication in general practice. Journal of the Royal College of General Practitioners 6

Liaw S T 1995 The computer-generated patient-held record. PhD thesis, Flinders University of South Australia, Adelaide

Liaw S T, Chan D C H 1993 MUFFIN: an approach to the computer-based patient record. Informatics in Healthcare Australia 2(1)

Mann N H, Brown M D 1991 Artificial intelligence in the diagnosis of low back pain. Orthopaedic Clinics of North America 22(2):303-314

McDonald C J, Gregory A W, McCabe G P 1980 Physician response to computer reminders. Journal of the American Medical Association 244(14)

Miller R A, Masarie F E 1992 The Quick Medical Reference (QMR) relationships function: description and evaluation of a simple efficient 'multiple diagnoses' algorithm. Proc MED-INFO 92, Geneva, Switzerland

Naranjo C A, Lanctot K L 1991 Recent developments in computer-assisted diagnosis of putative adverse drug reactions. Drug Safety 6(5):315-322

Patrick E A, Moskowitz M, Mansukhani V T et al 1991 Expert system learning network for diagnosis of breast calcifications. Invest Radiol 26

Pendleton D, Schofield T, Tate P, Havelock P 1984 The consultation. An approach to learning and teaching. Oxford University Press, Oxford

Read J D 1990. Read clinical classification. BMJ 305:45-50

Sager N, Lyman M, Bucknall C, Nhan N, Tick L J 1994 Natural language processing and the representation of clinical data. Journal of the American Medical Informatics Association 1(2)

Shortliffe E H 1976 Computer-based medical consultations: MYCIN artificial intelligence series. Elsevier Computer Science Library, New York

Shortliffe E H 1989 Testing reality. The introduction of decision support technologies for physicians. Methods of Information in Medicine 28

Timpka T, Hedblom P, Tibblin G 1982 A hypermedia document collection for primary care: why, what, and how? Artificial Intelligence in Medicine 2(4)

Van der Lei J, Musen M A, van der Does E, et al 1991. Comparison of computer-aided and human review of GP's management of hypertesion. Lancet 338

Weed L 1990. New premises and new tools for medical care and medical education. Proceedings of the International Symposium of Medical Informatics and Education, University of Victoria, British Columbia

Weed L L, Zimny N J 1989 The problem-oriented system, problem-knowledge coupling, and clinical decision making. Physical Therapy 69(7)

White R, Rigel D S, Friedman R J 1991 Computer applications in the diagnosis and prognosis of malignant melanoma. Dermatology Clinics 9(4)

15

Image management and communications technology

GARY F EGAN

The history of medical imaging can be dated from Röntgen's discovery and first clinical use of X-rays in 1895. These first X-ray images were humble portents of the increasingly important role which medical imaging has assumed, particularly in the last 25 years. In fact, diagnostic radiology continued more or less unchanged from Röntgen's discovery until digital computers were integrated with electronic imaging technology in the 1970s. After Hounsfield (1973) and Cormack's development of computerised tomography (CT) there was a rapid proliferation of new medical imaging technologies. These new technologies are now playing an increasingly important role in clinical diagnosis and patient management. With improvements in computing and com-munications technology continuing unabated, increased clinical use of digital imaging technologies seems assured.

Major medical imaging technologies

Diagnostic imaging non-invasively probes the interior of the human body to reveal the structure or functional condition of the tissue. The practice of radiology is based on the exquisite sensitivity of X-rays to variations in the density of different bodily tissues, e.g. bone and muscle. The variable attenuation of X-rays by different bodily tissues enables an image of the structure or the anatomy of the body to be generated (Table 15.1). Planar X-ray films provide projection images of the line integrals of the X-ray beam attenuation coefficients through an object. By using a computer controlled rotating X-ray tube and detector system many projection images from different views through the object can be acquired. By applying a mathematical transformation, known as the inverse Radon transform, to these X-ray projection images, tomographic *(tomo-slice,* from the *Greek)* images or transaxial views through the body can then be produced. The invention of computerised

Table 15.1 The most common non-invasive diagnostic imaging technologies categorised by probe type and distinguishing attributes

Modality	Quantity probed	Probe	Attributes
US	velocity[1]	sound	anatomical, functional, dynamic
X-ray	density	X-ray	anatomy, simple, static, high resolution
CT	density	X-ray	tomography, anatomical
MRI	proton	RF[2]	tomography, anatomical, some function
NM	-	γ-ray	simple, planar, function
SPECT	-	γ-ray	tomography, function, qualitative
PET	K[3]	β+	tomography, function, quantitative

[1] the velocity of sound is dependent on the adiabatic bulk modulus coefficient of the tissue

[2] RF denotes the radio frequency of the alternating magnetic field

[3] K denotes the metabolic rate constants of organ or tissue function

tomography (CT) revolutionised radiological practice and provided un–paralleled images of the interior of the body. Whilst both X-ray and CT provide anatomical images, nuclear medicine techniques based on the in-vivo administration of tracer amounts of radioactivity provide complementary images of bodily function.

Nuclear medicine (NM) evolved during the post Second World War period as probably the most universally condoned peaceful use of nuclear technology. Nuclear medicine is based on imaging the in-vivo bio-distribution of an administered radioisotope labelled pharmaceutical, which provides an image of the functional status of organs or bodily processes. The application of Hounsfield's work to planar NM images resulted in tomographic functional images, or single photon emission computed tomography (SPECT) images. More recently another radioisotope tracer technique positron emission tomography (PET), has provided quantitative non-invasive images of bodily function such as metabolism and blood flow.

Magnetic resonance imaging (MRI) probes the body through the use of high frequency magnetic fields which are tuned to be sensitive to the distribution of free protons within the body. Free or semi-free protons are most commonly found in water, and thus MRI is maximally sensitive to soft bodily tissues and to small variations between different soft tissues. Consequently, MRI images resolve finer anatomical detail, particularly in the brain and spinal column than CT images. More recently, MRI has been developed to image cerebral angiography (MRA) and functional imaging such as cerebral blood flow now appears to also be possible with MRI (Prichard & Rosen 1994).

Medical imaging technologies can be categorised according to their temporal resolution, with all of the above techniques essentially providing static images. In contrast, dynamic images are provided by ultrasound (US) where a continuously transmitting and receiving probe (transceiver) provides continuously varying anatomical images. Dynamic anatomical imaging using visible light is also performed using endoscopic techniques. Since these techniques use invasive video based technology they are generally considered separately from non-invasive imaging techniques and will not be discussed further. With the advent of digital ultrasound systems, three dimensional (3D) image visualisation as used in CT, MRI, SPECT and PET is now being developed for use in ultrasound.

The operation and management of medical imaging systems in large hospitals has traditionally been confined to radiology and nuclear medicine departments. In smaller private practices these departments are frequently combined. Digital integration of these systems using computer networks has until the last few years been fraught with difficulties due to the absence of networking standards for medical images. DICOM 3.0 is the most commonly accepted digital image communication standard (ACR/NEMA 1988) in medicine and now enables standardised exchange of digital images between imaging systems and other networked devices, including large data archives. Together with technological advances, standardisation makes possible the actual implementation of picture archive and communication systems (PACS), sometimes known as image management and communication systems (IMAC). With the major technological barriers to PACS now overcome, determination of the impact and cost effectiveness of these systems on patient care is now possible. PACS implementations are presently underway at a number of institutions including the United States Army, Madigan (MDIS project) and at the Hammersmith Hospital, London. Recently two Australian hospitals namely St. Vincent's Hospital, Melbourne and the Royal Children's Hospital, Sydney have embarked on staged implementation of PACS systems. Following difficulties with an earlier PACS project at the John Hunter Hospital, Newcastle the outcome of these two new projects will be pivotal to further expansion of PACS in Australia.

Image management and communication requirements

Television and cinema have proven that the production and distribution of images is extraordinarily influential. Generally new developments in imaging technology are rapidly incorporated into medical imaging systems, but the same has not been true for image distribution and display technologies. Surprisingly, digital medical images are routinely filmed for subsequent hard copy viewing by radiologists and nuclear medicine physicians. Films are also manually distributed to other internal or external hospital departments, and are used for permanent storage. Whilst electronic transmission, display and storage of images is possible most digital medical imaging systems produce film to perform these functions.

Digital image management and communication has not yet overtaken film because rapid clinical access to images requires communication bandwidth in excess of 100MHz, a very high degree of reliability of image availability, massive

Table 15.2 Typical image sizes, communication transfer periods and annual data storage requirements for a medium sized (500 bed) hospital

Modality	Data/ image (MB)[1]	Images/ study	Data/ study (MB)[1]	Transfer time (sec)	Studies/ day	Data/ year (GB)[2]
X-Ray	6	1-3	12	3	15	36
CT	0.15	30-60	7	2	20	28
MRI	0.15	60-120	13	3	20	52
US	0.1	20-30	2.5	1	10	5.0
SPECT	0.03	15-30	0.6	0.15	6	0.7
PET	0.03	30-60	1.3	0.3	4	1.0

1 = megabytes

2 = gigabytes

and rapid data storage capacity, readily accessible image viewing workstations, and most importantly significant changes in work practices throughout a health care institution. Technological solutions to most of these problems have now been developed but the cost effectiveness of an integrated system in a clinical setting is yet to be established. Rapid communication of images for clinical viewing remotely from an imaging department can be achieved using optic fibre technology operating at speeds of 100 MHz (100 Mbps). Actual data transfer rates of 30 Mbps (Rowberg & Zick 1992) result in image transfer times of three seconds or less for single patient studies (Table 15.2). The development of higher speed technology and a new communication standard called asynchronous transfer mode (ATM) will permit communications up to at least 600 MHz within the next few years. The communications requirements for PACS will then have been substantially exceeded.

The reliability of images via a PACS depends on the reliability of each component of the system. The central image database, which may consist of a number of server computers, must be continuously operational and accessible. Redundant arrays of inexpensive disks (RAID) permit data recovery in the event of a single disk failure. By stripping data across many disks, RAID disk technology allows for re-assembly of data in the event of a single disk failure. Consequently with rapid disk maintenance, data integrity can be assured to a very high level of confidence. RAID disk technology effectively assures the medico-legal requirement in various parts of Australia of maintaining diagnostic imaging results for seven years or more.

Computer network reliability has improved dramatically over the past few years, particularly for UNIX systems using the tcp/ip communications protocol. The security of data transmissions using tcp/ip has also dramatically improved, which is crucially important for non-isolated networks. The decreasing cost of diagnostic quality image viewing workstations permits groups of six or more monitors for comparative image viewing at reasonable cost. However monitor specifications are being tightened considerably to ensure that image interpretation is reliable and independent of monitor performance and characteristics. Multi-terabyte (1 TB = 1000 GB) optical disk storage units are also now available, albeit at significant expense. Finally, the significant benefits of a PACS system can only be realised when staff work practices fully incorporate the new technologies. Changes to work flow, staff skills, and actual staff numbers are necessary, as well as a financial commitment to continual system maintenance and development.

Medical IMAC systems

The earliest medical image management and communication systems date from the mid 1980s when the US Army funded PACS system development at the Washington University, Seattle and the Georgetown University, Washington DC. These systems have been progressively updated and are still in operation today. More recently there have been four major PACS projects installed and initial operational experiences with these systems have been reported (Irie 1991, Masser et al 1991, Glass & Stark 1991, Goeringer 1991).

The US Army has funded the successful medical diagnostic imaging support (MDIS) system at four army hospitals, of which Madigan, Washington is the most well known. The MDIS technical specification is extremely comprehensive and has been used to specify requirements at a number of other PACS projects (Goeringer 1991). Probably the largest PACS project is at Hokkaido University Hospital, Japan in which the PACS, hospital information system (HIS) and medical records are integrated (Irie 1991). Typical characteristics of the system are on-line image availability for one week, with image retrieval times of 40-60 seconds from optical disk library; twenty 1024 by 1024 pixel monitors for radiological image reporting; inclusion of echocardiography, endography, and microscopy images; and 200 terminals providing sub-diagnostic image quality access to the system. The clinical evaluation has concluded that from a users point of view the system is too slow, that the image quality is generally as good as film, and that workstations with more than two monitors are required.

The decision to implement a PACS system at the Hammersmith Hospital, London has been substantially based on their cost benefit analysis (Glass & Stark 1991). The cost benefit analysis included both direct components such as film, labour, and space utilisation, and indirect components such as improved productivity due to improved efficiencies, reduction of hospital in-patient stay, and reductions in repeated procedures. The system specification is based on the MDIS specification. Finally, the Vienna Hospital PACS project also incorporates the HIS and radiology information system (RIS) and has been developed jointly by Siemens and the hospital (Masser et al 1991). The communications architecture is a token ring topology using 100 MHz fibre digital data interchange (FDDI) protocol. Image display within radiology is based on high resolution (1024 x 1280 pixels) monitors, while elsewhere in the hospital PC based systems are used.

A number of other notable PACS systems have been developed including the Geneva DIOGENE system which integrated the PACS within the previously (in-house) developed HIS (Ratib 1992). All of the PACS systems described have multi-million dollar implementation budgets, and can generally be considered to be second generation systems. Third generation PACS systems building on the successes of the second generation systems are now in planning. Such systems benefit significantly from the recent rapid advances in PACS component technology (networks, storage, monitor) and may actually be cost effective in their implementation.

Australia's first PACS project was initiated with the construction in the mid 1980s of a new hospital in Newcastle, the John Hunter Hospital (Crowe 1990). Whilst state of the art technology such as optic fibre for communications was installed in the hospital, the project was hampered by the absence of standards for image data and high speed communications, the high cost at that time of the necessary technology, and most importantly the lack of functional applications and quality user interfaces. The project was partly promoted as a cost effective means of utilising building and staff resources, but even today with greatly decreased technology costs full PACS implementations are probably only just becoming cost effective. The failure of the John Hunter Hospital PACS project has undoubtedly retarded development of PACS elsewhere in Australia. Recently, an expanded project including telemedicine services between four hospitals in the region has been proposed (Osborne 1994). This project has greater emphasis on telemedicine services between Australia and South East Asian hospitals, anticipating a new revenue stream for these services to improve the cost benefit analysis of computer and communications investment in each individual hospital.

St Vincent's Hospital, Melbourne is planned to be filmless after relocation to new buildings presently under construction. The PACS system is planned to be implemented in four stages from mid 1994. Stage one involving installation of a computed radiography (CR) or digital X-ray system with image distribution from the Department of Radiology to ICU has already been completed. Stage two (expected in mid 1995) involves filmless operations within the Division of Medical Imaging. Data archive and intra-division image communication are required for the existing MRI, CT, SPECT, Ultrasound, digital subtraction angiography (DSA) and CR systems, with up to three additional CR systems expected within two years. Stage three is completion of the PACS system and is planned for early 1996, with filmless operations being extended throughout the whole hospital at that point. Finally stage four involves interconnection of the PACS with the RIS, but specific details of this stage are dependent on details of the PACS system chosen. The hospital is committed to a major investment in PACS and the project outcome will undoubtedly influence the development of PACS elsewhere in Australia.

Relocation of the Royal Children's Hospital (RCH), Sydney to a new site adjacent to Westmead Hospital in western Sydney has been the impetus for the installation of a partial PACS in that hospital. Telemedicine requirements play a major role in the design of the RCH PACS, with paediatric image transmission from rural and remote areas to the RCH an existing service (Crowe 1993). Expert paediatric radiological opinion is in many cases crucial to patient management prior to transfer to the RCH. CT and X-ray images are presently transmitted from hospitals in central and western New South Wales using ISDN and Fastpac communication links. Stage one of the RCH PACS implementation specifies distribution of CR images to ICU, with film continued to be used both within the Medical Imaging Division and the rest of the hospital. Later stages of the PACS implementation identify filmless operation with the Medical Imaging Division and then throughout the hospital.

The installation of state of the art PET and MRI scanners has been the impetus for PACS related developments at the Austin Repatriation Medical Centre (ARMC), Melbourne. The ARMC is a tertiary referral hospital with particular clinical strengths in the areas of neurology (epilepsy and spinal injuries), neuroscience, liver transplantation and cardiac surgery. A campus wide ethernet computer network was installed in early 1992, with internet access via an ISDN link to the University of Melbourne. More recently microwave links to other hospitals in the region have been commissioned. The network is presently utilised for image communication, email distribution, electronic information access, library CD-ROM catalogue searching, and a list server for hospital staff com–munications. Access to the HIS has been demonstrated. Presently there are over 100 computers and over 250 users on the network (Egan 1993a).

The initial PACS development at the hospital is a networked medical image database project (Egan 1993b). This project which is aimed at centralising neurosurgery patient image data from MRI, CT, PET and SPECT scanners is soon to commence clinical trialing at the hospital. The image database will provide co-registered images for multi-modality image viewing at neurosurgery patient contact locations within the hospital, as well as in the Division of Medical Imaging. Integration of the separate medical imaging and the hospital information networks is a key infrastructure component for any successful IMAC. The major concern at the ARMC in interconnection of the two networks has been the protection of patient confidentiality and the prevention of unauthorised access to patient related information (O'Callaghan & Egan 1994).

Advances in medical imaging technologies

Medical imaging technologies have evolved particularly rapidly over the past two decades. The 1970s and early 1980s witnessed the invention of CT, SPECT, PET and MRI. Since then the major advances have resulted from increasingly powerful computers and specialist visualisation software. It seems likely that future advances will follow this trend with computer based techniques providing more and more diagnostic information from existing imaging technologies.

Comparing or overlaying images directly from different imaging systems has until recently not been possible. Firstly, different tissue characteristics are generally displayed in different image styles. For example, whilst CT images of the torso show the chest wall and skin surface, PET images of the same region preferentially show the functioning organs such as heart and liver. Secondly, different orientations, magnifications, and distortions can exist in each different image type. And thirdly a common image format (DICOM 3.0) is only now becoming more widely accepted.

There have been two principal methods of over laying or registering medical images developed; the landmark technique (Evans et al 1991) and the surface matching technique (Pelazarri et al 1989). Both techniques determine a linear transformation of seven degrees of freedom (three translations, three rotations, and one magnification) between the two image types. Either image can then be transformed into the reference space of the other image for direct comparison. Registered image sets are being demanded increasingly by surgeons to enable them to unambiguously resect only those tissues implicated in a clinical problem. For example, thoracic surgeons at the Austin Repatriation Medical Centre now require registered CT and PET scans for lung cancer patients, so that only the metastatic nodes involved in the disease are identified and removed during surgery.

Registered image sets can also form the basis for computerised neurosurgery planning in which procedures can be practised by manipulating image sets prior to the actual surgery. A recent innovation is the neurosurgical computer wand or probe, in which the probe's movement in space is monitored by a computer (Peters et al 1993). The probe is initially oriented to the patient's scalp by simultaneously touching scalp points and controlling a computer joystick to identify the same points on the patient's images. Subsequently if the neurosurgeon uses the probe to point to a region within the patient's brain the computer image can show the exact probe location in cut away views. This can significantly enhance the neurosurgeon's spatial localisation for tissue resection or biopsy.

The conventional means of displaying an image is as a set of parallel slices, generally a set of transaxial slices perpendicular to the long axis of the body. Views from any direction can then be calculated and displayed as either a surface rendered object or as a volume rendered object. A surface rendered image is produced by determining along each line of sight through an object the first image voxel which has an intensity greater than a chosen threshold. Whilst surface rendered images greatly assist in applications such as craniofacial surgery where the external appearance is crucial, most other medical visualisation applications actually require volume rendered images. Volume rendered images are constructed by applying an opacity weighting function along each line of sight through an object. The intensity of each pixel in the resulting image is the summation of the product of the weighting function and intensity of each voxel along the entire line of sight. The weighting function can be adjusted to give greater weight to deep structures, enabling visualisation of internal structures whilst still retaining an overall perspective of the object.

Automated image segmentation and tissue classification tools have been developed by a number of groups (Collins DL et al 1992, Kamber et al 1992).

One technique uses computers to utilise the greater 16 bit dynamic range of digital images. The human eye is sensitive to 12 bit images, and generally to images having a lower dynamic range. An algorithm to segment an anatomical image into regions having different characteristic intensities was an early attempt to classify tissue types present in an image, since similar tissue types could be expected to have similar intensities. More recently machine vision techniques which use image segmentation algorithms together with knowledge based databases offer the possibility of automatically identifying normal and abnormal regions within an image. These tools can be used to enhance diagnosis and reporting of disgnostic images as well as providing objective analysis tools for medical research based on non-invasive imaging techniques.

REFERENCES

ACR/NEMA Publication 300-1988 1988 Digital imaging and communication. American College of Radiology/National Electrical Manufacturers Association, Washington DC

Collins D L, Peters T M, Evans A C 1992 Multiresolution image registration and brain structure segmentation. Proceedings IEEE EMBS 14th Annual International Conference, France

Crowe B 1990 International developments in PACS. Australian Institute of Health and Welfare, Canberra

Crowe B 1993 Telemedicine in Australia. Australian Institute of Health and Welfare, Canberra

Egan G F, O'Keefe G J, O'Callaghan D 1993a Computer networking and network applications at the Austin Hospital, Melbourne. In: Hovenga E, Whymark G (eds) Proceedings of the Inaugural Health Informatics Conference, HIC '93, Brisbane

Egan G F, O'Callaghan D, O'Keefe G J 1993b Networked medical image database at the Austin Hospital, Melbourne. In: Hovenga E, Whymark G (eds) Proceeding of the Inaugural Health Informatics Conference, HIC '93, Brisbane

Evans A C, Marrett S, Torrescorzo J, Ku S, Collins L 1991 MRI-PET correlation in three dimensions using a volume-of-interest (VOI) atlas. Journal of Cerebral Blood and Metabolism 11

Glass H I, Stark N A 1991 PACS and related research in the UK. In: Huang H K, Ratib O, Bakker A R, Witte G (eds) Picture archiving and communication systems in medicine, NATO ASI series F74, Springer, Berlin

Goeringer F 1991 Medical diagnostic imaging support systems for military medicine. In: Huang H K, Ratib O, Bakker A R, Witte G (eds) Picture archiving and communication systems in medicine, NATO ASI series F74, Springer, Berlin

Hounsfield G N 1973 Computerised transverse axial scanning (tomography). Part 1: Description of system. British Journal of Radiology 46:1016-1022

Irie G 1991 Clinical experience: 16 months of Hu-PACS. In: Hong H K, Ratib O, Bakker A R, Witte G (eds) Picture archiving and communication systems in medicine, NATO ASI series F74, Springer, Berlin.

Kamber M, Collins D L, Shingal R, Francis G S, Evans A C 1992 Model based 2D segmentation of multiple sclerosis lesions in dual echo MRI data. In: Robb R A (ed) Visualisation in biomedical computing. Proceedings of SPIE 1808, International Society for Optical Engineering, Washington

Masser H, Mandl A, Urban M, Hradil H, Hruby W 1991 The Vienna project SZMO. In: Huang H K, Ratib O, Bakker A R, Witte G (eds) Picture archiving and communication systems in medicine, NATO ASI series F74, Springer, Berlin

O'Callaghan D, Egan G F 1994 Connecting the Austin Hospital to the Internet — and still being able to sleep at night. In: Carter B (ed) Proceedings of the 2nd Australian Health Informatics Conference, HIC '94, Gold Coast, Qld

O'Keefe G J 1994 Personal communication

Osborne P 1994 Personal communication

Pelazarri C A, Chen G T Y, Spelbring D R, Weichselbaum R R, Chen C 1989 Accurate three dimensional registration of CT, PET, and/or MR images of the brain. Journal of Computer Assisted Tomography 13

Peters T M, Davey B, Comeau R, Henri C J, Munger P, Charland P, Evans A, Olivier A 1993 Online stereoscopic image guidance for neurosurgery. Nuclear Science Symposium and Medical Imaging Conference III:1805-1809, IEEE, New Jersey

Prichard J W, Rosen B R 1994 Functional study of the brain by NMR. Journal of Cerebral Blood Flow and Metabolism 14(3)

Ratib O 1992 Evolution of PACS concepts. In: DeValk J P (ed) Integrated diagnostic imaging, Elsevier, Amsterdam

Rowberg A H, Zick GL 1992 PACS: clinical evaluation and future conceptual design. In: De Valk J P (ed) Integrated diagnostic imaging. Elsevier, Amsterdam

16

Telemedicine

MALCOLM PRADHAN

Health care and telecommunication

Telemedicine can broadly be defined as health care services delivered through telecommunications networks. The concept of using telecommunication for patient care is probably as old as the telephone. Telemedicine, however, is more than simple voice communication over telephone lines; it includes the transmission of still images, video, and other forms of medical data.

Some of the earliest experiments using video and sound communication for health care were carried out in the space missions of the 1960s, by the US and Soviet space programs. Today telemedicine is predominantly seen as a way of delivering tertiary health care to rural centres that have limited health services, with the objective to provide equal health care services regardless of geographical location.

Telemedicine is undergoing a surge in popularity in many countries, with considerable interest and investment from the computer and communications industries. Most States in Australia now have some pilot or established telemedicine project linking major hospitals to rural centres. Several factors have been responsible for the recent interest in the field—the most important is the rapid fall of the cost of hardware required to build a telemedicine system, including the cost of connecting remote sites.

The reality of geographic and socio-economic barriers to health care access in rural communities has been recognised for many years. Despite this awareness, rising health care costs force many local hospitals to close, reducing access further. Health care workers in rural areas face professional isolation, and must deal with additional expenses for transportation when sending patients for referral. These problems outside urban centres increase the cost of health care to the individual patient, and therefore the entire system. It is believed that telemedicine can improve the standard of health care by providing medical intervention in a more timely manner, instead of the current practice of sending rural patients to urban hospitals resulting in delayed interventions.

Almost all medical specialties can be practiced via telemedicine. The most studied applications concentrate on areas in which there is a shortage of experts in rural communities, and in which the presence of visual data prevent telephone consultations from being effective. Examples include radiology, histopathology, dermatology, ultrasonography, and other imaging studies. Mental health care has also been one of the early applications of telemedicine.

Transmission of medical data

Telemedicine is a collection of technologies including computers, communication networks, video, and specialised medical equipment. The most common feature of a telemedicine system is the ability to transmit high quality medical images across a communication line. To understand how this is achieved it is important to understand the difference between digital and analog data.

Analog signals vary continuously. An example of an analog signal is an ECG which is recorded on a printout. Traditional sound and video data are also analog signals. Computers deal with digital data, so analog signals must be converted to digital signals that are stored in discrete units. The process is known as *analog-to-digital conversion* (ADC). An important advantage of digital signals is that they can be transmitted through a digital communication channel irrespective of the source of the signal, so digitised voice, video, ECGs, X-rays, and so on, may be sent through the same communication channel. In this section we will explore how various medical data can be digitised and transmitted.

Still images

When an image is digitised it is stored as a matrix of *pixels* (picture elements). Many computer screens can display at least 640×480 pixels. If each pixel is represented as a *bit* in the computer then it can be in one of two states, 'on' or 'off', which may correspond to two colours, say black and white. Almost all medical images require colour or many levels of grey so each pixel must be represented by more than one bit in memory. If a pixel is represented by n bits in memory it is said to have a pixel *depth* of n, and the pixel can take on one of 2^n colours. An example is a computer screen that can display 256 colours; such a display will require a pixel depth of 8 bits per pixel. Because computer images have this third dimension they are often described in terms of width $\times$ height $\times$ depth.

The amount of memory required to store an image varies considerably depending on the source of the image. A digitised X-ray is usually around $2000 \times 2000 \times 12$; that is, 12 bits per pixel with an area of 2000 pixels squared. The storage for such an image is about 6 Megabytes (Mb). In contrast a single CT slice requires about $512 \times 512 \times 12$, or about 400 Kilobytes (Kb).

Colour images require greater bit depth, around 24 bits per pixel, to represent smooth colour transitions. Fortunately clinical images or histopathology images can be around television resolution for most purposes, say $800 \times 600 \times 24$, requiring almost 1.5 Mb per image.

Video

Video images of the patient are often required for adequate patient assessment. In the simplest terms video can be thought of as transmitting still images 25 to 30 times per second to give the illusion of movement. The human eye is less perceptive to detail in moving images so video images tend to be around 300×200 pixels in size with a pixel depth of 16 bits for colour, or 8 bits for grey scale. Although 25 to 30 images, or frames, per second is the speed at which the television standard works (broadcast quality), lower rates of around 15 frames per second are adequate for many purposes not involving rapid movement. Frame rates below 10-15 are noticeably jumpy and can be irritating to view.

The data rate for raw video information is enormous. Consider that a $300 \times 200 \times 16$ still image requires about 120 Kb, but at a video rate of 15 frames per second the data transmission rate required is 1.8 Mb per second! Obviously transmitting raw video signal is not efficient, and compression techniques for still images and video will be discussed later in this chapter.

Telemedicine technologies

Telecommunication

Telemedicine is primarily concerned with the transmission of medical data between rural and urban areas, so it is important the technology takes advantage of existing communication infrastructure to be cost effective. Copper telephone wire is the most common form of communication channel connecting distant centres. Unfortunately telephone wires were not designed for fast digital communication and there is a limit to how fast data can travel through this medium. The capacity for information transmission of a communication medium is called *bandwidth*.

Modems (modulator-demodulators) are a common computer peripheral used for digital communication between two points using telephone lines. Modems convert digital signals into analog sound waves and transmit these analog signals to a receiving modem over a standard telephone connection. The receiving modem then converts the analog signals back into digital signals. The problem with this technique is that standard telephone connections are *noisy*—there is interference which limits the maximum bandwidth, especially to rural areas. Low-cost modems are available with speeds of 14.4 Kilobits per second (Kbps). Faster modems are now becoming available but it is not clear that speeds higher than 14.4 kbs are reliable over long distances due to line noise.

The unique conditions in Australia—a small population and large distances—have motivated some telemedicine projects to use satellite connections between tertiary centres and very remote regions (Watson 1989).

Integrated Services Digital Networks (ISDN)

ISDN improves the potential bandwidth of communication by transmitting data digitally from one point to another, for the most part, using existing telephone switches and wiring. Although the cost of ISDN has prevented its widespread use amongst home computer users (compared to modems) this technology is the most commonly used medium for telemedicine. The ISDN 'basic rate' provides 56 or 64 Kbps of data transmission, and two voice lines. ISDN lines may be aggregated to provide greater bandwidth, so two lines would allow 128 Kbps communication.

To put the limitations of ISDN using copper telephone wire into perspective, most universities and many businesses use twisted pair or coaxial wire cabling for data transmission rates between computers of around 10-16 Megabits per second (Mbps). Fibre optic connections can provide speeds of over 150 Mbps. The speed of ISDN communication is a major constraint when designing equipment to be used in telemedicine applications.

Compression

In a remote telemedicine consultation the time for image transfer must be minimised—it is not acceptable for busy physicians to spend a significant amount of time simply waiting for image data to arrive. If the technology interferes with the flow of medical practice the resulting poor user satisfaction will prevent its widespread use. It is clear that raw visual data cannot be sent through ISDN lines in an interactive fashion. Data compression is used to reduce transmission times by reducing the storage size of image and video data.

There are two general types of image compression: lossy and lossless. In general, lossless compression methods can compress data about 2:1 on average. Lossless compression guarantees that the process of compressing and decompressing an image will not change the image in any way (all the pixels will have the same value before and after compression). Although halving the memory required to store and transmit the image is good, much better rates of compression can be achieved by using lossy compression.

Lossy compression

Lossy compression techniques achieve much higher rates of compression than lossless methods by discarding some of the information in the image. Although this sounds alarming at first, most lossy compression techniques take advantage of the fact that the human eye perceives small colour changes less accurately than small changes in brightness. Therefore, by removing small differences in pixel colour much greater compression rates can be accomplished, usually in the range of 10:1 to 20:1 without much loss in image quality. The amount of compression, and therefore image degradation, can be selected by the user.

The most commonly used lossy compression technique is the Joint Photographic Expert Group (JPEG) image compression mechanism (Wallace 1991). The advantage of JPEG compression is that it is widely available on many computer platforms. JPEG compression has been used for teleradiology and for picture archive and retrieval systems (Kajiwara 1992). The standard JPEG compression technique compresses the whole image using the same compression factor, regardless of regions of interest that one might want to store in higher quality. Other methods of lossy compression exist but most are based on the same basic technique as the JPEG algorithm (the discrete cosine transform). Some variations of lossy compression have been customised for X-ray images—using lossy compression for areas of high contrast which will not be significantly affected by the information loss (Wilson 1992).

Video compression

Video is amenable to lossy compression because the eye does not have time to detect imperfections on a single frame. The largest gains for video compression derive from a technique known as *frame differencing*. Frame differencing calculates what parts of the image have changed between two frames and only transmits the differences instead of a whole frame.

The International Telegraph and Telephone Consultative Committee (CCITT) has recommended standards for transmitting compressed sound and video over ISDN connections (CCITT 1990). The standards, grouped under the name H.320, provide for up to a 352×288 image at to 30 frames per second, although the frame rate will depend on how many ISDN lines are aggregated. This standard was designed for teleconferencing and not specifically for telemedicine.

Interpretation of compressed images

A lossy compression technique can potentially reduce an X-ray image from 6 Mb to 600 kb with only a small loss of quality. An uncompressed image would take 12.5 minutes to transmit using a 64 kbps ISDN connection (assuming 100% efficiency), but if compressed at 10:1 using lossy compression the time required to transmit is under 1.5 minutes. Why not compress all data if there is such a significant time saving? Why not compress images at higher compression rates? The answer is, of course, image degradation.

The effect of lossy compression on clinical diagnoses has been studied in a few areas. Compression rates around 10:1 (Cosman et al 1994) up to 20:1 (Aberle et al 1993) did not change the detection of abnormalities in thoracic X-rays and CT scans, or in hand X-rays (Sayre et al 1992). At least one study has shown that there is a significant decrease in diagnostic accuracy when interpreting on-screen X-ray images of subtle orthopedic fractures (Scott et al

1993). These conflicting results indicate that further research is required to see what classes of image are amenable to lossy compression without significant loss of diagnostic information.

There is some early evidence that lossy compression methods in tele–medicine may not adversely affect diagnostic accuracy of images in remote consultation for ultrasonography (Beard et al 1993), histopathology (Weinstein et al 1992), dermatology (Perednia et al 1992), and other clinical disciplines.

Components of a telemedicine system

In the past most telemedicine systems were built specifically for a hospital and the remote site, usually at great expense. Today, there are numerous telemedicine hardware vendors providing 'off-the-shelf' systems. Each system varies in the exact specifications, but the basic components of a telemedicine system are similar.

A telemedicine system requires remote connections, usually through ISDN. Video and audio are provided using a high-resolution video camera, and a video-tape recorder. The analog image from the video camera is digitised using ADC hardware, after which the resulting image is compressed. Image compression is done by a hardware component called a *codec* (compressor-decompressor). Most telemedicine vendors have their own proprietary codec which is optimised for their own computer and display systems. It is very important to make sure that the proprietary codecs also support industry standards like JPEG and H.320 so systems from different vendors can inter-operate. The teleconferencing and image manipulation in telemedicine is controlled by a computer system.

There are numerous attachments that can be added to the telemedicine system to allow the remote physician to gather data about a patient. An electronic stethoscope is often provided to allow the heart sounds of a patient to be transmitted over the audio channel. Telepathology systems may include a facility for the consulting pathologist to control the movement of the stage and the zoom of a microscopy across the country, only relying on technicians to prepare and mount the slides. Direct control of remote equipment such as a microscope, endoscope, or other operative instruments requires even higher bandwidth communications and sophisticated user-interfaces because the control signal must appear to be synchronised with the visual feedback from the device (Keil–Slawik et al 1991).

If X-rays, ultrasound, ECGs, and other medical data are to be transmitted via a telemedicine system then specialised hardware is required to digitise the data, or transfer the data if it is already in digital form (for example, CT scans).

Usability and evaluation

Human factors

The technical problems of telemedicine are well recognised and solutions will improve as computers and networks become faster. It is not entirely clear how the use of telemedicine will impact the practice of medicine, or if in fact there are long-lasting cost and health related benefits to telemedicine consultations.

There are numerous changes to the way medicine is traditionally practised when dealing with telemedicine consultations. The most obvious difference is that all patient data is acquired through relayed images, with physical findings described by the local doctor or nurse who is carrying out the exam for the remote consultant. Consulting physicians now not only have to deal with uncertainty about the patient's condition, but they have to deal with added uncertainty of the quality of the data about the patient received via telemedicine. Some doctors feel possible defects in transmitted data may increase the risk of malpractice (Parsons 1994). Whether this problem will affect the use of telemedicine, and whether this added uncertainty results in an increase in the number of tests ordered, is yet to be shown (Holand & Pedersen 1993).

Several management issues concerned with the widespread use of telemedicine remain unresolved. Telemedicine requires that the consultant physician and the rural health worker be present with the patient at the same time. Because of the cost of communication and the staffing requirements to run the telemedicine system the efficient scheduling of the sessions at both sites is important. Another concern is the incentives for the physicians. Telemedicine consultations are more time-consuming than traditional consultations, and it is not clear if this difference will be reflected in the reimbursement structure for physicians.

The relative immaturity of evaluations in telemedicine give rise to concerns about its use. Some concerns are contradictory but exemplify the problems of introducing a technology into the medical system which does not simply make current work more efficient, but changes the practice of medicine. For example, doubts have been raised as to whether introducing more tertiary care into rural areas will actually reduce the cost of health care, and whether telemedicine consultations will reduce the incentive for specialists to work in rural areas. On the other hand there is great hope that telemedicine services will provide a source of continuing education for country doctors (Akselsen & Lillehaug 1993).

Evaluations

Despite the interest and investment in telemedicine there are surprisingly few evaluations of the field (Brauer 1992). At this stage the telemedicine literature has many pilot study reports and subjective evaluations but few generalisable studies.

What factors are important to evaluate in a new medical technology? First, a new technology must have proven safety and efficacy. Second, the system must have clinical utility (Perednia 1993); this is addressed with such questions as 'Is the system easy to use?', 'What effect does telemedicine have on the care of patients?', 'What is the most efficient use of telemedicine?' Lastly, telemedicine must be cost effective.

The issues of safety and efficacy require comparing the accuracy of diagnoses by telemedicine to some gold standard; for example, pathological diagnosis of biopsied material. This accuracy rate must be compared to the accuracy rate of 'live' consultations.

Most telemedicine projects do not attempt to address the points discussed above. Formal studies of these questions require a time frame beyond most pilot studies or proof-of-concept projects. The number of cases seen in most telemedicine projects is relatively small and it is hard, if not impossible, for one installation to collect a sample size of subjects that would produce statistically significant results (Allen 1994).

Another problem with interpreting telemedicine evaluations is the difference in technology that has been used over the years. Computer display, imaging, and compression techniques are improving rapidly so criticisms made five or more years ago may not be relevant today. It is difficult to apply lessons from many pilot projects that have been designed using 'ideal' systems, such as very fast networks and very expensive imaging equipment. It is unlikely that the majority of telemedicine connections will use fast network technology until new wiring and switching equipment is installed in rural areas.

Telemedicine co-operative ventures are now forming to pool data from multiple telemedicine projects in an attempt to answer some of the questions raised in this section (From et al 1993, Perednia 1993) It is likely that clinically relevant and statistically significant data will be available in the near future.

Security

Patient confidentiality and the security of patient data is often ignored in pilot studies. As yet there have been no breaches of security reported (Parsons 1994) but unless the issues of data encryption and user authentication are addressed telemedicine will be susceptible to security problems which could set the industry back many years. (It is interesting to note that paper-based records are inherently more secure than digital data because paper records are so difficult to find and search even when one is looking for them.)

Looking ahead

Computer technology is doubling in speed every 12 to 18 months, and with this increased speed brings the promise of faster and less lossy compression techniques. Colour displays are still very expensive but in the long term cathode ray displays will be replaced by some variety of liquid-crystal display technology which will not exhibit the same accuracy problems as tube-based displays when scaling up to larger sizes. High definition television (HDTV) promises a high-resolution digital standard for television which avoids the analog-to-digital conversion that is currently required. HDTV relies on image compression during picture transmission so the consumer production of HDTV systems will lower the price of large displays and compression hardware.

Networking technology is also increasing in speed very rapidly. Telephone systems are gradually being converted into fiber optical cable, and asynchronous transfer mode (ATM) appears to be the dominant networking technology of the future. ATM can deliver 155 Mbps to the desktop, and potentially deliver several gigabytes per second across wide area networks. Unfortunately it may be some time before rural connections are upgraded to provide ATM speeds. Another solution is to use copper-based T1 connections (1.5 Mbps) to major rural sites.

It is quite possible that the term 'telemedicine' will be replaced simply by 'teleconferencing'. Faster networks and cheaper hardware also mean that video and sound telecommunication is possible for non-medical businesses and consumers. As this technology becomes more widespread telemedicine may become a part of daily practice for many practitioners who have video and computer technology on their desktop, and connecting to remote physicians is as easy as a telephone call.

Conclusions

The growth of telemedicine has been hampered by high set-up costs, and by the paucity of quality data regarding many important questions which must be answered before the widespread introduction of the technology into the health care system. The rapidly falling prices of computer equipment mean that telemedicine projects are easier to initiate, but there are still valid concerns about the safety, efficacy, and security of telemedicine technology.

Telemedicine is an interesting case study in introducing a new technology that provides facilities not previously available; in this case, tertiary health to the rural sector. It is a mixture of many advanced technologies and the traditional practice of medicine.

Greater specialisation of medical graduates, and greater investment in tertiary centres has put pressure on the health care system to distribute services to rural areas which have been suffering a steady decline of health care resources. Telemedicine will be a useful tool in distributing services around the country, and possibly overseas. Until more evaluation data are available it remains to be seen how telemedicine must evolve to best suit the needs of medical practice.

REFERENCES

Aberle D R, Gleeson F, Sayre J W et al 1993 The effect of irreversible image compression on diagnostic accuracy in thoracic imaging. Investigative Radiology 28(5):398-403

Akselsen S, Lillehaug S I 1993 Teaching and learning aspects of remote medical consultations. Telektronikk 89(1):42-7

Allen A 1994 Evaluating telemedicine: the cooperative model. Telemedicine Today 2(1):8-9

Beard D V, Hemminger B M, Keefe B et al 1993 Real-time radiologist review of remote ultrasound using low-cost video and voice. Investigative Radiology 28(8):732-4

Brauer G W 1992 Telehealth: the delayed revolution in health care. Medical Progress Through Technology 18(3):151-63

CCITT 1990 Narrow-band visual telephone systems and terminal equipment No. H.320. International Telegraph and Telephone Consultative Committee, International Telecommunication Union, Geneva

Cosman P C, Davidson H C, Bergin C J et al 1994 Thoracic CT images: effect of lossy image compression on diagnostic accuracy. Radiology 190(2):517-24

From S, Stenvold L A, Danielsen T 1993 Telemedicine services integrated into a health care network: analysis of communication needs in a regional health care system. Telektronikk 89(1):12-22

Holand U, Pedersen S 1993 Quality requirements for telemedical services. Telektronikk 89(1):51-3

Kajiwara K 1992 JPEG compression for PACS. Computer Methods and Programs in Biomedicine 37(4):343-51

Keil-Slawik R, Plaisant C, Shneiderman B 1991 Remote direct manipulation: a case study of a telemedicine workstation. In: H-J Bullinger (eds) Proceedings of the Fourth International Conference on Human-Computer Interaction, Stuttgart, Germany, 1-6 Sept. Elsevier, Amsterdam

Parsons D F 1994 Telemedicine in New York State. Report nystelem. New York State Department of Health, New York

Perednia D A 1993 A brief introduction to telemedicine system evaluation and the Clinical Telemedicine Cooperative Group (CTCG). Oregon Health Sciences University

Perednia D A, Gaines J A, Rossum A C 1992 Variability in physician assessment of lesions in cutaneous images and its implications for skin screening and computer-assisted diagnosis. Archives of Dermatology 128(3):357-64

Sayre J W, Ho B K, Boechat M I et al 1992 Subperiosteal resorption: effect of full-frame image compression of hand radiographs on diagnostic accuracy. Radiology 185(2):599-603

Scott W Jr., Rosenbaum J E, Ackerman S J et al 1993 Subtle orthopedic fractures: teleradiology workstation versus film interpretation. Radiology 187(3):811-5

Wallace G K 1991 The JPEG Still Picture Compression Standard. Communications of the ACM 34(4):30-44

Watson D S 1989 Telemedicine. Medical Journal of Australia 151(2):62-6

Weinstein R S, Bloom K J, Krupinski E A et al 1992 Human performance studies of the video microscopy component of a dynamic telepathology system. Zentralbl Pathol 138(6):399-403

Wilson D L 1992 Compressed radiological images and workstation viewing. Journal of Digital Imaging 5(3):168-75

17

Physiological monitoring

BRANKO CELLER

Importance of physiological measurements in clinical medicine

The development of modern medicine has been characterised by the increasing application of scientific methods in the clinical setting. Following the defeat of most infectious disease by antibiotics, and the improvement in public health associated with improved housing, nutrition and education, the major challenges of modern medicine are now those associated with iatrogenic illness, chronic degenerative disease of major organ systems and those insidious slowly developing diseases associated with lifestyle habits such as smoking and excessive consumption of alcohol or with occupational hazards and environmental pollution.

As measurement is the essence of the scientific method it is not surprising that physiological instrumentation, measurement and monitoring has grown into an international multi-billion dollar industry, dominated by a number of multinational industries such as Hewlett Packard and Siemens, which for hospital based patient monitoring alone is approximately $US1.7 billion world wide (1992 figures).

It is also clear that future developments in clinical medicine and primary health care will depend ever more on sophisticated monitoring systems which will evolve out of the emerging technologies of semiconductor sensors, medical imaging, medical expert systems, micro-miniaturisation of computing power, advanced wireless communications and world-wide networking for access to clinical and epidemiological information. In this chapter we review the basis of physiological monitoring with reference both to a generalised instrumentation system and to applications in cardiology and hospital based intensive and coronary care.

General properties of medical instrumentation systems

Most instruments share a number of common characteristics. They all need signal conditioning to eliminate unwanted signals, computing power for control and analysis, display and hardcopy devices for output and memory for storage. Medical instruments essentially differ from other scientific instruments because of the source of the signal or the area of application, which is living tissue. This fundamental difference however imposes on the medical instrument industry the requirements for standards of safety, performance and quality only matched by the aerospace industry in cost and complexity.

In physiological monitoring the *measurand* is usually an accessible signal or quantity generated by an organ system, derived from a tissue sample or elaborated from some associated physical property. Of these, *biopotentials* originating from neural or neuromuscular activity and measurements of temperature, pressure, flow, displacement, impedance and chemical com–position are the most important. Some examples of physiological measurands include:

- electrocardiography (ecg)
- electromyography (emg)
- electroencephalography (eeg)
- phonocardiography (pcg)
- blood pressure
- blood flow
- respiratory flows, pressures and volumes
- blood gases, P_{O2}, P_{CO2}
- blood pH.

Many different techniques have been developed to measure these variables. Some measurements depend on the use of external electrodes. Others such as X-ray, ultrasound, and electromagnetic or doppler flowmeters depend on the application of external energy, whilst others require the collection of gas, liquid or tissue samples and the use of biochemical methods for the analysis of chemical composition and concentration.

The nature of the measurement and the range of its frequency content are major factors which influence the design of an instrument. Thus some variables change very slowly and may have a 24 hour circadian rhythm, others such as the ECG contain frequencies of clinical interest to approximately 300 Hz, whilst emg and nerve potentials have bandwidths extending to 3-10 kHz. Biopotentials are in the microvolt range and pressures are in the range of 0-300 mmHg.

Physiological signals may be affected by ambient and generated noise, dependence on other variables such as temperature, humidity and pH or by perturbations caused by emotional or physical arousal. All of these factors must be considered, and impose significant practical constraints on the design of medical instruments. Essential elements of a modern physiological instrument are shown in Figure 17.1.

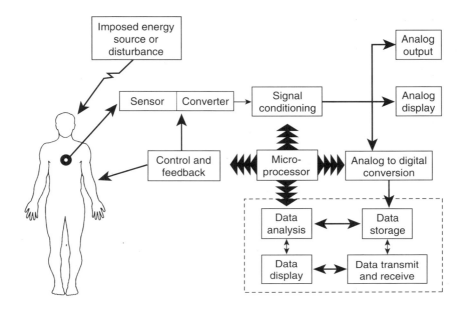

Fig. 17.1 Essential elements of a modern medical instrument for the measurement of physiological parameters

The sensor converts a physical quantity, such as flow or pressure to an electrical quantity. Sensors should be minimally invasive and should respond only to the desired measurand whilst providing minimum interference with the process being measured. An air flow sensor which provides an excessive resistance to flow could itself for example, influence the measurand. Microelectronic sensors, using the chemical and mechanical properties of semiconductor materials, and manufactured using microelectronic technology, are now revolutionising the industry because of their low cost, reliability and improved performance. Other sensors based on ion selective field effect transistors are now beginning to appear for the measurement of pH and gas and chemical composition. These will have profound effects as sensor elements in complex feedback control systems such as those required in metabolic demand driven cardiac pacemakers which can automatically change their rate in response to changes in pH or arterio-venous oxygen differences following increased physical activity.

Although sensors provide the primary sensing element, for example the displacement of a diaphragm by an increase in pressure, the conversion of this displacement to an electrical signal usually requires an externally powered conversion element, such as a strain gauge and bridge circuit. For biopotential recordings such as the ECG, currents carried by ions in tissue are transformed into electrical currents by electrochemical reactions taking place in surface electrodes. The design of innovative, reliable, accurate and robust transducers thus underpins the science of physiological monitoring and measurement.

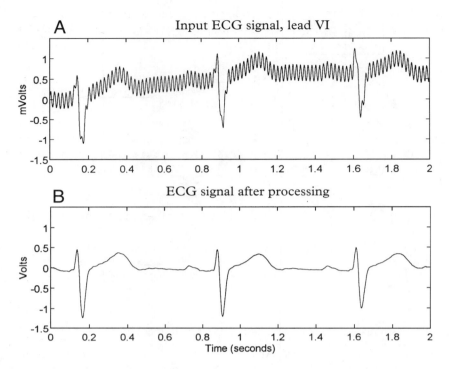

Fig. 17.2 (a) An ECG signal corrupted with mains frequency noise and respiratory artefacts. (b) The same signal as in (a) amplified 1000 times and digitally filtered

Transducers rarely have the inherent properties necessary for accurate and reliable operation. Signal conditioning is required to transform the signal produced by the transducer into a signal with reproducible stable properties and specified static and dynamic characteristics. These include adequate gain, insensitivity to external noise, a suitable frequency response, low inherent noise, good linearity and stability over time, and relative insensitivity to temperature or other environmental variables.

As an example, conditioning required for an ECG signal recorded with surface electrodes, would require amplification of approximately 1000 fold, elimination of unwanted noise frequencies produced by respiration or other skeletal muscle activity, and cancellation of mains frequency noise. The transformation of an unprocessed ECG signal, by signal conditioning techniques is shown in Figure 17.2.

Signal conditioning in modern instruments is usually a combination of analog processing at the signal source and digital filtering after the signal has been converted from a continuous (analog) signal to a discrete (digital) signal. Following signal conditioning and filtering the analog signal may be displayed on an oscilloscope or chart recorder, or directed through a loud speaker or other means depending on the particular nature of the measurand and its source. A calibration signal may be required for purposes of calibration and testing. This should have the same properties as the measurand and should be applied as close to the input signal source as possible. A signal of precise magnitude (2mV peak to peak) and known frequency (10Hz) for example can be used to calibrate an electrocardiograph.

Control and feedback may be required to adjust properties of the sensor or the signal conditioner, and to manage the flow of information for display, storage or transmission. These functions may be manual or automatic, but increasingly microprocessors are incorporated to carry out these and other functions. Thus once operator choices are made, control of the instrument and of data acquisition proceeds automatically, and data is collected, displayed and output in analog form to a video display or chart recorder.

In most modern instruments, analog (continuous) data is sampled electronically at an appropriate rate, typically 4-10 times the highest frequency content of the signal, and converted to discrete (digital) values which can be read and stored electronically. Control of this conversion process, acquisition of data, digital signal processing and analysis, storage, display, and transmission are all under the control of a microprocessor, which may be the Central Processing Unit (CPU) of a host computer or embedded in the instrument as a stand alone unit.

The digital mode of operation has many advantages. These include greater accuracy, repeatability, reliability and immunity to noise. Digital displays have largely replaced analog displays because of low cost and greater flexibility in mixing text data and signal data. Analog displays may however be preferred in situations where data is changing rapidly, or real-time display cannot be easily achieved.

The reader is encouraged to refer to texts edited by Webster (1988, 1992) for further reading in this area.

Performance standards and measures

As many clinical measurements rely upon empirical interpretation or the comparison of a result with statistically normal values, there is a requirement that electromedical equipment from different manufacturers adhere to minimum performance specifications. Standards are usually set by industry bodies or by professional associations such as the American Heart Association (AHA), the Association for the Advancement of Medical Instrumentation (AAMI), the American National Standards Institute (ANSI), and the International Electrotechnical Commission (IEC). Local national bodies such as the Federal Drug Administration in the US and the Therapeutic Goods Administration (TGA) in Australia are usually required to certify that specific instruments meet a required standard. Although there may be significant differences in standards originating from the USA or Europe, there is now an increasing tendency to standardise requirements and to develop joint guidelines.

As an example, Table 17.1 summarises the performance standards (ANSI-AAMI EC11-1991) that apply to electrocardiography.

Table 17.1 ANSI-AAMI EC11-1991 Performance requirements for an electrocardiograph

Input dynamic range	±5mV signal and tolerance for dc offsets of ±300mV
Gain accuracy	±5% for fixed gain selections of 20mm/mV, 10mm/mV and 5mm/mV
System error	For input signals limited to ±5mv and maximum rate of change of 125mV/sec, the maximum error permitted is ±10%.
Frequency response	Characterised relative to the response at 10Hz of a number of test signals. AHA recommends a bandwidth of 0.05Hz to 100Hz (+0.5dB, -3dB).
Step response	The device should respond to a step of 10mm, with an allowable overshoot of 10% and a decay time constant ≤3 sec when measured during the first 320ms.
Input impedance	A single ended input impedance of at least 2MΩ at 10Hz is required.
Direct currents	0.2µA in all patient electrode connections
CMRR at 50/670 Hz	Common mode noise rejection (CMRR) must be -90dB (1:30,000) with the reference (RL) electrode unbalanced by a standard impedance.
System noise	40µv when all inputs are connected together.
Patient risk currents	10µA in the event of specified mains power faults.

Patient safety

Use of electromedical equipment in the hospital environment involves particular patient and operator hazards associated with routine use of liquids, flammable gases and chemical agents in the vicinity of the equipment. Patients may be sedated or unconscious and may not react to painful stimuli, or be immobilised by connection to a number of pieces of equipment. Intravenous lines and in-dwelling catheters provide a low impedance path for electrical currents into the body which may prove fatal even at very low values. Because of this unique relationship between the equipment, operator, patient and treatment area, rigorous safety standards are required in the design of electromedical equipment.

Most countries have adopted the international safety standards for electromedical equipment developed by the IEC. As an example of these standards, IEC601-2-25 (1993) relates specifically to electrocardiographs. Major elements of this standard are given in Table 17.2.

Table 17.2 IEC safety standards for electrocardiographic equipment. IEC601-2-25 (1993)

Patient leakage currents	10µA. Under single fault conditions this may be relaxed to 50µA
Earth leakage currents	500µA from the mains to ground across insulation under normal operating conditions
Enclosure current	100µA from any part accessible to the operator or patient
Isolation	>3500Vac between the patient and the mains inlet to the device

Equipment which follows these standards may be classified either as body protected (BF) or cardiac protected (CF). The CF label signifies that equipment may be connected directly to the heart. If the equipment is designed to withstand high defibrillation voltages (>5000V), the BF and CF symbols are modified with the addition of two defibrillator paddles as shown in Figure 17.3.

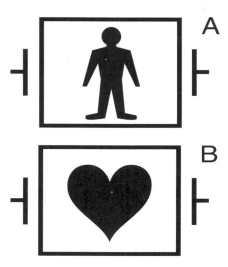

Fig. 17.3 International (IEC) symbols for (a) body protected (BF) (b) and cardiac protected (CF) equipment able to withstand defibrillation without damage

Design example: a 12 lead ECG monitoring system

The personal computer (PC) has become a de facto standard for many instrumentation applications because of its low cost, substantial power and the variety of third party products which support and enhance its functions. The Windows operating system and Graphical User Interface (GUI) has also contributed to an improvement in the user friendliness and ease of use of PC based instrumentation. Many specialist stand alone instruments are now offered as plug in cards for PCs or are designed to operate with specially modified PCs which satisfy CF standards for safety in areas such as intensive care units (ICUs).

An example of PC based clinical instrumentation is the PC-ECG, a 12 lead ECG system (PC-ECG) on a single card which fits into one of the PC slots (Celler et al 1994). The PC-ECG satisfies all international standards for performance and safety and has a sophisticated user interface and database for the collection, display, recall and comparison of 12 lead and Frank lead ECGs. Technical specifications for the PC-ECG are given in Table 17.3.

Table 17.3 Technical specifications for the PC-ECG electrocardiograph

Mode of operation	**12 lead clinical** Simultaneous recording of leads I, II, V1, V2, V3, V4, V5, V6. Leads III, aVR, aVL and aVF are synthesised. **Frank leads** Orthogonal vectors X, Y, and Z are derived from simultaneous unipolar recordings of leads A, C, E, F, I, H and M.
Input dynamic range	±5mV
dc offset voltage	±300mV maximum
Frequency response	0.05-300Hz
High pass filter	0.05 and 0.5Hz software selectable
Low pass filter	40, 100, 150Hz software selectable
Sensitivity	3µV
CMRR	>110dB at 50/60Hz
System noise	<30µV
Risk current	≤10µA
Overvoltage protection	defibrillator protected
Patient isolation	≥3500Vac

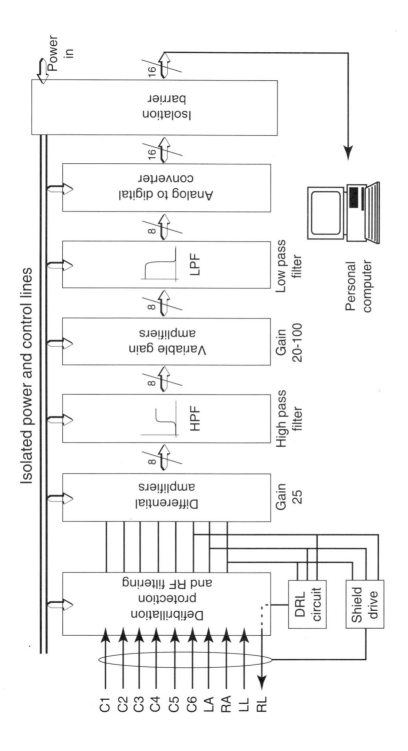

Fig. 17.4 Schematic diagram of the PC-ECG single card electrocardiograph system

A simple, front end patient management system is also incorporated for the registration of patient details, thus permitting stand alone use of the PC-ECG as a simple electrocardiograph. In applications where the PC-ECG must be integrated with an existing patient and practice management system, software links have been provided which allow the external application to directly operate the ECG data acquisition.

The schematic diagram of the PC-ECG shown in Figure 17.4 contains the following functional units:

Defibrillation protection and RF filtering. This circuit ensures that radio frequency (RF) signals are blocked out and that high voltages which may appear on the patient during defibrillation (cardioversion) do not damage the instrument.

Driven right leg circuit. This circuit reduces the common mode noise (principally mains frequency) on the body by approximately 50dB by cancelling out the noise voltage with another voltage of exactly opposite phase.

Shield drive. Reduces the capacitance of the electrical shields surrounding the patient cable thus improving high frequency performance, common mode rejection ratio (CMRR) and stability.

Differential amplifiers. These provide a very high CMRR (>120dB) and a gain of 25 which provides a tolerance to dc offsets of ±300mV which may be introduced by the skin to electrode interface.

High pass filter stage. Computer controlled to block the passage of dc voltages at the input, and to filter out frequencies below 0.05Hz or 0.5Hz. This circuit can also be activated automatically to provide a baseline restoration function under overload conditions.

Variable gain stage. Computer controlled to provide a variable gain of 20-100 in eight steps.

Low pass filter. A Bessel low pass filter which provides noise rejection for frequencies above 40Hz, 100Hz or 150Hz under software control. This is commonly known as an anti-aliasing filter as it stops the conversion of high frequency signals into low frequency signals by virtue of the sampling process.

Analog to digital converter. This circuit converts sequentially eight ECG analog inputs into digital numbers in the range of 0-4095 counts. The dynamic range is thus determined by the signal range at the input, the overall gain and the resolution of the conversion process which in this case is 12 bit (2^{12}-1 counts).

Isolation. This circuit provides the essential function of isolating all patient circuits from other circuits supplied by mains power. Isolation of digital data and control lines is carried out using optical means. Transformer isolation is more commonly used for the transfer of power across the isolation barrier.

PC Bus interface. This circuit provides the interface to the PC microprocessor for the transfer of digital data and the control of circuit function. The PC-ECG card needs to be identified by an address in the range of 120_H to 300_H which does not conflict with the address of other devices sharing the PC bus. Similarly an interrupt line (IRQ 2,3,10) must be selected, which the microprocessor uses for the reading, display and storage of data in real time. Key elements of the instrument are also controlled through this interface circuit. These include, highpass and lowpass filter characteristics, baseline restoration, amplifier gain and the rate at which the ECG signals are to be sampled and read.

Data display and output. One of the major advantages of using a PC as the dedicated microprocessor for the PC-ECG system is that all PC resources may be used for display, analysis and hardcopy output of the data. Thus ECG signals are recorded and displayed in real time on a high resolution (VGA 640 x 480) monitor. Once recorded, ECG signals may be subjected to further signal processing and filtering to eliminate unwanted disturbances such as mains frequency noise and baseline wander and then displayed as shown in Figure 17.5. Recorded signals may be viewed in high resolution for purposes of diagnosis or measurement as shown in Figure 17.6, before being printed out on a laser or bubblejet high resolution (300 x 300dpi) printer in the format shown in Figure 17.7.

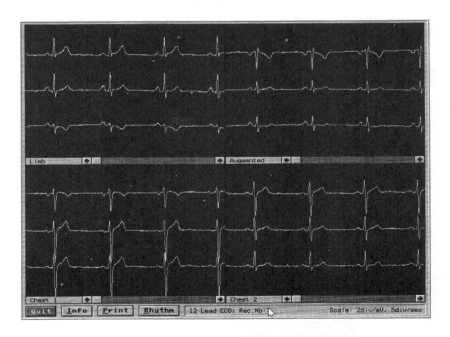

Fig. 17.5 Example of display of 12 lead ECG recorded with the PC-ECG

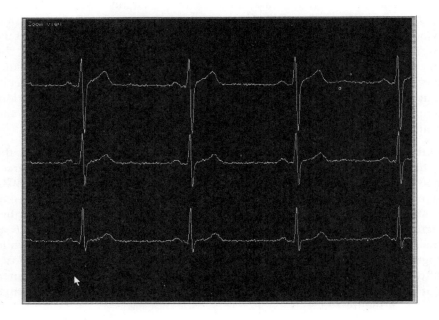

Fig. 17.6 High resolution display of three channels of the ECG in the PC-ECG system

Data reduction and data compression

ECG data is stored in a data base for future recall and online comparison. A ten second record of the eight ECG leads sampled at 500 samples/second (Hz) requires 80 kBytes of storage. A thousand ECGs could be stored on a 80 MByte hard disk. Very large applications may require removable optical WORM (Write Once Read Many) drives which can store many gigabytes on a single removable disc. Because of the large requirements for data storage a number of compression algorithms are available which seek to reduce storage requirements with little if any compromise of signal quality.

The turning point (TP) algorithm (Mueller 1978) reduces the sampling frequency by concentrating data points in the high frequency QRS region of the signal and selectively saving significant features such as peaks and valleys and turning points. A fixed reduction ratio of 2:1 is achievable without significant loss of signal detail. The AZTEC (Amplitude Zone Time Epoch Coding) (Cox et al 1968) decomposes ECG signal waveforms into zones of fixed plateaus or slopes. This algorithm produces an alternating sequence of durations and amplitudes which when reconstructed produces an ECG signal with stepwise quantization. This needs to be digitally filtered to produce a smoothed clinically acceptable signal. Data reduction ratios are not fixed but are typically in the ratio of 10:1.

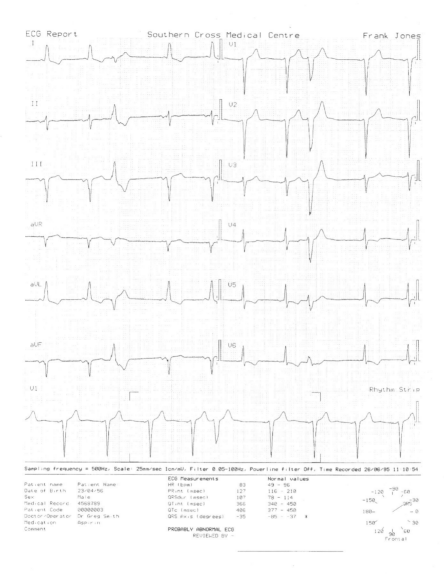

Fig. 17.7 Graphical printout of the 12 lead ECG produced by the PC-ECG system

Other codes derived from these two algorithms include the CORTES (Coordinate Reduction Time Encoding System) (Abenstein & Tompkins 1982) and the Fan algorithm (Bohs & Barr 1988). For the same reduction ratio, the Fan algorithm generally produces better signal fidelity than either the TP or the AZTEC algorithms.

Huffman coding exploits the fact that discrete amplitudes in a signal do not occur with the same probability. Thus variable length codes are assigned to different data sequences with short codes reserved for frequently occurring sequences. This gives a variable reduction ratio depending on the distribution of quantization levels in the signal. The Huffman coded original signal can be reconstructed without error, but transmission errors can be propagated to more than one sample. Other lossless codes derived from Huffman coding includes the Lempel-Ziv-Welch (LZW) algorithm, residual differencing and run length encoding. Signal processing of the ECG and encoding techniques for data compression are reviewed by Tompkins (1993).

The PC-ECG system uses run-time encoding and binary packing, to exploit the high degree of correlation which exists in adjacent samples of the ECG. This transforms a sequence of samples into a different sequence where each set of identical (correlated) samples are represented by the value of the sample and the number of repetitions. An average data reduction of 2:1 is achieved at high speed and without loss of signal fidelity. Blocks of ECG data are stored in the patient database as packed binary large objects (BLOBS).

Program languages

A program language is needed to provide an interface between human language forms and binary or machine code used by computers to execute instructions. Many languages (Fortran, Basic, Pascal, C, C++, Ada etc.) have been developed and continue to evolve to achieve improvements in program development time and to increase the reliability of complex software systems. Some of these languages provide exceptionally powerful utilities and functions which permit rapid prototyping and testing of algorithms for real time data acquisition, digital signal processing, graphical display, database design and data analysis.

These include ASYST a multitasking, FORTH based language which is device independent and supports a wide range of analog to digital (A/D), digital to analog (D/A), digital inputs and outputs (I/O), serial and parallel port communications as well as a complete set of statistical and scientific utilities for data analysis and signal processing. The language is highly pneumonic and complex functions can be carried out using simple commands as shown below:

```
DATA FFT       \Find Fourier Transform of DATA
ZMAG DUP*      \Square the magnitudes
CREATE.COPY    \Save as the Power spectrum
```

This small program carries out the relatively complex task of calculating the power spectrum of an input data file.

MATLAB is a powerful numerical package which together with Toolboxes for Signal Processing and other speciality functions, provides a wide range of functions for filter design and signal processing of both continuous and discrete data. Many of the filter functions used in the PC-ECG were developed and tested using MATLAB. The MATLAB programming language is written in an internal script format, and specific functions are made available as macros. Thus for example, an analog filter may be easily designed in the frequency domain, converted to discrete form and tested on a sample signal. The program code for the design of a digital Butterworth lowpass filter with a rolloff frequency at 40Hz and plotting out the result is shown below:

```
Fc=40;                    %  Cutoff frequency in Hz
Fs=500;                   %  Digital sampling frequency
[B,A]=butter(4,Fc/(0.5*Fs))  %  Design 4th order
                             Butterworth filter
freqz(B,A,200,Fs)         %  Plot out frequency response
```

New software development systems based on 4GL languages are now becoming available which retain many of the features described above but provide in addition a visual programming interface which uses standard or user defined graphical ICONS to describe even very complex functions. Once the program is designed graphically, the result is compiled into a program which may be linked to other programming languages such as C. Examples of these 4GL development systems are AmLab from Associative Measurements, LabView and LabWindows from National Instruments and Simulink from the Maths Works.

Notwithstanding the many advantages offered by these programming languages, most commercial products prefer to use C or C^{++} as their programming language. These languages are also the preferred languages for real time programming as they offer an excellent compromise between development time and run time performance. C is standardised and structured and provides many improvements over assembly languages without significantly reducing performance. C language programs are generally transportable and can be easily adapted to new host processors and architectures.

C^{++} attempts to overcome many of the problems associated with the system programming origins of C. C^{++} has become the language of choice for data abstraction and object oriented programming (Stroustrup, 1993). Its advantages include the ability to break down large applications into smaller pieces called objects, which closely match the underlying concepts of the application. Objects of user defined types contain information on that type and can be used safely in other contexts where their type may not be available during compilation. Objects may thus be re-used. Object based programs are usually quicker to develop, are shorter and easier to understand and are easier to maintain. Because the C language is also used for writing compilers and operating systems, significant advantages in speed and performance are possible by making low level function calls directly to the operating system.

The graphical library and most other routines for real time data acquisition, data processing and signal analysis in the PC-ECG are written in C^{++}, an object oriented language supraset of C.

Database design

With the increasing propensity towards computer based monitoring and diagnosis, efficient and robust methods of data storage, retrieval and archiving need to be implemented. The two key areas to be considered are the provision of mechanisms for information manipulation and the definition of structures for information storage. Most commonly, a database management system (DBMS) is used for these tasks. The primary data model for commercial data processing applications is that of the *relational model* where data and the relationships between data are represented by a series of tables. Each column within a table is known as a *field* and is given a unique name. Each database *record* corresponds to a particular row within the table. As such, each row represents a *relationship* among a set of values.

Importantly, from the viewpoint of medical informatics, DBMSs now have the capability of incorporating BLOBS of variable length. This is ideal for handling clinical measurement data as the size of the data record acquired is dependent on the type and duration of the measurement performed.

An example of a relational data model is shown in Table 17.4. Two tables are defined. The first 'Patient' table contains personal information. The second 'Procedures' table contains clinical measurement data relating to various procedures performed on a particular patient. There is a one-to-many entity relationship between the two tables based on the Pat_Code in the 'Patient' table and the Proc_code in the 'Procedures' table.

Table 17.4 A sample relational database

Table 'patient'

Pat_Code	Pat_Name	Pat_City
0001	Jack Smith	Brisbane
0002	John Doe	Sydney
0003	Susan Smith	Melbourne

Table 'procedures'

Proc_Code	Proc_Date	Proc_Description	Proc_Blob
0001	12/07/94	12 Lead ECG	"Binary Data"
0001	18/07/94	3 Lead ECG	"Binary Data"
0001	18/07/94	Spirometry	"Binary Data"
0003	13/07/94	12 Lead ECG	"Binary Data"

In order to retrieve database information, a number of languages for performing queries on the database have been developed. The most common query language for relational databases is Structured Query Language (SQL). This concise and efficient language can, depending on the implementation, perform retrieval of information either programmatically or interactively. A sample SQL query to retrieve patient procedures for the tables given above would be:

```
SELECT Patient.Pat_Name, Patient.Pat_Code,;
Procedures.Proc_Code, Procedures.Proc_Date,;
Procedures.Proc_Description;
FROM Procedures, Patient;
WHERE Patient.Pat_Code ==        Procedures.Proc_Code;
ORDER BY Patient.Pat_Name,       Procedures.Proc_Date;
```

Automated interpretation of ECGs

Automated interpretation of the ECG began more than 30 years ago (Pordy et al 1968, Pipberger & Stallman 1962) with the development of the Pipberger program (Pipberger & Stallman 1962) and the ECAN program (Caceres et al 1962). Since that time there has been continuous development of expert systems for automated interpretation of the ECG, and a number of programs are commercially available. These programs are now well accepted and approximately 30% of all ECGs recorded in the USA have computer based interpretations. The performance of these programs can vary but in general their result is in 75-85% agreement with a panel of specialist cardiologists. This is comparable to levels of agreement which are found between consulting cardiologists.

Automated interpretation of ECGs include two basic approaches. The first is based on decision logic where a rule based expert system is used to mimic the decision processes of a cardiologist. The second uses a multivariate statistical pattern recognition method to solve a pattern recognition problem (Klingeman & Pipberger 1967). New approaches based on neural networks (Rasiah & Attikouzel 1994) and on machine learning (Oates et al 1988) have been developed, but at present commercial systems are based almost exclusively on rule based expert systems which permit the operator to interrogate the machine logic and if necessary to review the full logic tree of the decision process.

The interpretation of ECG signals begins with feature extraction and measurement of key parameters. Principal parameters include the height, duration and morphometry of the P waves, T waves and the QRS complex in each lead. Figure 17.8 shows a typical ECG waveform and the range of parameters measured in the Hewlett Packard interpretation program (Doue et al 1985). ECG data are recorded and digitised data are examined by a *Quality Monitor* which identifies the presence of various forms of noise contamination. The *Data Conditioning Module* then applies a range of filters

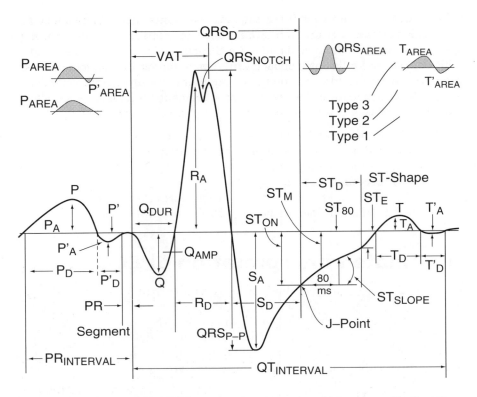

Fig. 17.8 A characteristic ECG beat showing the parameters measured in the HP automated ECG interpretation program (Reprinted with permission from Hewlett Packard)

designed to eliminate mains frequency noise and muscle artefact. The *Pattern Recognition Module* then adaptively filters the major P, QRS, ST and T regions and produces a comprehensive set of measurements as shown in Figure 17.8. These measurements are then sent to the *Criteria Module* which uses available clinical criteria to make a decision. As these processes are carried out on every beat in each lead, data must be correlated between leads, and comparisons made over time to identify rate related abnormalities. Other patient data such as age, sex, height, weight, smoking habits etc may also be used in making the diagnosis.

A medical knowledge base is also required which contains sets of rules for each diagnostic category much as are seen in the cardiology textbooks. Cardiac arrhythmias for example can be described according to their type class (event or rhythm), rhythm information and duration. Thus a normal beat is an event in which the duration of the QRS complex is between 60 and 110 milliseconds, and a premature ventricular contraction (PVC) is an event which has a duration

$0.8s \geq PVC \geq 0.4s$. Complex arrhythmias such as couplets, R on T, fusion beats, ventricular fibrillation or premature atrial contractions can be similarly classified.

Rules are typically formed as a large set of IF-THEN statements. An example from interpretation criteria developed at the University Department of Medical Cardiology at the Glasgow Royal Infirmary (Macfarlane et al 1989), which is currently used in the Siemens 44/700 series, is the following

IF
    (1) QRS duration $\geq 0.100s$ and $<0.120s$
AND
    (2) absence of Q wave in I and V_5 and V_6
AND
    (3) R peak time $> 0.060s$ in V_5 or V_6
THEN
Incomplete left bundle branch block

The advantage of rule based systems is that they are based on human knowledge and can therefore be interpreted relatively easily. An implied disadvantage however is that the automated system can never outperform the human expert as its knowledge is limited to that available to the expert.

An alternative approach is to recognise that many arrhythmias are defined in terms of other arrhythmias, and that if a sufficiently robust set of 'primitives' can be identified a syntactic language can be developed to describe the complete range of arrhythmias. Traditionally this has involved modelling these primitives as lines and simple curves using piecewise fitting and segmentation techniques (Trahanias & Skordalakis 1990). More recently these primitives have been modelled in terms of orthogonal polynomials and the polynomial coefficients passed to a probabilistic neural network for classification (Rasiah & Attikiouzel 1994).

Another approach (Oates et al 1988) which has been used with some success in real time monitoring of ischaemic changes in the CCU/ICU setting is to apply the principles of machine learning and inductive reasoning to parameters derived from a polarcardiographic representation of the orthogonal Frank lead ECG. In the application reported by Oates et al, the QRS plane of best fit is used as a reference for measurement of a new set of vectorcardiographic (VCG) and polarcardiographic (PCG) parameters.

An inductive learning program is then used to build a decision tree for the diagnosis of ischaemia, as a hierarchical set of comparisons between particular parameter values and a constant. This iterative process continues until a decision is made or no further divisions are possible. A decision tree based on both conventional ST parameters and QRS plane parameters gave a sensitivity of 96% and a specificity of 97% for the automated detection of ischaemia. This inductive reasoning approach is useful when new parameters are investigated for which no established expertise exists.

Case study II: The HP CCU/ICU Component Monitoring System

The Intensive Care Unit (ICU) or Coronary Care Unit (CCU) in a hospital provides the most complex and patient critical environment for physiological monitoring, and demonstrates the full range of integrated functions which are characteristic of present state of the art systems. The Hewlett Packard (HP) Component Monitoring system is an example of modular design where each element of the system, including instrumentation, display, communication and physical location can be tailored to suit the particular circumstance. The core element of this system is a modular rack system which can accomodate up to eight individual instrumentation modules for ECG, ECG/respiration, invasive blood pressure, non-invasive blood pressure, cardiac output, pulse oximetry, C_{O2}, TCGas, fractional inspired oxygen and temperature as well as a recorder module. Many of these modules can be transferred between racks without altering parameter settings. The measured parameters and associated alarm limits are displayed in numerical or graphical form on a 14" monochrome or colour display module.

A wide range of configurations are possible. The basic stand alone configuration is a computer and display module with a single component rack. Up to four satellite rack modules can be daisy chained to a single computer module over a physical distance of 30 metres. Larger remote data access networks can be formed using the HP CareNet interface. This digital network permits the interconnection of multiple modular component monitoring systems as well as analog bedside monitors. As information is a key element of patient management in any modern hospital a record keeping system is essential. The HP CareVue 9000 automates the task of documentation by providing Admit/Discharge/Transfer, Patient Admission, Flowsheets, Physician Data Sheets, Nursing Care Plans, Progress notes, Patient Reports and other forms on computer. Integration of this reporting data with data collected automatically at the bedside then makes the patient clinical record a valuable tool in the clinical management of the patient in an environment where responsibility for patient care is distributed over time between nursing staff, medical residents, visiting consultants and the patient's own physician.

Future trends in physiological monitoring in part already demonstrated in the HP monitoring systems, involve the widespread integration of modular bedside monitors, central basestation computers, telemetry systems for ambulatory patients, laboratory instruments, pharmacy data and medical records and accounting information in a local area network with gateways to other hospitals, general practioners and to sources of national and international medical and epidemiological information. Major developments can be expected in the near future in wireless communications and handheld instruments for patient monitoring. Monitoring systems will become smaller, more intelligent and self configuring. User interfaces will also change as the need to access clinical data quickly and easily will need to be balanced with considerations of security and confidentiality of patient data.

With the evolution of community based care, major teaching and specialist hospitals will form part of a network of specialist physicians, general practitioners, and community hospitals sharing patient information resident on distributed databases in each location. Multimedia applications involving the transfer of voice, data and video images will require interconnection of these sites with high speed optical fibre cables capable of bandwidths exceeding 10MBits/s. Information management will become ever more critical and intelligent means of handling the data volume and contents will need to be developed based on knowledge engineering and medical expert systems.

REFERENCES

Abenstein L P, Tompkins W J 1982 New data-reduction algorithms for real-time ECG analysis. IEEE Transactions on Biomedical Engineering BME-29:43-48

Bohs L N, Barr R C 1988 Prototype for real-time adaptive sampling using the Fan algorithm. Medical and Biological Engineering and Computing 26:574-583

Caceres C A, Steinberg C A, Abraham S, Carbery W J, McBride J M, Tolles W E, Ribli A E 1962 Computer extraction of electrocardiographic parameters. Circulation 25:356-62

Celler B G, Lim DeChazal K, Lovell N H 1994 Development of an integrated clinical workstation for general practice. Proceedings of the 2nd National Health Informatics Conference, Gold Coast Australia, August 1-2, pp 186-190

Celler B G, Lovell N H, Ilsar E, Lim K G 1994 Design of a clinical workstation for primary health care. 16th Annual Conference of the IEEE Engineering in Medicine and Biology Society, Baltimore

Cox J R, Nolle F M, Fozzard H A, Oliver G C 1968 AZTEC: a preprocessing program for real-time ECG rhythm analysis. IEEE Transaction on Biomedical Engineering BME-15:128-129.

Doue J Vallance A G 1985 Computer-aided ECG analysis Hewlett-Packard Journal, September 29-34

International Electrotechnical Commission 1993 International Standard 601-2-25, Medical electrical equipment, Part 2: Particular requirements for the safety of electrocardiographs

Klingeman J, Pipberger H V 1967 Computer classification of electrocardiograms Computers and Biomedical Research 1:1-17

Macfarlane P W, Veitch Lawrie T D 1989 Comprehensive electrocardiology: theory and practice in health and disease Vol 3, Pergamon Press, New York

Mueller W C 1978 Arrhythmia detection program for an ambulatory ECG monitor Biomedical and Scientific Instruments 14:81-85

Oates J, Celler B, Bernstein L, Bailey B P, Freedman S B 1988 Real time detection of ischemic ECG changes using quasi-orthogonal leads and artificial intelligence. Proceedings of the IEEE Computers in Cardiology Conference, pp 89-92, Bethesda, USA

Pipberger H V, Stallman F W 1962 Use of computers in electrocardiogram interpretation American Heart Journal 64:285-286

Pordy L, Jaffe H, Chesky K et al 1968 Computer diagnosis of electrocardiograms IV a computer program for contour analysis with clinical results of rhythm and contour interpretation. Computers and biomedical research 1:408-433

Rasiah A I and Attikiouzel Y 1994 A syntactic approach to the recognition of common cardiac arrhythmias within a single ambulatory ECG trace. In Press, Australian Computer Journal

Stroustrup B 1993 The C++ programming language, 2nd edn. Addison-Wesley, Reading, Massachusetts

Trahanias P, Skordalakis E 1990 Syntactic pattern recognition of the ECG. IEEE Transactions on Pattern Analysis and Machine Intelligence 12(7):648-57

Tompkins W J (ed) 1993 Biomedical digital signal processing. Prentice-Hall International, Englewood Cliffs, New Jersey

Webster J G (ed) 1988 Encyclopedia of medical devices and instrumentation. Wiley, New York

Webster J G (ed) 1992 Medical instrumentation Application and design, 2nd edn. Houghton Mifflin Company, Boston

ACKNOWLEDGEMENTS

The assistance of Dr Nigel Lovell in the preparation and review of parts of this chapter is gratefully acknowledged.

18

Remote access

WENDY MCPHEE

The delivery of primary health care in a rural setting is one of the most challenging and personally satisfying areas of medical practice. It is also, however, an under-serviced area and an unpopular career choice for many young medical graduates in Australia (Committee of Inquiry into Medical Education and Medical Workforce 1988, Piterman 1989). Remote access to technology is of significant concern not only to rural doctors but to all health professionals who supply health services in remote and rural Australia. Remote areas are generally serviced by Remote Area Nurses (RANs) and the Royal Flying Doctor Service. Reliable energy sources and technical backup services, both of which are of paramount importance, are often not available in remote areas. Furthermore RANs are not in an autonomous financial position to choose computer technology as a high priority in their practice. As full-time employees of governments RANs' access to the financial decision making processes and flexible leave arrangements for staff development are virtually non-existent.

The Primary Health Orientated Computer User's System (PHOCUS) is a collection of personal computers linked via telephone. It has been designed by a group of both country and metropolitan doctors in conjunction with Medical Informatics, Faculty of Medicine at Monash University. The system is intended to improve communication between general practitioners working in isolated rural or 'outback' areas and those working in often solitary urban medical centres.

This chapter will describe the background behind the PHOCUS project, the communication systems which have preceded it and the needs of the users. It also details the setting up and running of the system, its current functions and the scope for further applications in the future.

Background

Australia is a wide brown land with a green fringe. The majority of the population live in large cities along the coastline of the country. Smaller towns and farming settlements are scattered across the middle of the country in isolated rural and outback areas and often separated by hundreds of kilometres of desert. In many country areas, where the population is spread much less densely than in the cities, the general practitioner may be the only doctor in town. Such towns are often many hours away from the nearest hospital with specialist medical services.

Primary health care in a rural areas can therefore provide one of the few remaining opportunities for general medical practitioner to utilise the full range of skills acquired during undergraduate and postgraduate training. The proliferation of medical specialists in urban areas has made it increasingly difficult for city based general practitioners to practise anaesthetics, obstetrics, radiology and surgery without drawing criticism for being underqualified for the job. It is rare for urban general practitioners to even have admitting rights to public hospitals. In the country, however, the general practitioner is often the best qualified, indeed the only, doctor in the area who can perform multiple procedures. This emphasises the need for country doctors to be properly trained and well supported in their role. One of the major problems of rural medical practice is isolation. This isolation may be geographic, professional or intellectual.

Geographical isolation

The oft-quoted 'tyranny of distance' (Blainey 1966) has been an impediment to the development of Australia since the first aboriginal settlers arrived many thousands of years ago. It has been a credit to the various races of Australians that this tyranny has been reduced and often conquered in many cases. The motor car and the telephone have been two inventions with have vastly improved the ability to communicate and interact with neighbours, near and far. Rural doctors often complain that they spend an inordinate amount of time on the telephone and in their cars, incurring large expenses. Time spent travelling alone is also time away from family and patients.

Professional isolation

In many country areas the general practitioner may be the only doctor within a radius of many hundreds of kilometres. Even in towns with more than one doctor, communication between doctors may be compromised by the atmosphere of competition between what are, in effect, small businesses. Professional isolation also occurs in cities where a general practitioner may have no regular contact with other local doctors; the problem is often ameliorated for city doctors by the ease of access to other peer group resources and the occasional pharmaceutical company sponsored dinner. It is often difficult for country doctors to leave their towns to attend regional educational meetings or peer group social events. Such doctors often feel tethered to the town and this may engender feelings of resentment and eventual antipathy towards one's patients.

Intellectual isolation

Rural practitioners receive much printed material, such as medical journals and drug advertising, through the mail. It has been noted that a one way flow of information with little avenue for input can actually increase feelings of isolation. In a similar way, being the passive recipient of aid from a 'paternalistic' organisation can stifle any feelings of self-direction and motivation on the part of the recipient.

Larger country towns often have base hospitals which occasionally organise clinical meetings for doctors to hear a visiting specialist speak or discuss a current medical topic. These programs are popular and usually well attended but they tend to be sporadic and the fleeting contact with a city specialist may increase the emphasis on the country doctor's true isolation.

The advent of the facsimile machine has improved the lot of the country doctor. Many doctors use the fax to receive pathology results and send electrocardiographs to colleagues for a second opinion; however the slowness of transmission and the poor quality reproduction can be frustrating. The cost of transmitting large amounts of data over a large distance is expensive and the end product is greasy, flimsy, difficult to file and soon disintegrates. Nevertheless a telephone and fax machine do give a doctor a verbal link to millions of fellow telephone users around the world as well as the capacity to send and receive visual images of poor quality. High quality images can be summoned via the mail but a lag time of several days, at least, is unavoidable. Neither of these systems is totally adequate for the day to day needs of general practitioners.

Telecommunications and the needs of rural doctors

Telecommunication networks are not new. Most Australians have contact with one or more networks during the course of a single day whether it be while banking, telephoning or watching television. The term *networking* has been adopted into everyday usage to suggest a group of people with various skills who form a resource base for solving problems. The term implies the gaining of strength and breadth by interweaving single threads to form a more complex structure. In the situation of a computer network, the threads are usually personal computers which have been linked together to greatly increase their power and flexibility. This linkage allows communication between users and access to huge amounts of data and programs.

Similar communications networks have been developed in the past (Mason 1989, Meeks 1986) although none specifically address the needs of the rural practitioner in Australia. The advantages of such a telecommunication network to rural doctors is obvious and this has been confirmed at meetings of rural doctors around Australia where this proposal has received solid support and generated a group of keen participants.

Project establishment

A focus workshop was held with a sample group of ten country doctors each with some degree of previous experience in using a computer. This group was given the task of determining what was needed to improve the ability of rural general practitioners to communicate with their peers and with the community in general. The group decided that the ideal system would need to have these qualities:

- low initial purchase price
- enough usefulness to justify purchase
- economy of operation
- user friendliness
- speed of operation
- versatility to perform local functions.

The ten doctors then generated a list of what they would like to use on this telecommunications network. This list included electronic mail, bulletin board facilities, direct billing of the government health system, continuing medical education, access to databases of medical literature, drugs and travellers advice, generation of patient handouts, on-line pathology and radiology results, access to medical, research and computer consultants and sharing of software.

The ten doctors subsequently became the pilot group in the establishment of this Australia wide computer network for the use of primary health practitioners. The pilot phase ran for a period of four months. The users were supplied with the necessary hardware and taught how to log on to the network. Their usage of the network over the pilot period was monitored and they were involved in a continuing evaluation of the system and its facilities.

Modifications suggested by the pilot group were carried out on the system and it is now being expanded to involve 140 users. These are be the original 10 members of the pilot group plus 90 general practitioners recruited through advertisements in the medical press, by targeting doctors who have registered their interest in medical computing with the Royal Australian College of General Practitioners and by a Rural Health Support Education and Training (RHSET) grant obtained by Monash University.

Current functions

The first step of the pilot group was to establish electronic mail contact. A bulletin board facility was added. This was initially used for sharing clinical information and seeking consensus standards of management and ideas on office procedures. An electronic journal club has been established with users sharing details from interesting and relevant articles in a wide range of medical journals. Limited use of the system has been made by rural specialists who have made themselves available to discuss clinical problems in a form of electronic referral. Suggestions for the establishment of special interest groups among the users have been received.

The continuing medical education needs of the doctors has been addressed with the inclusion of computer based teaching programs on the network. Funding has been obtained to develop continuing medical education programs on therapeutics and the safe and rational prescribing of common medications. These programs will be evaluated through their use on this system.

Referral to specialists, using the system, has begun to occur. In one dramatic case, a solo doctor in a very isolated region received a quick response and advice from a paediatrician on the management of a sick child. The users have started to generate their own patient information handouts on common conditions and these are being used and refined by members of the group.

File transfer, primarily of word processing documents, has been widely utilised and the ability to transfer high quality graphic images is being developed. Doctors have also taken the opportunity to gain advice on research and medical computing by accessing the relevant experts within Monash University. At this stage, due to cost, limited use has been made of international bulletin boards and newsgroups.

The doctors are also able to use the system to assist with the commercial aspects of their general practice with access to electronic banking, electronic ordering of stock and direct billing to the government health service. It is interesting to note that the supervising group at Monash University is not acting as a central office, but rather as a systems maintenance and trouble shooting crew. This system is being developed by the users to address their own needs and Monash just acts as one of several information providers.

Future applications

The scope for future applications of this system is really only limited by the imagination and desires of the users. A register of specialists is being developed and our specialist colleagues are being encouraged to become involved in this project. The establishment of an electrocardiograph consultancy service is also being mooted. The opportunity to use this system as a gateway to other medical databases is being explored. Requested databases include poisons information, drug details and interactions and traveller's advice. The utilisation of on-line pathology and radiology reports is also being established with companies and laboratories serving rural areas.

One of the interesting, but not surprising, aspects of the project is that city based general practitioners have also shown a keen interest in getting involved. It seems that the problems of isolation are also shared by many doctors in small or solo practices and the system will be expanded to address the needs of these doctors as well.

Conclusion

With 140 users the network has become busy. The pre-pilot phase has demonstrated the areas of most interest and usefulness to the users and these areas are being developed preferentially. Further co-ordination and evaluation of the usage of the network by the supervisor is also allowing further modification and augmentation of the popular areas.

This project has been described at a number of health care gatherings around Australia and internationally and it has not only met with great enthusiasm but also with a strong desire for participation in the system by many health care workers.

Now that the project leaders have demonstrated the success of the network and identified the areas of prime interest, membership of the network is offered to all health care workers in Australia. It is believed that such potential users will not need to have any degree of computer literacy, or even computer interest, in order to derive benefit from using the ultimate system.

REFERENCES

Blainey G 1966 Tyranny of distance. Sun Books, Sydney

Committee of Inquiry into Medical Education and Medical Workforce 1988. Chairman: Doherty R. Australian Medical Education and Workforce into the 21st Century, Commonwealth of Australia

Mason S 1989 NHS family practitioner service data communications strategy. In: Barber B, Cao D, Qin D, Wagner G (eds) MEDINFO 89. Elsevier Science Publishers, Amsterdam

Meeks K B 1986 KARENET: Developing a multitiered network for rural health care delivery. In: Salamon R, Blum B, Jorgensen M (eds) MEDINFO 86. Elsevier Science Publishers, Amsterdam

Piterman L A 1989 Study of final year medical students', interns', junior resident medical officers' and senior resident medical officers' perceptions of rural training and practice in Victoria 1988. Monash University, Melbourne

19

Computerised education for health professionals

JENNIFER L HARDY, MOYA CONRICK, JOANNE FOSTER,
BILL MCGUINESS, ERICA BOSTOCK

As a result of the use of computers and information technology to support the management of health care information, it is essential that all health care professionals have a solid grounding in health informatics or information technology (IT). IT education is more than computer literacy, it also includes the concepts of information science and how it can be best used by health providers and consumers. IT education can be learnt via computer based education and it offers learning opportunities provided by no other teaching medium. Therefore, it is critical to identify, develop, implement and evaluate educationally sound computer based education programs that support and enhance education and practice. These programs must reflect educational theories and instructional design principles and be applicable to current practice.

Why is computer based education important?

Research into how students learn, the consequence of different styles of learning and the effect of instruction on the learner has lead many researchers to seek innovative solutions to education and training. Educators in many fields have, and are, exploring alternative teaching strategies to obtain prescribed learning goals and an increase in student performance outcomes. Among the educators who have recognised the need to examine alternatives to traditional teaching methods are the health professionals. These educators believe the challenges of the future in health will not be served by rigidly structured, group based education (Jacobs 1976), but rather individualised modes of instruction accommodating students of different academic background and learning styles (Conklin 1983). Some researchers believe that technology has provided such a panacea (Mouton 1990). Following technology advances and a decrease in the cost of computers, educators have begun to examine computer based approaches to education more closely (Hamby 1986, Butcher & Greenberg 1992).

Over ten years ago educators advocated instructional computing, citing the benefits of individualised, self directed learning, the inexhaustive nature of computers, the capacity of expanding students participation in the learning process, and the availability of immediate feedback (Thomas 1986). The name given to this type of instruction is known as computer aided instruction (CAI) or computer based education (CBE), and the learning process as computer assisted learning (CAL) (du'Jardin 1992). CBE was developed over twenty years ago using time sharing computers, mainframe or minicomputers. However, the disadvantages of transportability and costs of the programs prevented the spread of CBE until the availability of microcomputers (Ball et al 1988).

Emerging multimedia technologies such as video images, CD-ROM, advanced graphics, sound and animation programs and the use of the telecommunications network (Kidd et al 1992a, Procter 1991), have made available interactive media driven by computer technology (Zelmer 1992). The transfer of educational and professional knowledge can also be enhanced through other computer mediated communication technologies like bulletin boards, electronic mail, computer conferencing, online systems, imaging and Hypertext (Taylor 1992).

The principle of student interaction is a basic component in any CBE program. The types of CBE used include drill and practice, tutorials, problem solving, gaming, testing and simulation. In 1970 De Tornyay indicated the distinctive capabilities of computers for health simulations, pointing to the variety of experiences provided in a given time and the safety aspect of not practising on real patients. Students can therefore make mistakes and receive immediate feedback on the consequences of their decisions. Programs can be repeated, providing opportunity for revision and assistance in retaining information (Kidd et al 1992b).

CBE can be used by all disciplines within the health care sector. Distance education, hospital orientation, continuing education or professional development are all areas where computer technology can be used to strengthen knowledge and skills (Spector 1986, Arnold & Bauer 1988, Shehee 1989). The establishment of computer networks to provide instruction for health care providers and patients is another example of the use of CBE. This is of particular significance in rural and remote geographic areas, where health care providers are unable to be given educational leave to attend seminars and conferences (Marten & Conover 1990).

CBE, particularly in the simulation mode, offers tremendous potential for health education. Decreasing length of stay, bed closers and increasing competition for clinical places has meant the total opportunities afforded students in the clinical environment is decreasing. Computer simulation provides one avenue for students to gain insights into problems posed by real clinical practice without having to directly access clinical agencies. Computer simulation also enables students to experiment with care options. Within the clinical environment any inappropriate decisions exposes the patient to possible detrimental outcomes. Computer simulation encourages students to experiment, safe in the knowledge that no real risk exists. Equally drill and practice packages provide health educators with immediate assessment of rudimentary competencies (e.g. drug calculations) prior to clinical placement. Such tests could be provided by the computer, randomly assigning questions, with results being presented immediately to the student, and potentially, the educator at the desk.

Evaluation of any software should be seen as an integral part of the development and implementation of CBE. An awareness of the effectiveness of CBE is best obtained through the evaluation process. Evaluation includes the assessment of students learning style preferences, attitudes towards CBE, the value of CBE for individual disciplines and the recognition of skills required to develop and implement CBE (Koch et al 1990, Franco et al 1991, Billings & Cobb 1992, Byrum 1992, McCormac & Jones 1992, Ward 1992). The evaluation process is applicable to both commercially produced or self developed CBE packages. One of the first questions to ask is how educational theory has been applied in the development of the CBE package.

Applying educational theory to CBE

Techniques proposed by theory and supported by research form the foundation for effective CBE. Most techniques applied to computerised education have their foundations either in behaviourism, systems theory or cognitive educational theory.

Behaviourism

Behaviourism, Thorndike's connectionism, Pavlov's classical conditioning and Skinner's operant conditioning (Skinner 1953, Thorndike 1969) were the theoretical underpinings used by the early researchers examining the impact of CBE on behaviour. Behaviourism is based on the principle that instruction should be designed to produce observable and quantifiable behaviours and behavioural change in the learner. So when using CBE, behaviourists would expect to change the student in some obvious and measurable way. However, Pavlov's work on the 'psychic stimulus' led to the realisation that higher order conditioning was the result of building complex chains of stimuli that control behaviour. This promoted the belief that when designing educational instruction the process should be organised from the simple to complex.

Skinner's work expanded on this, and he espoused the use of reinforcers following a response or reinforcers produced by a response. He regarded the reinforcer as responsible for behavioural change. Behaviourism also uses the strategy of breaking the content into chunks (chunking), the use of frequent practice activities and provision of immediate feedback. Positive reinforcement is also used as is the practice of keeping the learner informed of progress and success in a lesson (Dreber & Caputi 1992). This theory was the design basis for many CBE packages.

Systems theory

The systems theory conceptualises the organisation and structure of a whole organism. Measurement and identification of the relationships of factors and events that affect the organism's stability is an essential component of the systems theory. The application of the systems theory in education and particularly to instructional development of CBE lies in the approach taken to design the learning activities. The systems approach consists of a series of steps that guide the developer through systems definition, systems design/development systems evaluation (Simonson & Thompson 1990).

Cognitive theory

Cognitive theory moves from behaviourist theory to the internal processes which influence learning. Cognitive psychologists focus mainly on the way in which learners receive, organise, retain and use the information. They emphasise the more complex intellectual process such as thinking, language and problem solving; these they feel are important aspects of the learning process (Snelbecker 1985) and needed for the performance of actual tasks (Montague 1988).

According to Simonson and Thompson (1990) cognitive theory has many guidelines for the development of CBE programs:

- Instruction needs something to get it started, to keep it going and to keep it from being random.
- Before learners can understand abstract experiences, they require a sufficient depth and breadth of more realistic experiences (Dale 1946).
- Sequencing instructional material is important.
- The form and pacing of reinforcement must be considered.
- Discovery learning is an important technique when using cognitive theory.

However, the three theories considered above do have some commonality in that all advocate feedback and all look at sequencing instruction. But that is where common features end. As the behaviourists consider student outcomes, the advocates of systems theory look at entire systems, while cognitive theorists centre on the learner.

CBE package design

In any educational program, planning the environment in which the learning takes place is almost as important as the content itself. In CBE the screen is the primary interface between the user and computer, producing and setting the learning environment. Four specialised areas are readily identified in CBE package design: instructional design, content specialist, graphic design and programming. Only instructional design will be considered here.

Instructional design

An instructional design model gives a framework to help designers keep on target, it serves to organise thinking and ideas, ensures the inclusion of important steps in the developmental process and ultimately helps to produce instructional products. The approach used by Romiszowski (1986) is based on systems theory and uses a four level model of instructional design applied to a framework of a five-stage problem solving process (Fig. 19.1). This provides an easy to use approach to the task.

Using CBE: expositive

Romiszowski (1988) refers to the use of computers for testing, drill and practice and programmed tutorials as a programmed or expositive use of the medium. These formats are cost effective, can be made user friendly and the content can be easily changed by adding another data base. However, they also foster a surface approach to the learning task in which students are rich with information but do not increase their knowledge or understanding.

Drill and practice

The Suppes-Atkinson computer education model, based on Skinner's theory of operant conditioning was introduced in 1963. It consisted of computer programs that presented randomly generated problems, elicited a response, provided immediate feedback and then proceeded to the next question. The model allows students to stay with the same type of problem until a level of proficiency is attained, before progressing to problems of a more difficult nature. This became known as drill and practice (Simonson & Thompson 1990).

The packages can be individualised allowing students to work at their own pace with the computer determining mastery before more complex questions are posed. The advent of intelligent computer aided instruction (ICAC) which incorporates the use of artificial intelligence has meant that the computer can also analyse mistakes and explain the problem to the student. By the early 1990s the ICAC technology was viewed as difficult, time consuming and expensive (Simonson & Thompson 1990).

The research on use of drill and practice has met with a mixed response. Limitations include the loss of motivation when the novelty is lost, lack of learner challenge and lower level learning and rote learning (Meadows 1977, Koch & Rankin 1987, Digital Equipment Corporation 1983). Whereas quality drill and practice packages can hold student attention much longer than the traditional methods (Simonson & Thompson 1990). The effectiveness in the analysis depends on the objectives set for the package and the learning approach taken.

225

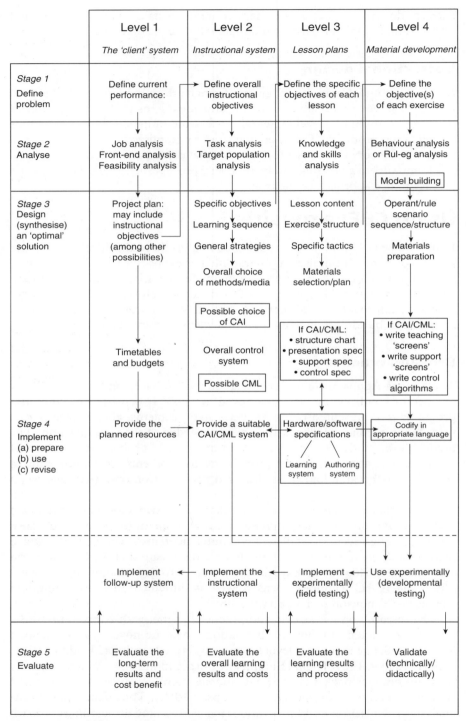

Fig. 19.1 Matrix for overall instructional design process. *Source:* Romiszowski 1986

Tutorials

Self teaching programs abound, these give a short passage of information then question the user. As with the drill and practice programs the quality is variable. Some of these programs can adjust the level of knowledge exhibited by the student and therefore give a degree of individualised teaching (Koch & Rankin 1987). Other programs are simply electronic page turners which are repetitive by nature and also become boring (Simonson & Thompson 1990). These also reward surface approaches to learning.

However, well designed tutorial programs can offer one-to-one, in–dividualised instruction which is impossible in the large classroom. The program can adjust the level of and complexity of the tutorial to suit the level of knowledge displayed by a student as the tutorial progresses. The student, by having to drive the package, becomes an active participant with some control over the rate of advancement and of their own learning. The introduction of ICAC has the potential to expand the tutorial and to take the learning from the surface approach to a greater depth.

Using CBE: adaptive

'Simulation, dialogue tutorials, and inquiry type database searches are referred to as adaptive or experiential uses of the computer in education' (Romiszowski 1988). These have encouraged an increased shift to a theoretical base in computer educational package design which will foster deeper approaches to learning.

Simulation

Simulation is described as a representation or model of an event, an object or some phenomenon. In clinical nursing terms, it refers to the verbal or pictorial description of a real-life patient care situation but, in reality it is generally an incomplete model that contains only the essential elements of what is being simulated. Nevertheless, simulation is recognised as one of the more effective methods of managing clinical teaching. Simulation encourages the student to become an active participant, to think more deeply and to become part of the educational environment (Conrick 1993).

In nursing, clinical simulations have developed around patient management problems and have been described by many writers (Dincher & Stridger 1976, Holzemer et al 1981, Holzemer et al 1986). Although most reports in the literature are subjective and anecdotal, they catalogue a variety of advantages for using simulations in teaching clinical nursing. 'A serendipitious advantage of using simulations to teach clinical nursing is that simulations tend to simultaneously teach in two or more domains, such as psychomotor and cognitive or cognitive and affective' (Hanna 1991). de Jong and Njoo (1992) also regard simulation as having much to offer and they explain three reasons for the popularity of simulations using computer technology:

1 Computers used for skills or procedures have very practical advantages; for example, being able to introduce catastrophes by means of flight simulators or laboratory experiments: reduction of stress in treating patients and cost effectiveness.

2 Simulation by means of dynamic models allows natural time scales to be altered so that processes may be sped up or slowed down to make them more visible to the learner.

3 Models from the real world can be simplified to match the prior knowledge and level of cognitive development of the learner.

There are disadvantages of simulation not the least of which is the considerable time and effort needed for design and the cost in dollar terms. There is also little evidence supporting the relationship between clinical simulation performance and the clinical setting (Henry & Holzemer 1993).

Dialogue CBE

Dialogue CBE is the 'intelligent' use of CBE in which the student may either ask or respond to questions. These programs have a common element of adaptation to the individual learner and they actually 'learn about the learner'. Because of difficult programming, time constraints and cost there are few dialogue CBE programs available.

Some dialogue packages however, are built on deep questioning techniques and multi-faceted analysis of the responses given by the student. These packages have the potential to take student learning from the surface approach to the deeper learning approaches (Conrick 1993).

Implementation of CBE

Implementation is equal in time and energy requirements as the development process and lays the groundwork for a smooth efficient transition from a developed concept to a working productive tool (Smaldone & Greenberg 1992).

Developments in computer and information technology during the late 1980s and early 1990s have enabled greater power and ease of use (Alessi & Trollip 1991). This extends to networking, multimedia and virtual reality and their application to education. Mikan (1992) states there are twelve components to the implementation process and they are:

1 Establish need
2 Organise early adopters
3 Survey and utilise local resources
4 Establish computer support groups
5 Conduct faculty development sessions
6 Determine administrative and faculty commitment and support
7 Prioritise computer applications
8 Select hardware and software
9 Plan for computer user interface

10 Provide computer support services
11 Evaluate benefits and effectiveness
12 Expand computer applications

These components form the framework of a process which is useful, flexible, relevant and applicable in establishing or enhancing computer based education.

Types and uses of tools available for use in CBE

Contemporary educators have skills in the use of blackboards, white boards, overhead projectors, slide projectors and video players. Likewise, CBE demands a rudimentary understanding and skill in the use of computer devices and the software that makes them work. Both elements fall into one of two major categories development requirements and implementation requirements. Before describing the various tools used for CBE production, it is pertinent here to examine the task at hand and to offer a few words of warning on costs.

While, it is true that some types of CBE can be produced using modest resources, the quality of the final product must be acceptable to the user. This may not be as simplistic as it sounds. It must be remembered that the users of CBE are sophisticated audiovisual consumers having spent their lifetime being exposed to broadcast quality television productions and in some cases complex computer games, so in order to engage this audience in educational tasks using a computer, similar high quality production is necessary.

This quality does not always come cheaply and may require the services of video production personnel, script writers, graphic artists and instructional designers. The initial outlay for the necessary hardware and software for development and production of CBE can also be quite high as is the time needed for development. The latter is mooted as approximately one hundred hours of production time to one hour of delivery. An alternative to in-house development is to contract a software design house but once again the costs can be very high. With these issues in mind, it can be argued that the choice to develop CBE should only be made once an exhaustive search of the available software has been found wanting.

On the positive side however, there are a number of educational institutions which have and are continuing to develop the resources necessary for CBE production. Most of these institutions are willing to negotiate the use of these resources by other individuals and institutions. This can reduce the costs of equipment and the educator's time while creating potentially fruitful networking.

Tools to develop CBE

Before beginning the foray into the tools required to develop CBE it is important to note that the specific brand names mentioned here are current at the time of press, are examples of the packages available and are not specifically recommended by the authors. The tools and packages selected will depend on the institutional needs, developers' need, personal preference and budget. These should be discussed and packages trialled before purchase.

The following is offered as a guide to requirements only and not as a panacea for CBE production.

A workstation should be equipped with:

1   A computer with substantial memory and speed capacities; able to accept sound and video cards, and peripheral devices such as scanners. This will vary depending on the nature of the package developed and the technology of the day. At the time of press, 16-20 megabyte (Mb) of RAM and hard disc capacity or 600 Mb-1 Gb is not an unreasonable request.

2   The graphic software comes in one of two major groups; image creation or image editing. The first group facilitates the creation of images by providing drawing and painting tools (e.g. Adobe Illustrator, Corel Draw, Aldus Freehand). Drawing packages allow the user to add text and draw a variety of shapes (e.g. squares, circles, polygons and curves). Once the image has been created individual objects within the image can be manipulated (e.g. changing position, size or shape). Painting packages provide similar features as drawing packages but include tools that simulate painting and the ability to edit individual pixels. This enables minor changes to be made to the shading or lines of an image. The second group of graphic software, image editor, (e.g. Adobe Photoshop) enables these images to be manipulated. Still images can be captured by scanning photographs or line drawings, or direct from video tape, or disc, via video capture cards. Changes can be made to colour hues, brightness, or size of the image. These packages also enable visual effects to be added to the image. 'Filters' provide a variety of visual effects such as blurring, sunglare, diffusion, solarisation, or sharpening. A number of image editing software programs allow editing of video motion (e.g. Adobe Premiere, Video for Windows). Small clips of video can be captured then edited into one sequence of video display much the same as video productions are edited. It should be noted here that video motion requires large amounts of memory storage and are therefore limited to short clips (15 seconds up to 2 or 3 minutes).

3   Animation software, as the name suggests, enables a number of images to be integrated into an animation sequence (e.g. Macro Mind Director). This is particularly useful for health education. Simulating physiology, demonstrating procedures, or describing the function of equipment can all be enhanced with animation.

4   A colour scanner enables images to be stored digitally for use in the production. They are available as both black and white or colour and in a range of sizes from hand held devices to A3 size models. Slide scanners are also available. However before beginning scanning check copyright issues. To some extent scanners are being superseded by digital cameras or photo CD. These devices allow images to be captured as digital images direct circumventing the need to scan them in.

5   Colour and movement are enhanced by the inclusion of sound in multi media productions. Sound recording devices and software that facilitates the manipulation of the sound are therefore essential inclusions in any development work station (e.g. Sound Wave). Sound recorders provide the interface between the sound and the computer. They may be as simple as a microphone or as sophisticated as a sound studio. Audio editing software allows alteration to pitch and tone, as well as joining a number of sounds into one sequence. The sound is usually represented graphically on screen to facilitate subtle editing.

6   Authoring software facilitates the development of resources for CBE and provides the means of combining these resources into an educational package (e.g. Authorware Professional, Tool Book, Macro Mind Director, Hypercard). Screens can be designed, interactions with the user created, and navigational attributes developed in the authoring environment. Some authoring systems enable a 'run time' to be attached to the final version or provide a 'player' that can be distributed with the final version. Both enable the user to access the educational package without having a copy of the authoring software that developed it.

Authoring systems reduce the programming skills needed to develop and educational package. The author simply directs the computer, (e.g. put text here, link this button to this screen) and the software performs the necessary programming to create the package. While authoring systems are capable of performing many detailed tasks and can be used by the novice to produce basic packages, to achieve more complex interactions requires advanced understanding of the package's capabilities. In some cases it may be advisable to have some understanding of basic computer programming and/or access to a programmer.

Resources additional to the work station would include:

1   Video production facilities. A multi-media production will require some video motion. This will need to be scripted, shot, edited, and compressed before integration into the computer package.

2   Facilities to master a laser or compact disc. Computer packages that include still and motion graphics plus sound require a large storage capacity. Large hard disks are one option (600 Mb to 1 Gb) but increasingly optical storage devices such as laser or compact discs are being used. Commercial companies will press, or master, final versions of a package to both media.

Delivery needs

When selecting delivery hardware the rule of thumb is to buy the fastest machine the budget will support and ensure that it is equipped for multi media packages. The latter will include sound and video cards, facilities to accept an internal or external CD player, and stereo speakers. Monitors should be colour and as large as the budget will support. The larger the screen the more features/ options that can be included in each screen. Attached to each machine should be a CD or laser disc player, amplified speakers or two sets of quality head phones. The CD player should be multi session and triple speed. These need not be included in the original purchase but the option to add to the basic machine should be available.

The number of machines, their location and laboratory configurations will depend on the intended use, number of students and budget. Laboratories can be arranged with the computers in rows or around the walls. Rows enable more machines to be placed in the same area while the wall configuration allows the teacher to visualise the computer screens. When performing 'follow along' teaching this is useful to ensure all students are keeping up.

Ergonomics also needs to be considered. Appropriate work station desks, seating, lighting that does not reflect on the monitor screens, and security for the hardware need to be considered and incorporated into the budget. The budget should also cover maintenance and replacement of the equipment. Accidental damage and the inevitable updating of equipment and software is a reality for any institution involved in the ongoing development of CBE.

Evaluation of CBE

The increasing use of computer and information technology in health care is creating a greater demand on educators to utilise the technology in education. Evaluation is the critical step in the process to ensure high quality computer based education.

Effective evaluation incorporates evaluating the development tool, content, lesson, delivery systems and learning outcomes. Theoretical aspects of cognitive psychology can guide the process of evaluation and design of computer based education. There are eight major aspects which can be applied and these are summarised below:

1 Perception and attention

Effective computer based education is dependent on presentations that are designed for easy and accurate perception. For perception to occur student attention must be gained and maintained. This can be affected by factors such as past experience, level of student involvement, personal interests, difficulty of lessons, novelty format, timing and variety.

2 Memory

Efficient storage and retrieval of information is a critical element.

3 Comprehension

Information must be perceived, interpreted and integrated into current knowledge not just stored and retrieved.

4 Active learning

Learning is achieved by observing and by doing.

5 Motivation

Motivation is critical to learning.

6 Locus of control

Refers to whether the control of the content, methodology and any other instructional factors are determined by the teacher via the lesson, student or a combination. The success of the lesson depends on which aspects are controlled by the student and which aspects are controlled by the teacher via the lesson.

7 Transfer of learning

This refers to the extent to which student performance has improved from the lesson and the application to real situations. Transfer of learning is the critical outcome of computer based education.

8 Individual differences

Students do not all learn alike and therefore some methods of instruction are better for some students than for others. One advantage of computer based education is that instruction can be individualised by utilising appropriate methodologies and lessons (Alessi & Trollip 1991).

Evaluation of the lesson incorporates the above aspects but has three distinct phases and these are:

Quality review

- Language and grammar
- Surface features of the displays (e.g. displays, presentation, text quality, input devices)
- Questions and menus
- Other issues of pedagogy (motivation, locus of control, interactivity, animation and graphics)
- Invisible functions of the lesson (records and data, security, accessibility)
- Subject matter
- Off-line materials (manuals, auxiliary materials, other resources)

Pilot testing

Pilot testing is a process of testing the lesson by utilising representatives of the target population for use. It has seven steps:

1 Select the helpers
2 Explanation of the procedure
3 Find out how much of the content they already know
4 Observe them go through the lesson
5 Interview them afterward
6 Assess their learning
7 Revise the lesson

Validation

This phase is the process for checking of the lesson for authenticity in real situations. It is sometimes referred to as field testing. There are two reasons for this process. Firstly, the real situation for the lesson can be quite different from the pilot test. Secondly, the helpers utilised in the pilot testing may not have covered all ranges of abilities from the target population (Alessi & Trollip 1991).

This process of evaluation is summative, very comprehensive and can be adapted to suit many varied situations in health care education. There are many guidelines and checklists available in the literature but individuals can develop specific tools to meet specific needs (Alessi & Trollip 1991, Smaldone & Greenberg 1992, Discenza 1993, Posel 1993).

Evaluation is probably the most important step in the process of computer based education as it ensures successful effective outcomes of the development process. It is critical to apply and evaluate the theoretical underpinings of cognitive psychology, teaching and learning, computer and information technology and instructional design to computer based education. This brief summary of the process of evaluation will give the reader some basic guidelines. The area of evaluation of computer based education in health care is limited and is an area that must be expanded to ensure high quality educational outcomes and ultimately patient care.

The reader may contact the authors for details about specific educational packages developed in Australia.

Glossary

Courseware	the actual materials that students use.
Hypercard	an authoring tool for the Macintosh computer
Hypermedia	links between different types of media, e.g. sound, graphics and text
Hypertext	words linked by key words, e.g. from text on a screen, click on a word which will then be linked to a variety of interrelating functions.
Interactivity	the relationship between the stimulus of the presentation, and the response of the user. There are five levels of interactivity which reflect the success of interactive projects. Level 1 (passive) is a forward-backward, predetermined and linear

sequenced instruction; level 2 (hierarchal) is a predefined set of options, much like a menu; level 3 (update) relates to computer generated problems and update and feedback on user responses; level 4 (construct) is an extension on update interactivity, where the learner has to manipulate components to reach a goal; level 5 (simulation) provides the learner with more control over the instructional sequences.

Multimedia   any combination of two or more different types of media, usually made interactive through computer controlled technology.

REFERENCES

Alessi S, Trollip S 1991 Computer based instruction: methods and development, 2nd edn. Prentice Hall, New Jersey

Arnold J M, Bauer C A 1988 Meeting the needs of the computer age in continuing education. Computers in Nursing 6(2):66-69

Ball M J, Hannah K J, Gerdin Jelger U, Peterson H (eds) 1988 Nursing informatics, where caring and technology meet. Springer-Verlag, New York

Billings D M, Cobb K L 1992 Effects of learning style preferences, attitudes and GPA on learner achievement using computer assisted interactive videodisc instruction. Journal of Computer-Based Instruction 19(1):12-16

Butcher P G, Greenberg J M 1992 Educational computing at the open university: the second decade. Education and Computing 8:201-215

Byrum D C 1992 Formative evaluation of computer courseware: an experimental comparison of two methods. Journal of Educational Computing Research 8(1):69-80

Conklin D N 1983 A study of computer assisted instruction in nursing education. Journal of Computer Based Instruction 9(3):98-107

Conrick M 1993 The development of computer based learning courseware for teaching clinical decision making in nursing. Unpublished Major Project. University of New South Wales

Dale E 1946 Audio-visual methods in teaching. Dryden Press, New York

De Tornyay R 1970 Instructional technology and nursing education. Journal of Nursing Education 6 3 8 34-35

de Jong T, Njoo M 1992 Exploratory learning processes. In: De Corte E, Linn M, Mandl H, Verschaffel L (eds) Computer based learning environments and problem solving. Springer-Verlag, Berlin

Dincher J, Stridger S 1976 Evaluation of a written simulation format for clinical nursing judgement; a pilot study. Nursing Research 25:250-285

Discenza D 1993 A systematic approach to selecting and evaluating instructional materials. Journal of Nursing Staff Development 9(4):196-198

Dreber M, Caputi L 1992 The integration of theoretical constructs into the design of computer assisted instruction. Computers in Nursing September/October: 219-224

Digital Equipment Corporation 1983 Introduction to computer-based education. The Corporation, Marlborough

du'Jardin R 1992 Computers in nursing education. Informatics in Healthcare Australia 1:(3):29-33

Franco A, King J D, Farr F L, Clark J S, Hag P J 1991 An assessment of the radiological module of NEONATE as an aid in interpreting chest X-ray findings by radiologists. Journal of Medical Systems 15(4):277-287

Hamby C S 1986 A study of the effects of computer assisted instruction on the attitude and achievement of vocational nursing students. Computers in Nursing 4(3):109-113

Hanna D 1991 Using simulations to teach clinical nursing. Nurse Educator 16(2):28-31

Henry S, Holzemer W 1993 The relationship between performance on computer-based clinical simulations and two written methods of evaluation: cognitive examination and self-evaluation of expertise. Computers in Nursing 11(1):29-34

Holzemer W, Schleutermann J, Farrand L, Miller A 1981 A validation study: simulations as a measure of nurse practitioners' problem solving skills. Nursing Research 30:139-144

Holzemer W, Reskin B, Slichter M 1986 Criterion-related validity of a clinical simulation. Journal of Nursing Education 25:286-290

Jacobs R M (ed) 1976 A flexible design for health professions education. John Wiley & Sons, New York

Kidd M R, Cesnik B, Connolly G, Carbon N E 1992a Computer-assisted learning in medical education. The Medical Journal of Australia 156:780-782

Kidd M R, Hatchings G A, Hall W, Cesnik B 1992b Applying hypermedia to medical education: an author's perspective. Educational and Training Technology International 29(2):143-151

Koch E W, Rankin J A, Stewart R 1990 Nursing students' preferences in the use of computer assisted learning. Journal of Nursing Education 29(3):122-126

Koch B, Rankin J 1987 Computers and their applications in nursing. Harper & Row, London

Marten Y, Conover K P 1990 Automated continuing education and patient education. Computers in Nursing 8(4):144-149

Meadows L 1977 Nursing education in crisis: a computer alternative. Journal of Nurse Education 16:13-21

Mikan K 1992 Implementation process for computer supported education. In: Arnold J, Pearson G (eds) Computer applications in nursing education and practice. National League for Nursing, New York

McCormac K, Jones B T 1992 The content and the context of Nursing CAL: an evaluation of the use of computerised nursing knowledge. In: Lun K C, Degoulet P, Piemme T E, Rienhoff O (eds) MEDINFO 92. Elsevier Science Publishers, Amsterdam

Montague W 1988 Promoting cognitive processing and learning by designing the learning environment. In: Jonassen (ed) Instructional design for microcomputer courseware. Lawrence-Erbaum, New Jersey

Mouton H 1990 Some thoughts about computers in training and instructional design. In: McDougall A, Dowling C (eds) Computers in education. Elsevier Science Publishers, Amsterdam

Posel N 1993 Guidelines for the evaluation of instructional software by hospital nursing departments. Computers in Nursing 11(6):273-276

Procter P M 1991 Using telecommunications to teach information technology. Nursing Educators Microworld 5(5):34

Romiszowski A 1986 Designing auto-instructional material. Kegan Paul, London

Romiszowski A 1988 The selection and use of instructional media, 2nd edn. Kegan Paul, London

Shehee A 1989 Extensive use of CAI for hospital orientation and continuing education. Nursing Educators Microworld 2(6):44

Simonson M, Thompson A 1990 Educational computing foundations. Macmillan, New York

Skinner B 1953 Science of human behaviour. McMillan, New York

Smaldone A, Greenberg C 1992 Nursing software: develop your own. In: Arnold J, Pearson G (eds) Computer applications in nursing education and practice. National League for Nursing, New York

Snelbecker B 1985 Learning theory, instructional theory and psycho-educational design. University Press of America, Lanham

Spector A F 1986 Continuing nursing education in computer technology. Journal of Continuing Education in Nursing 17(4):134-135

Taylor A 1992 The impact of electronic publishing on nursing education. In: Lun K C, Degoulet P, Piemme T E, Rienhoff O (eds) MEDINFO 92. Elsevier Science Publishers, Amsterdam

Thomas B S 1986 Instructional computing in American nursing programs. International Journal of Nursing Studies 23(3):221-229

Thorndike E 1969 Educational psychology. Arno Press, New York

Ward R 1992 Interactive video: an analysis of its value to nurse education. Nurse Education Today 12:464-470

Zelmer L C A 1992 A multimedia primer. Informatics in Healthcare Australia 1(2):31-39

20

Computerised education for consumers

ROHAN JAYASURIYA, MARK HARRIS, GURPAL K SANDHU

Prevention involves action to reduce occurrence of disease or disability, or action to minimise the damage that may result from it. There has been an increasing prevalence of chronic disease such as cardiovascular disease, cancer and mental illness which is associated with behaviour and lifestyle. At the same time, due to the increasing cost of institutional health care and medical interventions, patients and their families are being encouraged to use self care and services are being provided to support this outside hospitals.

Many activities related to patient education have traditionally been carried out in institutional settings (i.e. hospitals and clinics) and using mass media approaches (i.e. posters, radio and television). The current trend is to target the message and activity to the individual and at their home. The emergence of information technology as an accepted part of the lifestyle of society has paved the path towards this goal.

Patient education

With the chronic nature of many health problems today, educating patients about their condition and management is becoming an essential aspect of their management. Education has been shown to influence the degree of patient involvement in their own care (Hansen 1990). This is desirable in itself but it is also associated with improved health outcomes as a result of behaviour change or compliance with therapy (Greenfield et al 1985). This is especially important in the elderly who are likely to suffer from multiple chronic diseases, be on multiple medications and who may also suffer impaired cognition.

Opportunities for patient education exist throughout the health system. Most hospitals in Australia conduct some patient education programs. These programs cover chronic health problems such as diabetes, cancer and heart diseases. Community health services are another important venue for patient education especially in aged, diabetes and palliative care, mental and early child health.

General practice is an important setting for patient education. Over 86% of the population consult with a general practitioner (GP) at least once a year (Australian Bureau of Statistics 1991). GPs perceive themselves and are perceived by patients to be an appropriate source of health education and information (Ford & Ford 1983). Patients not only expect to hear health promotion messages, but they welcome them and change their behaviour as a result (Sullivan 1988). Counselling or advice was given in about 25% of encounters with general practitioners in Australia in 1990 (Bridges Webb et al 1992). This was especially common in consultations with the 15-44 year age group and much of this advice concerned treatment. One study identified opportunities for problems-related patient education in a quarter of all consultations but only a small proportion of these were taken up by GPs (Boulton & Williams 1983).

Written materials and methods

Lack of health worker time is perceived to be a major constraint on patient education. In general practice lack of time and remuneration are major barriers to health promotion. Other identified barriers include patient acceptance and compliance, lack of resources and special skills in health promotion and education (Bauman et al 1989, Wilson et al 1992).

Patients also frequently fail to understand information given to them and may forget the information even when it was understood at the time. These factors diminish patient satisfaction which in turn diminishes compliance with advice or management as a whole (Ley 1985).

Written information may compensate for the lack of time in the consultation by providing information in addition to that given verbally. It also acts to reinforce the message and provide a record of the information given both for the patient and their family to review later and increases satisfaction with care (Laher et al 1981, George et al 1983). Printed materials can also serve to document that informed consent procedures were followed and that follow up instructions were given (Carr 1989).

Written patient education materials also vary widely in their readability with many requiring reading ages at least five years higher than the average patient (Davis et al 1990, Glanz & Rudd 1990, Bradly et al 1994). Most word processing packages now include readability and reading age scores and can be readily applied to patient education materials. Guidelines suggested (Kitching 1990, Albert & Chadwick 1992) for written patient education materials are as follows:

- Reading age of 8–9 years
- Avoid jargon and 'unless'. Use short concrete rather than abstract words and avoid too many participle phrases.

- Use headings and subheadings or questions as prompts for text.
- Short sentences, active rather than passive
- Positive rather than negative messages
- Order of mention the same as the sequence of actions or events followed by the patient
- Instuctions specific rather than general
- Personal style and personalised message
- Avoid unnecessary capitals.

The use of illustrations improves the readability of health education materials (Michielette et al 1992). Simple labelled line drawings have been demonstrated to be more useful than coloured, complex pictures or cartoons especially among high risk populations (Doak et al 1985).

Written materials should be customised to the consultation, the health worker and the patient so that they are relevant and all concerned have a greater sense of ownership (Richards 1991). They should also be regularly updated and need to be translated into the language which the patient and their family most readily understands. All this may create problems with storage and ease of access to the materials in a busy practice or service.

Computerised patient education materials

Computerising patient education materials offers a solution to the problem of storage although leaflets with graphic images may be relatively memory intensive. It also may allow the materials to be adapted by the health worker both to their own practice (e.g. putting practice details on the leaflets) and to the individual patient (providing advice for specific problems of patients at the time of the encounter) (Kahn 1993).

Some computerised patient education materials have been designed to be accessed during the consultation acting as an aid and prompt to verbal education and providing a record of advice given (Harris et al 1993). Characteristics of such material are:

- Easy to use requiring few keyboard or computer skills
- Specific information of relevance to one situation or problem; not confusing the patient with information not relevant to them
- Able to be adapted to the health worker, patient and the encounter
- Provide accurate and reliable information (where possible validated by appropiate authorities).
- Available in a number of languages
- Provide a record of use for each patient
- Follow guidelines for all written materials
- Compatible with databases, record systems, operating systems, modems and printers.

Efficacy and effectiveness of computerised patient education

Computerised patient education materials have been demonstrated to improve comprehension and follow up especially where combined with face to face education (Sumner III 1990).

Patient education programs run in institutions require the patient to come back to the facility, and require staff time to repeat the same message to a number of groups. A project in Aberdeen for asthmatics addressed this issue by using a computer based system to generate personalised health education booklets. A computer system was used to merge patient risk factors with relevant blocks of information on prevention. In addition answers to questions made to the consultant were included in the quarterly booklet. Assessment of the project showed that the patients given the computerised booklets had fewer hospital admissions and sleep disturbance due to asthma (Osman et al 1994). The results suggest that the booklets made patients aware of warning signs and reinforced advice and management instructions for controlling symptoms.

The main obstacle to the wide spread use of computerised patient education materials is the fact that few primary health workers have computers available for use during consultations. Another obstacle is unfamiliarity with computers and keyboards by health workers, especially general practitioners. This may be overcome by more user friendly programs and pen based computers. Training is also of great importance and is an important task for academic departments, the college based training programs, divisions of general practice and other professional organisations.

There are a number of computer patient education systems designed to give information independent of the health worker. These involve patients accessing information with the use of a keyboard or touch screen technology (Mitchell 1993). Some studies have shown that these have the acceptability of face to face education while providing the recall comparable with written format leaflets (Deardoff 1986). In particular such systems may allow the patient time to ask questions which they were unable or unwilling to ask during consultations (Roter 1977) or are intimate and embarrassing to ask from a care provider. There have also been suggestions that such systems may be used as a supplement to face to face education.

Health risk appraisal

Health goals and targets in many countries also have included proposals for preventing death and disability due to major illnesses by reducing the prevalence of health risk factors (Health Targets Implementation Committee 1988). Current interests in preventive actions have created a corresponding interest in development of strategies and techniques to foster personal health behaviour change. Thus, health risk appraisal (HRA) programs were developed. These personal risk assessment programs are used to convey the impact on mortality and morbidity risks of clients' personal characteristics, family history and health related behaviours. HRA is used as a framework for client education about determinants of health and for motivating them to modify the behaviour to reduce health risks and adopt healthy lifestyles (Schoenbach et al 1993).

Health risk appraisal instruments developed as a prospective medicine practice tool were popularised by Robbins and Hall in 1970, initially to prevent cancer by identification and reduction of cancer precursors at an early stage of disease process and prevent progression. Computerised health risk appraisal has been used in the USA and Canada since the mid 1970s and a number of studies have been conducted for its efficacy and effectiveness (Schoenbach et al 1993).

Risk factor intervention strategy at an individual level has been viewed as a reflection of the 'medical model'. On the other hand, directing efforts for risk factor reduction by accumulating information on a computer database and implementing a preventive intervention for risk factor reduction at a total community (e.g. mass screening for cardiovascular risk factors, a North Coast experience in NSW) has received special attention by broadening the community approach to stimulate change (Lefebvre et al 1988, Van Beurden et al 1993).

The traditional model of HRA uses mortality data of major causes of death to estimate a person's risk of death/disease based on person's current profile of age, sex and risk factors in the next ten years. Developers of the instrument used United States epidemiological data for calculation of average risk which have been replaced by Australian mortality data to develop an Australian version by the Shephard Foundation (Larsen 1987). HRA provides in–dividualised risk assessment based on:

- major causes of death for people of the same age and sex category
- the health related behaviours and personal characteristics of that individual as recognised precursors for specified diseases
- risk factors for that person in order of importance
- the estimated risk of death in the next ten years and an average risk for that person (appraised risk) and the risk level of that individual after reduction of specific risk factors for that person (achievable risk) adjusting for the effects of changes in health (Ruth 1985).

However, it is not always possible to reduce the risk factors such as those contributed by family history and environmental factors over which an individual has no control, except for its raising awareness and potential for early detection and possible treatment. Therefore achievable risk can become a source of frustration in some clients. Advocates of socio-environmental factors impact upon health, consider this approach to be 'victim-blaming'.

243

Computerised health risk appraisal

During the last two decades, the growing use of HRA instruments has been facilitated by expanding the initial model and include lifestyle inventory and fitness evaluation for example. An Australian microcomputer based program developed by the Shepherd Foundation included positive aspects of good health such as high cardiovascular reserve, stress handling ability, abstinence from tobacco, alcohol and drugs, nutritional awareness, personal life goals and prevention of common chronic disease (Larsen 1987).

Since their early development stage, most HRA instruments have expanded the range of applications while continuous refining and extending of technological aspects of the measurements goes on. More recently, the educational component particularly for uni-focus instruments such as alcohol, drugs and AIDS/STD risk appraisal is accompanied by correct information provided with effective and interesting visual computer techniques. The range of applications in current programs available include:

- comprehensive health assessment
- a personalised computer report of positive health aspects and those needing improvement
- interactive lifestyle appraisal
- identification of areas for counselling
- accumulated data on groups for population based studies.

Efficacy and effectiveness of HRA instruments

The major questions to assess the efficacy and potential effectiveness of HRA instruments that may be considered are:

- How accurately does the instrument assess the individual's risk factors?
- How effective is the instrument in motivating behaviour change?

Some of the guidelines have been developed through research to assess the HRA instruments. The guidelines may be considered for future research or when selecting a HRA instrument for a program (Beerby et al 1988).

The assessment of a HRA tool should gauge the interest and participation of clients, the effectiveness in communicating the relationship between lifestyle and health risk, and the information on risk behaviour (Seydel et al 1990). Other criteria include its ability to develop a database and provide an index for health risk and health related behaviours.

While the efficacy of HRA instruments has been challenged (Smith et al 1987), many proponents of HRA have fostered unrealistic expectations about the role of HRA in effecting behavioural change. It has been indicated to be a priority as a motivational tool to stimulate such change (Beerby et al 1988), which need to be tested in future research. When used along with counselling, HRA can serve as a fulcrum upon which users of the instrument can balance both the health assessment and behaviour change efforts in a health promotion program. Computer assisted instruments of risk appraisal are low in cost and easily accessiblity to the participants, are personalised and assist the health promotion practitioner in processing essential information quickly to enable effective counselling.

Consumer education

In recent times consumers are more vocal towards their rights to be involved in decisions that affect their health. Types of information required by consumers relate to the acuity and stage of the condition. For acute conditions this information is mostly on action they need to take to obtain medical services, while for chronic conditions more information is needed as usually there is more than one problem and increasingly the patient has to be empowered to direct their own care. In some cases patients require information on the alternative choices available for treatment (e.g. breast cancer) and their implications on their future life style. Such information is necessary to ensure that informed consent is given.

Typically most of this information is provided to patients during consultations with their practitioner. A vast amount of information needs to be transferred to a patient who may not be in the most receptive state during a consultation. Patients also need time to reflect on this new information before taking decisions. There is also evidence that the lack of time has led to only a fraction of the opportunities for health education being used by GPs (Boulton 1983).

On the other hand some consumers who require information that concerns their health have been reticence in asking their doctor and have had to depend on sources such as newspaper agony columns, help lines and phone-ins (Grunder & Garrett 1986). This leads to the postponement of what is usually a preventive action until it becomes an issue that needs a visit to the doctor. Socially underprivileged groups may be most disadvantaged, especially in countries where health is not provided under social welfare.

A project that illustrates many of these concepts is based in Cambridge, Massachusetts. The Harvard Community Health Plan, an HMO type of health service which envisages that over 5000 of their clients will have a home terminal connected to the health centres. In a pilot study of 150 households, consumers received medical advice and general health information from the centre via a modem. The computer collects symptoms directly from the patient using an interactive protocol and generates advice, either recommending home treatment or to make an appointment. The information provided by the client is also channelled to alert staff to contact the home if there is a possibility of serious illness (Bergman 1993, Winslow 1992).

The advantages of this system are that it allows consumers to access the centre without delay, the patient's information is captured in the centre's electronic medical record and in a high percentage (30%) of times a visit is not required thus saving time and money for both the consumer and the Health

Plan. In addition the system allows consumers access to a computer library to research over 250 relevant topics.

A similar concept of home terminals have been used in Minneapolis for patients diagnosed with cancer. This computer connection allows the patients to sieve information on options for treatment and prepare questions when they next visit the consultant (Gustafson 1992).

A public computer network is utilised in Cleveland to allow home-bound individuals to reach peers and professionals. Two ComputerLinks (sets of specialised programs and utilities residing in the network) were provided, one for persons living with AIDS and the other for caregivers of persons with Alzheimer's disease (Brennan 1994).

In the eastern suburbs of Sydney a disability information and referral center has developed a computerised database that assists disabled persons (and service providers) to find services they need. This database has also enabled proxy measures of community needs for planning and indicators of consumer expectations and satisfaction to be ascertained (Ousman 1994).

Efficacy and effectiveness of consumer education

The main benefits of IT for consumer education are due to its ability to store large amounts of data (Bergman 1993) to allow manipulation by the user and to address specific concerns (Tongue & Stanley 1991). In addition information is accessible to consumers without restrictions in time. Advances in telecommunication has made it possible for consumers to access information from their home and networking has allowed the exchange of information among consumers (Milio 1992).

Computers are being used as repositories of community information. In Mersey Regional Health Authority access to health education material in computers in patient waiting areas is used to monitor health concerns and determine health education needs for populations (Tongue & Stanley 1991).

The ComputerLinks in Cleveland were evaluated through randomised field experiments. This showed that it lead to improved confidence in decision making and facillitated the participation of clients in the health care delivery process (Brennan 1994).

Future developments

Major advances in IT may have a considerable impact on computerised education for preventive action in the future. The main areas where potential is seen are advances in:

- telecommunication technology
- data storage technology
- artificial intelligence
- use of multimedia.

Advances in telecommunications would provide the backbone for carriage of digitalised information from consumers to central health units or providers. Networking capabilities would enable consumers requests to be transferred to the appropriate node. Consumers would benefit from computer conferencing between providers and from access to large databases that would suit their information needs. In a similar manner to the Educational Technology Network (ET net) where the US National Library of Medicine offers access to health professionals, a number of disease/disability specialty libraries could be made available for special groups of consumers. Consumer managed bulletin boards would enable them to exchange information including their experiences. Some of these have already been realised. On the other hand when such massive overload of information is easily accessible to consumers, protocols need to be developed to guide consumers in using them efficiently.

The advances in data storage including optic disk technology would enable not only alphanumeric information but high quality graphics to be available for patient education and consumer education. Increasingly, computer games are developing the capability of providing children with visually appealing messages. A project utilised this concept even before such quality software was available to teach children how to manage their asthma by using a computer game called Asthma Command (Rubin et al 1986).

Developments in artificial intelligence, especially in expert systems and neural networks also have potential for preventive health. Typically they have been used to provide non-experts with the knowledge of experts in decision making. A great advantage expert systems possess is their ability to feed back the reasons (decision rules) and assumptions used. Consumers can be provided this information to verify whether these assumptions are correct for decisions taken regarding their treatment choices. Such systems therefore have the potential to empower the consumer in decisions regarding their health. The acceptance of such systems is slow and limited with less working artificial intelligence systems in use than might be expected.

REFERENCES

Albert T, Chadwick S 1992 How readable are practice leaflets? British Medical Journal 305:1266-1268

Australian Bureau of Statistics 1991 National health survey 1989-90. ABS, Canberra

Bauman A, Mant A, Middleton L, Mackertich M, Jane E 1989 Do general practitioners promote health? A needs assessment. Medical Journal of Australia 151:262-269

Beerby W, Schoenbach V, Wagner E 1988 Health risk appraisal: methods and programs NCHR. DHHS Publications No (PHS) 86-3396

Bergman R 1993 Computers make 'house calls' to patients. Hospitals 5:52

Boulton M G, Williams A 1983 Health education in the general practice consultation: doctors' advice on diet, alcohol and smoking. Health Education Journal 42(2):57-63

Bradly B, Singleton M, Li Wan Po A 1994 Readability of patient information leaflets on over-the-counter (OTC) medicines. Journal of Clinical Pharmacy and Therapeutics 19:7-15

Brennan P 1994 Community health information networks: reaching the client directly. In: Carter B, Walker D (eds) HIC'94: Proceedings of the Second National Health Informatics Conference. HISA, Melbourne, 1-3

Bridges Webb C, Britt H, Miles D, Neary S, Charles J, Traynor V 1992 Morbidity and treatment in general practice in Australia 1990-91. Medical Journal of Australia 157: special supplement

Carr M J 1989 Patient education. Dimensions of Critical Care Nursing 8(4):258-259

Davis T C, Crouch M A, Willis G, Miller S, Abdehou D M 1990 The gap between patient reading comprehension and the readability of patient education materials. Journal of Family Practice 31:533-538

Deardoff W W 1986 Computerised health education: a comparison with traditional formats. Health Education Quarterly 13(1):61-72

Doak C, Doak L, Root J 1985 Teaching patients with low literacy skills. J B Lipincott, Philadelphia

Ford A S, Ford W S 1983 Health education and the primary care physician. The practitioners perspective. Social Science and Medicine 17(20):1505-1512

George C F, Waters W E, Nicholas T A 1983 Prescription information leaflets: a pilot study in general practice. British Medical Journal 287: 193-1196

Glanz K, Rudd J 1990 Readability and content analysis of print cholesterol education materials. Patient Education and Counselling 16:109-118

Greenfield S, Kaplan S, Ware J E 1985 Expanding patient involvement in care: effects on patient outcomes. Annals of Internal Medicine 102:520-528

Grunder T H, Garrett R E 1986 Interactive medical telecomputing: an alternative approach to community health education. New England Journal of Medicine 314:982-985

Gustafson S 1992 Personal communication

Hansen B W L 1990 A randomised controlled trial on the effect of an information booklet for young families in Denmark. Patient Education and Counselling 16:147-150

Harris M, Zakinthinos P, Celler B 1993 Computerised patient education for general practice. Presentation to 1993 HIANSW Conference

Health Targets Implementation (Health for All) Committee to Australian Health Ministers 1988 Health for All Australians. AGPS, Canberra

Kahn G 1993 Computer-generated patient handouts. MD Computing 10(3):157-164

Kitching J B 1990 Patient information leaflets: the state of the art. Journal of the Royal Society of Medicine 83:298-300

Laher M, O'Malley K, O'Brien E, et al 1981 Educational value of printed information for patients with hypertension. British Medical Journal 282:1360-1361

Larsen L 1987 Computer programs for health promotion projects. The Journal of Occupational Health and Safety–Australia and New Zealand 3(1):75-77

Lefebvre C, Lasater T, Assaf A, Carleton R 1988 Pawtucket heart health program: the process of stimulating community change. Scandinavian Journal of Primary Health Care (Supplement) 1:31-37

Ley P 1985 Doctor-patient communication: some quantitative estimates of the role of cognitive factors in non compliances. Journal of Hypertension 3(Suppl 1):51-55

Michielette R, Bahnson J, Dignam M B, Shroeder E D 1992 The use of illustrations and narrative text style to improve readability of a health education brochure. Journal of Cancer Education 7(3):251-260

Milio N 1992 New tools for community involvement in health. Health Promotion International 7(3): 209-212

Mitchell D 1993 Point of contact. Nursing Times 89(48):66-67

Osman L M, Abdalla M I, Beattie J A G et al 1994 Reducing hospital admission through computer supported education for asthma patients. British Medical Journal 308:568-571

Ousman R 1994 Personal communication

Richards R N 1991 Preparation and mechanics of patient instruction sheets. Seminars in Dermatology 10(2):96-97

Robbins L and Hall J 1970 How to practice prospective medicine. Methodist Hospital of Indiana, Indianapolis

Roter D 1977 Patient participation in the patient-provider interaction: the effects of patient question asking on the quality of interaction, satisfaction and compliance. Health Education Monographs 5:281-315

Rubin D H, Leventhal J M, Sadock R T et al 1986 Educational intervention by computers in childhood asthma: a randomised clinical trial testing the use of a new teaching intervention in childhood asthma. Paediatrics 77(1):1-10

Ruth D 1985 A review of health risk assessment (unpublished)

Schoenbach V, Wagner E, Karon J 1993 The use of epidemiologic data for personal risk assessment in health hazard/health risk appraisal program. Journal of Chronic Diseases 36(9):625-638

Seydel E, Tall E, Weigman O 1990 Risk appraisal outcome and self-efficacy expectancies: cognitive factors in preventive behaviour related to cancer. Psychology and Health 4:99-109

Smith K et al 1987 The validity of health risk appraisal instruments for assessing coronary heart disease risk. American Journal of Public Health 77(4):11-16

Sullivan D 1988 Opportunistic health promotion: do patients like it? Journal of Royal College of General Practitioners 30:24-25

Sumner III W 1990 Computer-assisted patient education. Family Medicine 22:92-93

Tongue B, Stanley I 1991 ELFIN: a computer terminal providing health information and monitoring health concerns among general practice populations. Health Promotion International 6(4):269-279

Van Beurden E, James R, Montague D et al 1993 Community-based cholesterol screening and education to prevent heart disease: Five year results of the North Coast cholesterol check campaign. Australian Journal of Public Health 17(2):109-116

Wilson A, McDonald P, Hayes L, Cooney J 1992 Health promotion in the general practice consultation: a minute makes a difference. British Medical Journal 304:227-230

Winslow R C 1992 Desktop doctors. The Wall Street Journal, April 6

21

Health consumer issues

DEBRA O'CONNOR

It may seem self evident that consumers should be placed at the centre of any new development in health care practice. However they are frequently the last people to be consulted or included in discussions.[1] Health care has traditionally been practiced by experts who know what is best for their patients, and have felt that it may even be counterproductive to share knowledge and ideas with them. This attitude still prevails in many areas of health care and medicine today, but it is increasingly being attacked and challenged by a growing movement of health consumers who feel they have the right to have a say in their health care. This movement has some supporters within the health professions who attempt to influence their more conservative colleagues.

The consumer perspective includes belief in certain rights: the right to information; the right to safe products and services; the right to equal opportunities to obtain services; the right to fairness; the right to participate as an active partner in the doctor-consumer relationship (CHF 1993).

The health consumer movement in Australia gained momentum in the 1970s and 1980s, growing out of international consumer, feminist and human rights movements (Baldry 1992). The movement operates on several levels: there are individual consumers who may or may not be a member of a group; specific groups concerned with a particular disease or condition; state or national umbrella organisations; and consumer representatives on diverse working parties or standing committees.

There is, therefore a shifting philosophy of care that is gaining both international and national acceptance. Consumers are being allowed to have a voice in and some influence on health policy and practice. At an individual level of care patients are being encouraged to be more assertive and expect more information and say in decisions that affect them; and there is a gradual but sometimes a grudging acceptance that individuals and communities may have some responsibility for their own health care policy and services.

Ultimately the consumer should be able to assess the benefit derived from any changes in their terms. It may not always be the same as the assumptions made by professionals. For instance, issues of quality and choice are important considerations. Draper states:

> How quality is defined matters...for health service users, the health product is both process (how I get treated) and outcome (whether I benefit). The experience of quality is also about a continuous, whole process, not just about a part of the body, or what happens in the hospital ward. When health care users define quality, as opposed to health care providers, it may look quite different (HIC 1992).

One of the goals of health informatics is the improvement in communication and management of information. Communication can be rapid and accurate. Important decisions about patient care can be made quickly on the basis of transmitted photo images etc. Due to the rapid development in this field, a number of issues which have been discussed broadly by consumers in the last few years have gained a more immediate relevance. Privacy and security in relation to personal information held by another party are obviously the most crucial and overriding concerns. Related considerations are the nature of informed consent, control of information, ownership, and consumer access to medical records.

Information is of vital importance to consumers. They need to know about their health status or treatment, to have access to their records, and to have a say about what happens to their records (e.g. consent and control over transfer and usage).

The use of computers in health, particularly medicine, means that a lot of data can be communicated to many different people, for many different purposes in a very short space of time. This process obviously leaves many people feeling very concerned about security and access issues. The fear that a mass of data are being collected and stored about individuals with the potential for cross linking with government departments, and other bodies, stirs up images of 'Big Brother' and loss of civil liberties. The ease with which data can be sent and accessed could make it easier to become careless about consent procedures. It can no longer be assumed that professional ethics and guidelines will be enough to control the use of personal health information.

Privacy and the consumer

Although computer technology in health will be used to send and access a wide variety of data—educational, research, drug information, community information, marketing etc.—it is obviously the ability to send personal information relating to individuals that is of most concern to consumers. Consumers who have been advocating to strengthen privacy controls in terms of manually compiled medical records, now have to tackle the more complex privacy aspects of personal information held on computer based records.

Privacy legislation in Australia is currently piecemeal when it comes to protecting health information. *The Privacy Act* (1988) (Cwlth) only covers Commonwealth government departments and funded bodies. Although states generally have privacy clauses in their Health Acts, they do not cover private practitioners and organisations. Professional codes of ethics provide some protection but are not enforceable and do not give the consumer legal right of redress. A working party of the Commonwealth privacy commission has drawn up privacy guidelines relating to HIV/AIDS patients and has recommended that these be adopted more broadly.

The relationship between patient and doctor has long been based on trust, where the patient trusts the doctor not to disclose any personal information without their permission, and where it may cause them harm. Exceptions exist when information is subpoenaed or there is the likelihood of harm to a third party. For the consumer to feel secure therefore, privacy principles need to be extended to make sure that they take into account the increased risks associated with computers. Privacy also covers notions of access, control, ownership and consent.

Access

Who can access information depends on the nature of the information and the terms of consent. Patient access to files has only been possible under the various forms of Freedom of Information (FOI) legislation, and only in the public system. Even then information may be edited or summarised for patient consumption. Other countries have recognised a patients right to access medical records; for instance, the UK has recognised this right for computerised records, both public and private since 1984 (1990 for manually created records) (Carter 1994).

Consumers argue that access to files enable them to be more informed about their condition and care and play a more active role in their own health care. Research by the Health Issues Centre has shown that far from being upset and confused by such information, consumers are less anxious and more co-operative with treatment when they know why certain decisions are made (Loftus Hill 1993). Access to personal records can therefore enable consumers to be more responsive and to make informed choices. Health providers and professionals have generally opposed consumer access fearing possible litigation as well as holding the assumption that patients will become too anxious and will not understand the information. These outcomes have not proved to be the case in other countries, where patients have been able to alter inaccuracies in the files, gain peace of mind, and work in partnership with doctors (Southgate 1991). In fact there is probably less likelihood of litigation where consumers can amend and comment on their own file (Carter 1994). However these paternalistic attitudes are still ingrained in the Australian medical fraternity. According to Carter the Australian Medical Association (AMA) is concerned about the possibility of litigation and is opposed to complete access to files and suggests that doctors may end up keeping two files, one for the doctor and one for the patient (Carter 1994). These arguments were also put forward when FOI legislation was being developed, but there does not seem to be any evidence to support them. Certain groups may require added protection and a different approach to access; for instance children, or severely mentally ill patients.

Patient held records and smart cards

The optimum access arrangement for consumers would be to allow patients to hold their own records. Consumers groups and some professionals support the concept of patient held records (Evans 1994). There are useful precedents already in the pharmaceutical area, where patients hold information relating to the pharmaceuticals they use.

The advent of computer technology makes this more practical and possible through the use of integrated circuit cards, or smart cards. Such cards, would be able to process and store the personal health records of the consumer, in a card similar to an electronic banking card. Providers could access this information when allowed to do so by a consumer during a consultation. Consumers would hold certain access codes, or a PIN number. Such a system has the obvious advantage for a consumer as it gives them control over, access to and some degree of ownership of the information. Consumers would therefore be able to ensure consistency and continuity of care. However there are reservations by consumers at present as to how accessible and under-standable these would be to consumers. Consumers would need to see that they are consumer friendly. These cards are being trialled overseas at present, and contrary to expectations, relatively few problems have been reported.

Paradoxically a need to prevent abuse of the system may also indicate a need for a centralised personal identification number for verification. An attempt at a national identification system (the Australia Card) has been resisted in the past. The community has felt that tax file numbers and Medicare numbers are more than sufficient methods of government control.

The smart card also raises issues over who can change it, and who has the technology to read and access it. It is difficult to envisage a medical profession ready to give up a perceived right to keep information collected by them about their patients. There is a danger, therefore, of multiple sets of information residing in a number of sites, e.g. with the GP, specialist, hospital, etc.

Control

Just as in the past it was recognised that knowledge represented power today control over information represents power. It is difficult to encourage people to relinquish power, and all professionals are very reluctant to do so. It is, after all, the basis of their position in society. Computers represent an extra dimension to this power, as information has the potential to be hidden and only accessible through highly complicated processes.

Smart cards may be a way to overcome issues of access but they do not remove control of the input away from health professionals. Data that are encoded or transformed in some way are harder for consumers to have any control over. It is also harder for consumers to be able to amend or retract information from computerised records. It is understandable therefore that consumers feel that there is a risk of losing any gains so far achieved in accessing their records.

Choice is a further aspect of control. It is important that the use of computer technology is not used to limit choice of consumers in terms of how much and to whom they disclose information, and that the availability of second opinions is not determined by information already recorded.

Consent

There are several common circumstances where patient information may need to be shared with a third party:

- for direct referral and continuity of care purposes, e.g. GP to specialist/ hospital; hospital to GP on discharge
- for research. The information may or may not be identified and collectively passed on for research purposes.
- for a registry of conditions or procedures, e.g. for breast screening purposes, or where a new drug or treatment was introduced
- where a condition is a notifiable disease
- for consultation, when a doctor may need to confer with a colleague
- for teaching and learning purposes.

These circumstances would as a rule require consent of the patient before communication could take place.

Consent must be informed; that is, a person must understand why the information is being passed on, and also no undue pressure or coercion should be applied. Sometimes pressure can be subtle or consent assumed by implication. Practitioners need to be aware of the effect of the power imbalances between a health provider and consumer. Patients are generally vulnerable and anxious to please and they may later regret a decision. Opt out clauses in registries are important, as they give consumers a greater degree of control. Reassurance and an opportunity to review consent (if the process is long term) would ensure less initial anxiety and greater trust. Most consumers are happy to allow this information to be transferred, especially when it will lead to better care for them, or the community in general.

It is also important that the content of medical records is relevant and succinct, free of unnecessary social, personal information and subjective opinions, and it must be accurate. The Health Services Commissioner in Victoria receives complaints about accuracy, where treatment and ongoing care is based on the wrong assumptions and information. Both the Commonwealth and several State governments are preparing privacy guidelines that relate directly to medical records.

Consent is not always sought in cases of risk to an individual or third party and when legally subpoenaed. Files may also be accessed for fraud control and professional standards monitoring.

Confidentiality

The opportunity and temptation for Government departments and other bodies to cross link information or adopt surveillance techniques is also of concern to consumers. At present information from the Department of Social Security can be cross referenced with taxation information to overcome welfare fraud. If this is extended to health there are concerns that insurance, superannuation etc. may be affected, and represent a gross personal violation.

'Function creep' is a term coined in America to describe how information collected for one purpose may eventually be used in other ways. Obviously there will have to be strict guidelines and administrative procedures to make sure that there is no unauthorised or unnecessary access to data on all levels. There is a well founded fear of unauthorised access to data banks. According to Kidd (1992) the World Health Organization resolved that medical data banks be only available to the medical profession, and not linked to central databanks.

In an attempt to identify health care policy and practice, and provider views on consumer access and privacy the Health Issues Centre conducted a survey of public health agencies in Victoria. Results showed that although most centres were aware of the need for privacy and security of medical records, few could give a clear account of their procedures, and were not aware of all the relevant legislation and guidleines. They did however support in principle the notion of patients having a right to view their records (Loftus Hill 1993).

Ownership

It has until recently been generally accepted that providers own the health information they enter into records to help their patients. Under FOI legislation consumers have had access to this public system information for several years. They have demanded the right to comment and change this information. However in many cases only summaries or selections of files have been released. There appears to be no way of enforcing complete access. In the private sector this is even more difficult. The laws around ownership appear to be vague and ambiguous. In a case recently heard in Victoria it is not even clear whether records belong to individual practitioners or to a practice where he worked. Relatives of deceased practitioners maintain they own records. In a Health Issues case study a woman with a genetic disorder, possibly related to a drug taken by her mother (DES), was unable to access files held by the widow of her late doctor (Vickers Kerr 1986).

With the advent of medical entrepreneurship some private practices are now owned by non-medical business men. It has not yet been established legally to what extent these practice owners own or have access to medical records. Consumers are very keen to see anomalies around ownership resolved.

Consumers and research

Consumers are keen to encourage productive research, and are in general, very willing to consent to allowing access to personal information for these purposes. The NHMRC have ethical guidelines (currently being trialled and under review) which must be adhered to by researchers. Proposed research in health must be passed by an ethics committee. Requirements include the necessity to obtain consent from all individuals and strict practices governing the handling of personal data. Research may involve accessing files re–trospectively and cross matching data, or conducting longitudinal studies. It is important for consumers that results of research is made available to them. This also provides accountability and recognises the contribution of consumers.

The use of computers has obvious benefits for research; far more data can be collected on a national level, and the opportunity for good public health research is therefore much improved. For example, a researcher may wish to look at whether a particular medical procedure or drug is associated with a disorder occurring at a later period in time. Computers enable faster and more comprehensive cross matching and analysis. Whether or not research data should be de-identified in all cases is problematical: obvious research problems of replicability and reliability must be addressed. Consumers are divided on this issue and the debate will continue for some time.

The establishment of national registries should also help both the individual consumer as well as the community. Breast screening registries should aid in the regular recall of women, as well as show general trends and problems. According to a worker at the Victorian Breast Screening Program only 10 women out of approximately 80 000 have refused to have their name on a registry in the first two years of screening. Health consumers cautiously support the access of researchers to data that may be seen to be for the good of public health when it is not possible always to obtain consent, but only if assured of good quality assurance procedures. This means that consumers would expect to participate in the monitoring of the research and involved in decisions about defining the nature of the public interest and health being presented.

Coding

Coding practices are necessary to enable data to be transmitted and accessed appropriately. At present there seems to be difficulty in developing a coding system that is not too unwieldy but can capture the complex nature of health information and enable accurate and unambiguous decoding. It is clear to consumers that coding is of major importance, but they are concerned that it doesn't dehumanise the consumer, or affect the nature of the patient-doctor contact. They share the professionals concern about security of encryption codes and the need to understand the technology to a level that enables them to have input into discussion and implementation. Like professionals, consumers need to work with software manufacturers and academics to fully ensure that coding meets everybody's needs.

257

Health informatics and general consumer issues

The health consumer movement is also vitally interested in quality assurance, accountability and evaluation issues. Applied to health informatics, consumers are anxious to see proper quality assurance mechanisms in place, where professionals have to take account of the nature of outcomes in relation to their practice. This could be by peer review, but preferably by boards or panels representing a cross section of perspectives, including consumers.

Evaluation of technologies in terms of outcomes should always include some account of the impact on consumers. This will help avoid the tendency to become taken with or carried away by the glamour of the technolology. Measures need to be developed that show the nature of improved patient care.

Benefits for consumers

For the individual patient, improved communication between providers of health care should only improve continuity and consistency of care, as long as confidentiality and consent procedures are respected. It should relieve them of having to undergo repeated tests with different providers. (Often a patient has been forced to undergo the same tests in a hospital that they may have just had with their GP. This can be particularly harrowing with some procedures.) On discharge they should be sure that follow up care is co-ordinated and consistent. Community support agencies, such as the Royal District Nursing Service and Community Health Centres, as well as GPs, should be able to be more easily co-ordinated to offer appropriate post-hospital care.

Information technology should enable better quality drug prescribing; doctors could have access to on line data bases which could inform them of the most recent allergy or adverse drug interaction information. Better quality research should be possible. Consumers should also be able to use this research to inform their own self-management, and access data banks and information for their own research

Indirect benefits for consumers are obvious through having providers better informed about current medical findings and other relevant information such as changes in government requirements and guidelines.

Consumers should benefit from better education opportunities offered to them and practitioners by computers. It may also be possible to link either seriously ill or isolated patients at home together for support, and/or to health providers for ongoing monitoring or education.

The ability to offer rapid and appropriate care to a seriously ill or injured patient in an isolated geographical area is often cited as one of the major advantages for consumers. Isolated practitioners could also confer and consult with colleagues to improve their own practice. This of course assumes the use of appropriate consent protocols.

Other indirect benefits for consumers will be that costs of health care could be better tracked which would increase efficiencies and reduce the overall costs of health care to the communuity.

Summary and conclusion

It is important that the patient or consumer is placed at the centre of any discussion about health informatics. The ultimate goal of any new development in health is an improved health outcome for consumers. Information technology promises many benefits for consumers but not without some serious hazards. There are no easy solutions but it is important that there be continuing dialogue between all parties concerned. In order for this dialogue to take place there has to be an acceptance of the consumer as a serious player with a right to be fully informed about the technology and its application in health care services. This has to occur at all levels, from the individual doctor and his/her patient, to policy makers, professional associations, consumer and advocacy groups.

The advent of information technology in health represents an opportunity to transform the traditional paternalistic doctor patient relationship to one of mutual co-operation, with the patient gaining a greater degree of responsibility in managing their own health care, due, in part, to the right to contribute to and access their own health information.

NOTE

This chapter refers mainly to consumers who represent and advocate from a particular perspective as distinct to providers and professionals who represent the needs of an industry. Consumer may also refer to one individual, or the collective voice. It is a term with less implication of power differences than the term patient. However occasionally the term patient is used where it feels more appropriate.

REFERENCES

Carter M 1994 Consuming health information: telecommunications, computers and health records. Health Issues 39
Consumers Health Forum of Australia Inc 1993 Guidelines for consumer representatives, 3rd edn.
Evans R 1994 Why you should start keeping your own health records. Health Voice 4
Health Issues Centre 1992 Casemix quality and consumers. Prepared by Mary Draper, Health Issues Centre, Melbourne
Loftus-Hills A 1993 Medical records: consumers rights to access and privacy. Health Issues 35
Southgate J 1991 For your eyes only: health records, access and privacy. Health Issues 26
Vickers Kerr M 1986 Medical records: the DES experience. Health Issues March/ April

FURTHER READING

Baldry E 1992 The development of the health consumer movement and its effect on value changes and health policy in Australia. Unpublished PhD thesis. University of New South Wales

Health Issues Centre 1993 The power of information: health providers, consumers and treatment records. Prepared by Alison Loftus-Hills and Jan Southgate, Health Issues Centre, Melbourne

HIANSW Discussion paper 1993 Patient held medical records. Informatics in Healthcare Australia 2(5)

Kidd M 1992 Information in health care: what does it mean for the consumer? Health Issues 33

Teng Liaw S 1994 Patient held health records or patient held medical records? A South Australian perspective. Informatics in Healthcare 3(2)

22

Medico-legal issues

GERALDINE MACKENZIE

It may be obvious that there is a need for privacy and confidentiality of the patient record, but the legal implications of a breach of either of these are not always considered and understood. Medical records are by their very nature intensely personal, and a patient must be able to have trust in the privacy and security of this information in order to provide it with confidence. Breaches can lead to serious consequences for a patient and the health professional.

Because of a computer's increased capacity for storage, its enhanced ability to retrieve information quickly, and the potential to network large numbers of computers, it is possible for a large number of people to have access to the patient record. Not only is there the possibility that this would result in the leakage of sensitive information, there is also the possibility that electronic records could be altered by unauthorised persons. Although this is also the case with paper records, the potential for harm is not so great. For further details on system security refer to Chapter 8.

This chapter examines some legal issues in health informatics; in particular the privacy and confidentiality issues in the electronic storage of health records.

The right to privacy

It is probably fair to say that members of the general public would be of the opinion that they had a right to privacy of their confidential health records. In general ethical terms they do, but in legal terms it is another matter. The 'right to privacy' is somewhat of a misnomer. Generally speaking there is no such thing as a legal right to privacy in Australia. There has been limited recognition of such a right in, for example, the *Privacy Act* 1988 (Cwlth) which establishes rights in certain circumstances.

Most breaches of privacy will also be breaches of confidentiality, for which there are other remedies available (see below). The *Privacy Act* was passed by the Commonwealth Government in response to the OECD Guidelines on the Protection of Privacy and Transborder Flows of Personal Data. It applies only to 'agencies' which are established under the Commonwealth, and therefore applies only to bodies such as Commonwealth hospitals, the Health Insurance Commission, and the like.

Central to the Act are the 11 Information Privacy Principles which are contained in section 14. They specify such things as the reasons for which information can be collected, how the information shall be stored, how access can be gained to the records, the use to which the records can be put, and the limits on disclosure of personal information. Principle 11 which is particularly relevant, states:

> A record-keeper who has possession or control of a record that contains personal information shall not disclose the information to a person, body or agency, (other than the individual concerned) unless...

A number of grounds upon which the information may be released are then stated, including: (b) the individual concerned has consented to the disclosure.

The Act creates the office of Privacy Commissioner (s. 19), who has the power to investigate complaints under the Act. If the Commissioner finds that a complaint is made out, he or she has the power to make various orders, including an order that the complainant be compensated for any loss or damage suffered.

There have been concerns expressed that the Act is not broad enough in its jurisdiction, and also that it may no longer be appropriate to cover computerised record keeping. (O'Connor 1994). There is a need for some sort of legislation to cover medical records more generally, i.e. records held by State bodies and private bodies, rather than just Commonwealth agencies as is the case under the *Privacy Act*.

Further to the *Privacy Act*, it is also an offence under s. 70 *Crimes Act* 1914 (Cwlth) for a Commonwealth Officer to disclose information they had a duty not to disclose.

So far, the only State to attempt similar legislation is New South Wales, which has a Data Protection Bill presently before the Parliament, and, when passed, will be similar in content to the Commonwealth Privacy Act.

The duty of confidence

Breach of confidence in a minor matter concerning a patient may be bad enough, but when the breach, for example, reveals that the patient has HIV/AIDS, the consequences for that person can be catastrophic.

A duty of confidence can arise in a number of different ways. It can arise by virtue of the ethics of a profession. For example, the Australian Medical Association (AMA) Code of Ethics states:

In general, keep in confidence information derived from your patient, or from a colleague regarding your patient, and divulge it only with the patient's permission, except where a court demands.

There are also guidelines set down by the various health departments.[1] These type of guidelines can sometimes have a quasi-legal effect, as the courts have examined them when determining whether a duty of confidentiality exists.[2] There are also statutes in the different jurisdictions which create obligations for confidentiality of health records.[3]

Furthermore, a duty to keep personal patient information confidential may be an express or implied term of contract which a patient enters into with the health provider when care is provided.

The law also imposes duties in other situations where there is an obligation of confidence arising from the circumstances in which the information was obtained. In order to succeed in this type of legal action, the plaintiff (i.e. the person taking the action) first must show that the information has the necessary quality of confidence about it in the sense that the preservation of its confidentiality or secrecy is of substantial concern to the person taking the court action.[4] This would almost certainly be the case in a doctor-patient relationship, and other health professional-patient relationships. Secondly, the information must have been imparted in circumstances importing an obligation of confidence; and thirdly, there must have been an unauthorised use of that information to the detriment of the party communicating it.[5]

Negligence

Depending on the nature of the breach, the patient may be able to take other legal action against the person responsible. This may be, for example, because of the negligence of the record holder in releasing confidential information. Taking such an action can be very difficult, take a long time, and be very expensive. This can be a deterrent in a lot of cases.

According to the law of negligence, a health provider would be liable if he or she owed a duty of care to a patient, if the duty of care was breached by the health provider, and if damage resulted which was causally linked and not too remote. As part of this test, the health provider would be liable if he or she failed to take the necessary steps to eliminate reasonably foreseeable and significant risks of injury to the plaintiff (Trindade & Cane 1993).

Avoiding legal action

The key to avoiding legal action is to ensure that proper precautions have been taken. This will include putting in place such things as proper procedures for record keeping; adequate staff training on an ongoing basis; close and regular monitoring of these procedures, including adequate staff supervision; and review of these procedures making sure that they are sufficient.

Taking these precautions will minimise the exposure to liability for the health professional. It is probably impossible to completely eliminate the risk.

What security measures are needed?

The question of what security measures have to be put in place to safeguard patient records is a difficult one to answer. At the time of writing, there are no standards which apply generally to give guidance in this matter. Implicit in this is the need to not only provide an appropriate level to cover all known risks, but also to have a level of security which is sufficient to minimise the risk of legal action.

What precautions must be taken depend on the concept of foreseeability of the breach. The courts have held that even though the risk may be unlikely to occur, it should still have been foreseen, provided that it is not far-fetched or fanciful.[6]

This means that a record holder must take all reasonable steps to safeguard the security of the information. This involves taking proper security measures, such as password protection and not leaving files open on the screen when there is the possibility of access to them by unauthorised persons.

If a record holder takes all reasonable steps to provide proper security, and a breach of security still happens through an event which could not possibly have been foreseen, the record holder would probably not be negligent. This could be contrasted with the position where the record holder has not taken proper precautions e.g. staff have not been properly trained, and a breach of security occurs. In these circumstances, the record holder probably would be negligent. Whether or not the record holder actually is negligent is a question which has to be answered in every case and the above examples are a guide only.

Medical records held in networked computers are particularly vulnerable. The potential for outside interference e.g. by hackers, is real, and must be taken into account. It would be prudent therefore to seek advice from an appropriate computing professional in order to determine the security measures necessary. It must also not be forgotten that these measures will be subject to change as time passes, due to the changing nature of the computing industry. What is adequate protection today may not be so in one year's time, and almost certainly will not be adequate in five years' time.

If no alterations are made to computer security measures to take account of the changes in information technology and changes in known risks, a person who has suffered harm by the release of the confidential information would have a far greater chance of establishing negligence than would otherwise be the case.

Standards for the keeping of medical records

Although at this time there are no standards which apply generally, these issues are being addressed by a number of bodies. For example, the Royal

Australian College of General Practitioners have an *Interim Code of Practice for Computerised Medical Records in General Practice* which was adopted in February 1993 and is to be piloted over two years. The limitation of this Code is that it does not cover all general practitioners, as not all are members of the RACGP.

Standards Australia in mid 1994 released the *Draft Australian Standard on Information Security and Personal Privacy Protection in Healthcare Information Systems* for public comment with the intention that the Standard would be adopted by various organisations, who will use it as a base for their own standards. This standard was adopted in August 1995.

Although the implementation of standards such as these is to be applauded, record holders adopting them are not automatically guaranteed immunity from legal action. There is still a need to be vigilant, and to note that information technology changes at such a rapid pace that what is an appropriate standard now may not be so in the future. On the other hand, a failure to comply with these sorts of standards would leave a record holder vulnerable to legal claims should a breach of security occur.

When can confidential information be disclosed?

There are exceptions to the rule that patient information must be kept confidential, and mandatory HIV/AIDS reporting is one of these. There are other times when access to the patient record is sought, e.g. for medical research, raising both ethical and legal issues. Thomson (1993) points out that disclosure of information in medical records for medical research without consent involves a breach of the duty of confidentiality. He then notes three exceptions to the general rule that confidential information cannot be disclosed: (1) where the patient has consented to the disclosure; (2) compulsion of law, where for example there is a compulsion to disclose information as part of judicial proceedings, or the mandatory reporting example given above; and (3) where the disclosure would be in the public interest.

An example of the third category occurred in the UK in the case of *X v Y*.[7] In that case information was supplied to a newspaper that two doctors were carrying on general practice despite having contracted AIDS. One of the issues in the case was whether it was in the public interest that the information be published. The court held that the public interest in preserving the confidentiality of medical records in identifying AIDS sufferers outweighed the public interest in publishing the information, and that this was necessary so that victims would not be deterred from seeking treatment.

A court in the United States has held that in certain situations there is a duty to disclose confidential information in order to warn others who may otherwise be at risk.[8] This has not yet been followed in Australia although it is possible (but unlikely) that it could be adopted here one day.

Access to information

Contrasting with the situation previously where patients had limited (if any) access to their medical records, there is now much greater access available with the advent of Freedom of Information (FOI) legislation, although the situation is unchanged in that the record is still owned by the person who created it.

Freedom of Information Acts are now present in every Australian jurisdiction except the Northern Territory.[9] They operate to allow access to information held by certain specified bodies. In most instances this does not apply to private bodies such as private hospitals, or to medical practitioners in private practice. In some jurisdictions, there is no need to rely on procedures under FOI legislation, as administrative access to records is possible. For example, the Queensland Health Department in 1994 issued their revised policy *Administrative Access to Health Records*. This allows patients access free of charge to their medical records held by Queensland hospitals.

Conclusion

The electronic storage of patient records is increasing in popularity, and before long will be commonplace. It needs to be acknowledged that this brings additional problems of privacy and security of the information stored in those records. These problems raise the threat of legal liability to the record holder if confidentiality is breached.

The only way to minimise legal liability and comply with duties of confidentiality is to be aware of the issues, and put in place appropriate mechanisms to address them. It will be necessary in doing this to seek advice from computing/data protection professionals, and where appropriate, take precautionary legal advice. Not only should the legal issues be considered, but also the ethical and moral issues, because the information contained in the patient record is sensitive and it is clearly the obligation of the record holder to safeguard that information. Only then will the health profession continue to maintain the confidence of the public that it presently enjoys.

NOTES

[1] See Health Commission of NSW Circulars No 82/369 and 84/82; Department of Health NSW (Hunter) *Policy for the Management of Acquired Immune Deficiency Syndrome and Hepatitis B*, 1 July 1988; Department of Health NSW *Infection Control Policy for HIV, AIDS, and Associated Conditions* 1992, *Queensland Privacy Guidelines for Hospitals*, Department Standing Committee on Privacy and Health and Medical Records, April 1986; WA Health Department *Guidelines for Release/Access to Health Records 1986*; SA Health Department *Guidelines Regarding the Release of Information*.

[2] See the case of *W. v Egdell* [1990] 1 Ch 359 where the UK Court of Appeal relied on the General Medical Council's *Advice on standards of professional conduct and of*

medical ethics when determining whether a doctor had breached his duty of confidence.

3 See *Health Act* 1937 (Qld) s.49(1); *Health Services Act* 1991 (Qld) s.5.1; *Public Health Act* 1991 (NSW); *Health Administration Act* 1982 (NSW); *Public and Environmental Health Act* 1987 (SA) s.42; *South Australian Health Commission Act* 1976 s.64; *Public Health Act* 1962 (Tas); *Health Act* 1958 (Vic); *Health Services Act* 1988 (Vic) s.141; *Health Act* 1911 (WA) s.314; *Health Services Act* 1990 (ACT); *Health Services (Consequential Provisions) Act* 1990 (ACT); *Notifiable Diseases Act* 1981 (NT).

4 *Moorgate Tobacco Co. Limited v Philip Morris Limited* (1984) 156 CLR 414, at p 438.

5 *Coco v A.N. Clark (Engineers) Ltd.* [1969] RPC 41, at p 47.

6 *Council of the Shire of Wyong v Shirt* (1980) 146 CLR 40, at p 48.

7 *X v Y* [1988] 2 All ER 648.

8 See *Tarasoff v Regents of the University of California* 17 Cal 3d 425, 551 P 2d 334 (1976).

9 *Freedom of Information Act* 1982 (Cwlth); *Freedom of Information Act* 1992 (Qld); *Freedom of Information Act* 1989 (NSW); *Freedom of Information Act* 1982 (Vic); *Freedom of Information Act* 1991 (SA); *Freedom of Information Act* 1989 (ACT); *Freedom of Information Act* 1991 (Tas) *Freedom of Information Act* 1992 (WA).

REFERENCES

O'Connor K 1994 Emerging information privacy issues in health care. Proceedings of the Second National Health Informatics Conference Melbourne, Australia, Health Informatics Society of Australia 21-25

Thomson C J H 1993 Records, research and access: what interests should outweigh privacy and confidentiality? Some Australian answers. Journal of Law and Medicine 1:95-108

Trindade F, Cane P 1993 The law of torts in Australia, 2nd edn. Oxford University Press, Melbourne

4

Informatics and health care management

23

National strategy for information management

J MICHAEL BRITTAIN

Information management in the health services has been with us ever since we have had health services! As soon as one records patient details, there is some, albeit elementary, need to manage information. The use of information technology (IT) to manage information is of much more recent origin. With the advent and widespread availability of affordable mainframe computers in the 1960s, the health services, along with other major organisations, quickly used them for a limited number of tasks—in the first instance, mainly for the payroll. In the beginning information technology and computers affected relatively few administrative staff in the health services. Clinical and medical staff gradually developed their own departmental computing facilities and acquired the skills necessary to use computers as they went along.

In the last decade information, information management, and the use of IT to manage information affects over 90% of the workforce in health services. There is now multi-billion dollars spent on IT in health services throughout the developed world. It is generally recognised that the health services are behind other sectors of business and industry (e.g. airlines, service industries, some government departments) in the deployment of IT to assist in the management of information.

Education and training for the use of IT for information management has been relatively neglected, perhaps more so in the health services than in other sectors of the economy. But even outside the health services, education and training was usually the last line in the corporate budget for many decades; and in times of cut back and scarcity it was the education and training budget which suffered first.

It is now a familiar cry that there is an enormous wasted investment in IT in all sectors of the economy, particularly in health care. Stories about IT equipment lying idle, underutilised, and inefficiencies in its use are legion (Warden 1993). It's paradoxical that the increasing amounts spent on IT, accompanied by increasing claims of IT suppliers about its efficacy and cost benefits, occurs at the time of documented studies on wastage and in–efficiencies. We are still waiting for the definitive study that proves without doubt that investment in IT is cost effective! (Walker 1993). At one extreme, most people would agree that the airline industry today could not function without the deployment of computers and communication technologies; and more recently the same can be said of some manufacturing processes. However, in many other service industries, in government departments, in the administration of universities, and in the health services, the benefits that have been promised for so long have yet to be fully documented and substantiated.

For many, investment in IT in complex administrative environments is still an act of faith and the take up of IT and EDI (Electronic Data Interchange) is slow (Pugsley 1994). We live in a world in which computers are regarded as a good thing, an indication of modernity, and a necessity for us all to know about. We have been told for a long time that everybody will be effected by computers during their life time. Until about thirty years ago it was generally accepted that the learning of Latin at school was a good thing. We were told that it would help us learn other languages, help with spelling, and all sorts of other goodies were paraded. But there was little evidence to back up these claims. Universities demanded that all applicants had school leaving qualifications in Latin. Such demands are unthinkable today. The overselling and the over enthusiasm of the past decade for IT and computing will no doubt be unthinkable in twenty years time (Greenes & Shortliffe 1990). In the future we shall not invest in IT unless there are demonstrable benefits to be gained. A better educated and trained workforce will ensure that this is so!

In the health services the public knowledge that now exists (Warden 1993) about the wasted millions of dollars on IT investment has had a beneficial effect. There is more caution about IT investment, and a better planned approach to IT is absolutely essential for most of the health care workforce.

The information intensive health services

The provision of health services has always been an information intensive activity. Medical and health care knowledge, data and information continue to grow at a great pace: patients generate information, more patients than ever continue to be seen each year in hospitals and within the community, and the management of health care continues to grow in complexity world-wide (MacDougall & Brittain 1994).

There are many factors, both within and outside health care that are influencing the generation, capture, processing, storage, and use of information for health care management and for clinical practice, as well as for accessing health care requirements and meeting the increasingly sophisticated information demands of patients, their relatives, and, indeed, the general public

(MacDougall & Brittain 1992). Health promotion as an allied activity is also predominantly information intensive (Gann 1991).

Activities and factors of the last few years that have had a tremendous influence upon the development of new information systems for health care include:

- Resource allocation formulae
- Cost centre and accrual accounting for costing and cost modelling
- Relative Stay Index
- DRGs
- Patient Classification: e.g. Nurse Dependency; Health Insurance; Nursing Homes (RC1)
- Medicare Benefit Scheme, and Pharmaceutical Benefits Scheme
- Medical audit
- Assessment of health care needs of populations
- Performance indicators
- Care Evaluation Program (CEP)
- Clinical Indicator (CI)
- Inaugural National Clinical Data Evaluation System (INCIDE)
- Outsourcing/contracting
- Health data dictionary
- Health information agreements between Commonwealth and States
- Development of a National Health Information Plan.
  (For more details see Brittain & MacDougall 1995.)

Performance indicators in medical audit, as well as assessment of outcomes, are all part of the new culture of quantifying activity and performance, both at the aggregate level and also in terms of individual performance. These activities form part of a new management culture which can only operate successfully with the aid of a new generation of information services. Many of the measures and performance indicators listed above are included in the Australian Council on Healthcare Standards (ACHS) Care Evaluation Program (CEP), which aims to improve the quality of patient care by measuring the processes and outcomes of patient care. Lawson and Callopy (1993) describe the progress made with the national Clinical Indicator (CI) and the CEP Inaugural National Clinical Indicator Data Evaluation System (INCIDE). All these measurements, indicators, and databases could have been recorded and constructed by hand, at least in principle, before the advent of computers and information technology; but in practice, it would have been impossible.

The long term value of the CEP and INCIDE systems (as indeed is the case with all performance indicators) is the potential to provide feedback to health care professionals about levels and efficacy of practice. The ultimate value to both practitioners and patients is the educational value of feedback: as McIntyre and Popper (1983) note knowledge grows more by the recognition of error than the accumulation of new facts. Health care professionals continue to be suspicious and resistant to new, so called, management information systems.

The educational and training spin offs of new information systems have been played down. There are good reasons to support education and training programs aimed at the basics of data collection, storage, retrieval, and presentation, but if the programs can in addition address the spin offs for better and more informed practice, the value of information management education and training will be seen as essential, rather than desirable.

When education and training was still seen as an expendable resource that could be dispensed with in difficult economic times, this is just what happened. But when the skills, competencies, and knowledge in information management are seen to be part of the key ingredients of a successful health care strategy, training and education likewise are placed high on the corporate agenda.

Many senior managers in health have resisted the wide scale introduction of IT. But in recent years, in many countries, outsourcing and contracting of services (sometimes between sectors of the health services) have increased the perceived need for IT to facilitate the outsourcing and contracting processes. In the early days of outsourcing and contracting it soon became evident that inadequate information systems could be extremely costly. Thereafter, senior management that was formerly cool towards information management and a new generation of information systems began to embrace them enthusiastically!

Why a strategy?

Strategies (of any nature) are often resisted by an organisation's workforce. It is necessary in such cases to enumerate the reasons for developing, and subsequently implementing a strategy. Some attractions of a strategy are given below:

- enables a detailed plan of activity to be agreed, facilitates financial planning, and allows progress to be assessed against objectives
- assists in justifying expenditure of large sums
- provides a vehicle for publicity
- helps develop local ownership and motivation
- reduces the chance of duplicated effort and wasted resources
- provides coherence to a national, state, or international activity
- helps plan for future direction.

In many organisations the single most important aspect of a strategy is that it enables organisations to devote large amounts of money to specific plans, and sometimes to obtain considerable funds, which no government department would agree to allocate in the absence of a strategy.

Elements of an education and training strategy

A training strategy, in its most simple form, addresses the following factors:

- the skills, knowledge and competencies required of health care workers

- the existing distribution of skills, knowledge and competencies across the workforce
- the training needs, ordered according to priority levels, for different groups of employees
- training plans, over time periods; e.g. immediate, middle term and long term training plans
- delivery of training, both from within the health services, and also from outside
- types of training and education currently available
- evaluation of training and education
- evaluation of the strategy
- dissemination of information about the strategy
- the development of a local training infrastructure.

Strategies and plans range from the very general through to the very detailed and explicit. Certainly, at some stage in the implementation of an education and training strategy it is necessary to produce a detailed assessment of training needs and existing provision, and a detailed plan for the local delivery of training and education. In large organisations local ownership and local plans are essential. The task is too large to be operated at a national/federal level. However, a general strategy provides guidance and motivation, and can be instrumental in the development of a local training infrastructure, and also in the allocation of both central government funds and local health authority funds.

A case study—the IM&T training program of the UK National Health Service

The work is known as the IM&T Training Program for the NHS (UK NHS 1989). The program addresses the training needs of clinicians, professionals allied to medicine, administrative, clerical, technical and auxiliary staffs, at all levels from the most senior to the most junior. There are over one million employees in the NHS and all are in some way affected by one or more aspects of the information cycle of data capture, storage, analysis, presentation and use for management and clinical purposes. The IM&T Training Program is part of the wider information plan known as the IM&T Strategy. In the discussion below it is important to note the difference between the IM&T Strategy and the IM&T Training and Education Strategy; the latter is designed to help implement the human resources aspect of the former.

The IM&T Training and Education Program covers all awareness, training, education, and development needs relating to:

- collection, coding, storage, analysis and use of information for clinical, managerial, and operational purposes, and
- the procurement, operation and use of information systems in technology.

In addition to covering the major NHS workforce, it also addresses, for the 6000 specialists IM&T staff in the NHS, the issues of:

- workforce planning and supply
- graduate staff recruitment
- code of practice
- the development of nationally recognised qualifications which meet the needs of the NHS.

All projects are managed using PRINCE project management methodology, which provides clear mechanisms for ensuring that projects are completed to explicit time scales, cost and quality standards. All training packages and all major events from 1993 onwards are evaluated using specially designed questionnaires.

The program is financed in terms of a phased reduction in central funding, which makes explicit the need to build expertise delivery infrastructures at a local level, so the need for central development work will reduce. The policy also acknowledges that given the rapid pace of change for IM&T and the new skills needed, a residual level of activity at a central level will be required for the foreseeable future. Since 1989 the program has been funded to the level of approximately £4.5 million per annum, with expenditure in the 1993/94 year of approximately £4 million falling to £1 million in 1996/97.

The work of the IM&T training program is organised into five major program areas as follows:

- Training and awareness to support the IM&T strategy
- Program for managers
- Education and training for doctors, nurses and professionals allied to medicine
- IM&T specialist staff
- Training infrastructure.

Each of the five parts are described briefly below.

Training and awareness to support the IM&T strategy

The aim of the IM&T Strategy is to help clinicians and managers make better use of information to achieve better patient care. The overriding principle is that management information must be derived from operational systems. The strategy includes major activities such as introducing a new NHS number for every person in the country, setting up a new IT network linking the whole of the NHS, introducing common clinical terminology and data standards, and providing guidance on data security and confidentiality.

As part of the training program it is necessary to:

- identify the implications and requirements for training, and also or–ganisational development
- develop and disseminate materials to raise awareness of the IM&T strategy for all NHS staff—materials include videos, briefing packs, and overview guides

- for each major component of the IM&T Strategy to 1) design specific awareness training materials; 2) produce good practice guidance in planning and implementing; 3) work with software suppliers to ensure that hands-on technical training manuals that they produce are of good quality and meet current standards of practice
- produce a handbook which details all training that is or will be available to support the IM&T Strategy.

Manager program

The program consists of high profile briefing events for chief executives, general managers and non-executive directors. These provide an opportunity for the participants to hear about the latest developments in, and benefits of IM&T.

The program also consists of *Focussed learning sets*. These are a form of action learning aimed at top management teams. Participants have the opportunity to work on problems they have identified, experiment with solutions, evaluate progress and adopt new approaches. Typically, the management team might decide to devise an information strategy in support of the organisation's business plan. However, experience has shown that existing business plans are not usually robust enough for use as a basis for determining information requirements. As a result, much work is being done in management teams to help strengthen or refocus their business plan.

Also, as part of the program for managers, 'corporate strategy workshops' have taken place. They provide an alternative to the focus learning set approach, and enable top management teams to address information and IT issues in a more intensive and structured way.

The managers' program is supported by a series of computer assisted learning packages. These include LEARN-IT and Spreadsheets for Managers. These packages develop managers' skills in information management, resource use, decision making, and planning. They can be used as stand alone packages by individuals, or delivered to groups of about ten managers by local trainers.

Education and training for doctors, nurses and professionals allied to medicine

The aim of the program is to ensure that IM&T is integrated into the education curriculum for doctors, nurses and professionals allied to medicine and becomes an integral part of their professional training.

IM&T specialist staff

There are approximately 6000 IM&T specialists in the NHS and two major initiatives have been taken as part of the IM&T Training and Education Program.

First is the development of a *Statement of recognition* for IM&T specialists. This is a new professional qualification which has been developed by the NHS in conjunction with professional associations and educational establishments. There is a new professional association—ASSIST—which will take an increasing responsibility for awarding the *Statement of recognition* (Le Maistre 1994).

The second initiative is the *Code of practice* for IM&T specialists.

Training infrastructure

In order to ensure that the guidance, training materials and packages that are developed centrally reach the people they are aimed at, much effort has been given to the development of local infrastructures for training. This has taken place in three ways: first by setting up and supporting a network of IM&T training coordinators—currently one per regional health authority. Second by funding (on 50/50 basis) a wide variety of IM&T centres, usually based in local hospitals, and there are over two hundred centres now in operation. Third by producing and disseminating a range of guidance and support materials for trainers at the local level. These packages include:

- IM&T training resource pack
- a blueprint for setting up an IM&T learning centre
- case studies of a wide variety of local training activities
- directories of training available from commercial suppliers and the educational sector.

Overview

The IM&T Training and Education Program for the NHS is centrally funded, directed and evaluated. No individual health authority or department (or indeed, university) could fund or operate such a wide ranging and extensive program. However, the emphasis has always been upon the eventual local responsibility for training.

The central program has been successful in stimulating, guiding and supporting training at the local level. It has done this by way of:

- identifying the key target groups for training
- helping to define training needs
- developing and designing training materials, courses, computer assisted learning packages and good practice guides, particularly where central development can achieve economies of scale
- building the training infrastructures at local level by part funding a wide range of activities, including local IM&T learning centres
- identifying examples of good and innovative training practice (not just in the health services), documenting the experience in the form of case studies and making it available throughout the NHS with the aim to spread good practice, and also to avoid wasteful duplications of effort

- providing information and advice, by way of directories and a computerised database, on the large number of training courses available from suppliers in the commercial and educational sectors
- supporting curriculum development in universities to meet the longer term IM&T training needs of the health services in IM&T.

The IM&T training program began in 1986. At the time few people could have predicted that eight years later the total expenditure of approximately $50 million, with a further $10 million allocated for the 1994-1997 period, would be forthcoming. The success has been due in large measure to the development of a viable strategy in the first instance. In the early years many said that a strategy without finance to implement it was useless : all agreed. The other cry that we hear so often: 'We don't need a strategy, give us the money and we'll get on with it' would not have produced such an extensive and systematic program. The finance would have been dissipated and spread thinly across a large NHS : also it is inconceivable that a central government body would provide $10 million per annum in the absence of an agreed and documented program!

Many of the issues covered by the IM&T Training and Education Program deal with generic issues; and those that do not could relatively easily be modified, at a fraction of the cost of the original development, to meet Australian needs. All the products of the IM&T Training and Education Program can be made available to anyone (or any group) in Australia, at the normal selling price to the NHS. The selling price in no way reflects the development costs! For example, LEARN-IT cost over $400 000 to develop and is sold, as a set of floppy disks, plus guidance and materials for trainers and trainees, for $90.00.

The future?

The delivery of training in the future will be an interactional activity, capitalising upon economics of scale, high quality training materials, and multimedia delivery of training through open and distance learning modes. Already the delivery of IM&T training and education for health services is a multifaceted activity, involving many suppliers both within and outside the health services (Brittain & Abbott 1993, Brittain & Maggs 1993).

The full impact of health informatics is only just beginning to be realised world-wide. The fact that so many activities in medicine and all forms of health care are extremely information intensive makes the implementation of information technology and communication essential in today's health services. A new generation of information systems specifically designed for use in health care will be implemented during the next few years, facilitating increased efficiency and reducing costs of healthcare generally. The development and implementation of international standards for data exchange and definition, coding of medical terminology, and effective electronic networking will enhance global co-operation and sharing of expertise. Equally, the application of performance indicators for health care services will ensure the cost effectiveness and consumer satisfaction now demanded by health care users and providers. These factors, together with new university courses in healthcare informatics offered world-wide, will guarantee the emergence of a critical mass of well educated and experienced health informatics personnel over the next decade. These many and diverse developments will transform the delivery of health care at all levels, benefiting health consumers and leading to improve health for all.

REFERENCES

British Journal of Healthcare Computing (Editorial) 1994 Empire of the future: déjà vu. 11(4):12

Brittain J M, Abbott W (eds) 1993 Information management and technology training and education in healthcare. Taylor Graham, London

Brittain J M, MacDougall J 1995 Information as a resource in the National Health Service. In: International Journal of Information Management 15(2): 127–133

Brittain J M, Maggs J 1993 Ships in the night: training and education. British Journal of Healthcare Computing and Information Management 10(7):20-22

Gann R 1991 Consumer health information: the growth of an information specialism. Journal of Documentation 47(3):284-308

Greenes R A, Shortliffe E H 1990 Medical informatics. Journal of the American Medical Association 263(8):1114-1120

Lawson M J, Collopy P C 1993 Australian Council on Healthcare Standards care evaluation program. In: Hovenga J S, Whymark G K (eds) HIC '93: Proceedings of the Inaugural National Health Informatics Conference, Brisbane, 2-3 August 1993. Health Informatics Society of Australia, Melbourne

Le Maistre J 1994 News: grand nationally. British Journal of Healthcare Computing and Information Management 11(6):9

MacDougall J, Brittain J M 1992 Use of information in the NHS. British Library Board. London (Library and Information Research Report 92)

MacDougall J, Brittain J M 1994 Healthcare informatics. In: Williams M (ed) Annual review of information science and technology 29:183–217

McIntyre N, Popper K 1983 The critical attitude in medicine: the need for a new ethic. British Medical Journal 1919-1923

Pugsley W 1994 Ready for EDI? British Journal of Healthcare Computing and Information Management 11(6):26-27

United Kingdom National Health Service Training Authority and Information Management Group 1989 IMT strategy for training and staff development. National Health Service, Training Authority, London

Walker D 1993 Editorial: to succeed, computers need to be 'irresistible'. Informatics in Healthcare Australia 2(5):5-6

Warden J 1993 The Wessex fiasco. British Medical Journal 306, 1292

24

Preparing staff for information technology

PETER FEENEY

The health system is expanding the use of IT. To manage the accompanying changes staff education, staff attitudes and the management of change require addressing.

There are many barriers in the path of information technology. The health system relies heavily on the visible print and paper culture, the Gutenberg Culture. The key to overcoming this is the recognition that computers merely act as a mechanism for the storage and retrieval of information (Biscoe 1986). Other factors that influence the health system stem from the fear of losing control over the power of knowledge and confidence. To succeed, computers need to be irresistible (Walker 1993).

Staff education

It is essential to the success of an IT implementation that all staff obtain sufficient training to quell the fear of losing control and the loss of confidence. The health sector has recognised this (Purcell 1994). The education not only encompasses training in the new software, it also includes the introduction of new terminology and basic computer skills to all staff. On commencement of employment, new staff are introduced to computer terminology or jargon. Terminology education relevant to the hardware configuration in use is provided for new employees through the orientation program.

The first session does not require hands-on participation but aims to alleviate some of the technophobia that relates to computer jargon. A second education session involves hands-on experience for the participants. This second session introduces first time computer users to concepts and terminology specifically related to the hardware environment, including the logging on procedure. Switches and lights on a terminal and personal computer are described together with what these mean to the user. A practice session using the keyboard allows the users to put into practice what they have learnt. Troubleshooting problems is also covered; for example, how to solve problems with printing and when to contact the Help Desk and what to tell them. Data security and privacy consideration such as password security and detecting security violations are covered, as are ergonomic and occupational health and safety issues that relate to computers.

Advances in information technology provide exciting opportunities for education in the health sector (McPherson 1994). Future courses must direct user education at several levels. The emphases being on courses that provide a practical, hands-on approach (Purcell & Feeney 1993).

Change

Change is becoming a more common event in the work place. Change is continuous and necessary to respond to internal and external changes in technology, attitudes, organisational structures, policies, consumer expectations and many other internal and external factors. These factors initiate change. The changes in technology in the past twenty years have been enormous: technology has realised such wonders as penicillin, open heart surgery and the birth control pill (Kotler et al 1989). Changes in the size and cost of computers allow users to have a computer in the work place or at home. The changes in technology have occurred with increasing frequency and speed: 'every new technology is a force of creative destruction' (Kotler et al 1989). Transistors displaced the vacuum-tube industry and videos have displaced the movies. It is, of course, futile to fight the fact that change is going to occur.

External forces for change like government cutbacks, rapidly increasing costs of labour, and services can impact on the health system. Internal forces, particularly from new strategies and technologies are pressures for change (Stoner et al 1985). Service changes influence organisational changes. Some service changes 'involve radical reconfiguration of the service' (Kotler et al 1989). For example, the Domiciliary Midwifery Program has remodelled obstetric nursing, changing its focus from the traditional health institution to caring for the patient at home (James et al 1987). The introduction of fresh business ideas such as day surgery has radically changed the face of health services by decreasing the length of stay (DHHCS 1991). This has relieved some of the time pressures that are prevalent in society. 'All of these forces for change come about because of changes in the business requirement' (Ferraby 1991).

Many changes in the health system are coming about because of the development of an increasing number of clinical computing systems. The systems range in size from a PC stand alone to a full scale hospital information system. Recognition of the changes by the health system is already evident (Sittig 1993). The technology revolution has traditionally brought in technology to fit around the work. Now work practices need to change to maximise the potential benefits of technology. In conjunction with information technology changes to the health care system can be radically rethought, from the current work practices to the delivery of service (Fitzpatrick 1993).

Attitudes

Resistance to change has not lessened with the introduction of information technology. Indeed the pace of the technology revolution has heightened fears that users are becoming subservient to machines and stiffened user resistance to technology (Hussain & Hussain 1988). Detecting resistance to a computer environment may be noticed by a drop in service, failure to meet service requirements, increased absenteeism, high staff turnover, complaints, low morale and a reluctance to learn new job skills. Resistance to information technology at the managerial level can be that managers feel hemmed in by information technology, and that the computer systems limit their choices because they are central to important decision making.

The use of behaviour alteration strategies facilitates the changes in attitude. The first of these is the directive change, imposed by management: compulsory sessions performed that all staff are to attend; resistors co-opted to play an active role, for example, identifying problems and planning solutions. A climate receptive to change is vital when new information technology is being introduced to an organisation (Hussain & Hussain 1988). Without human co-operation, the new technology is unlikely to live up to its productivity potential.

Organisational culture

The philosophy that underlies organisation policy determines organisational culture (Vecchio et al 1992). There are three levels of organisational culture and each has its own interaction with the organisation. Every organisation, regardless of size, has a formal and clearly defined set of relationships (Fulmer 1989). The first level of an organisation's culture is its artefacts and creations. This includes the physical layout of the premises, the technology, the signs, rituals and stories. The second level of organisational culture consists of the values. These being the sense of what ought to be, as distinctive from what is. The third level of organisational culture reflects the basic underlying assumptions. These assumptions develop when organisational values become entrenched, taken for granted, and assumed to be unchanging. To achieve an understanding of the organisation's culture there is a need to collect information. Efficient and effective communication is a requirement for the gathering and distribution of information (Vecchio et al 1992).

Fact finding tools

The most important element of an information system is people (Whitten et al 1989). More important than anything else, people want inclusion regarding things that are going to effect their work. Consulting the staff on decisions (Thorn 1990) prior to implementation is the reason for interviewing employees. As employees are most knowledgeable about their work, they have many good ideas that need acknowledgement and respect. In this process one needs to determine who performs the work, what and when the work is being done, where the information goes, why does it happen that way, and how complete it is.

There are many different evaluation tools employed to effect the gathering of information. There is no single source that describes in detail the steps and numerous tools available to help the investigator carry out and interpret the documentation collected (Sittig 1993). Some of the tools available are:

- sampling existing documentation, forms, and files (Burch 1992)
- research and site visits
- observation of the work environment
- interviews and group work sessions (Whitten et al 1992).
- time-motion analysis
- personal record of activities
- subjective evaluations (Sittig 1993).

The documentation required to gain an understanding of workflow includes documents that describe the business function being studied. These documents may include policy manuals that place restraints on the information flow; completed forms that represent transactions at various points of the process; and standard operating procedures, job descriptions, and task instructions from procedure manuals that specify day-to-day operations.

The second fact-finding tool includes the researching of the processes. This involves visiting other sites, other companies or departments that have completed implementation to assess potential for implementation in the health system. The objective of the visit is to document the delivery of patient care and monitoring quality of delivered patient care (IRMC-Nursing Consultants 1992). Observance of the work environment is one of the most effective tools for data collection and for obtaining an understanding of the work flows. The use of this technique is to validate data collected through these methods. Complex tasks are often difficult to explain clearly. The use of observation to identify the complex tasks of workflow alleviate the difficulty of clear oral explanation. At this time the collection of data describing the physical environment such as physical layout, traffic, lighting, and noise level will complete the observation study. Workflows identify how and by whom the system is used and how much time is spent using the system. Before commencing any observation permission from the appropriate supervisor or managers should be obtained. Inform the people that you are intending to observe and state the purpose of the observation.

There are three rules to follow strictly when observing workflow. These are:

- Do not under any circumstances interrupt individuals at work.
- Do not focus on trivial activities.

284

- Do not make any assumptions (Whitten et al 1989).

Interviews are another beneficial and often used fact-finding technique. The purpose of interviews is for fact verification and clarification of workflows; to generate enthusiasm and get the user involved; and to identify user requirements and solicit ideas and opinions from users. The structured interview has some planned questions and others are spontaneous to clarify the answers provided by the interviewee.

Time-motion analysis provides a direct measurement of activities (Sittig 1993). There are a number of work measurement techniques available. The benefit of time and motion study is that these provide accurate time values regarding how long a qualified worker should take to perform the selected activity to achieve the desired result. The disadvantages of time and motion studies are that they require qualified people to conduct them.

Alternatively the self reporting of activities and the time required to perform them rely heavily on the subject's memory and are prone to error. This method is a subjective evaluation of time estimates. Self reporting and the use of questionnaires are useful for job analysis purposes and relatively easy to administer, interpret and obtain valuable information concerning work activities. Such methods provide imprecise measurements of work activities but the use of questionnaires in conjunction with one or more of the other fact finding methods, do provide important information (Sittig 1993). It is essential that the user provides the most appropriate and relevant information using one or all of the methods discussed.

Business process re-engineering

The health system is endeavouring to take full advantage of the potential offered by new technologies. One method that provides an opportunity to radically rethink health care delivery is *business process re-engineering* (Fitzpatrick 1993). This uses an enterprise wide approach to identify key business outcomes and to determine both the value and the quality of services (Fitzpatrick 1993). Business process re-engineering approaches projects from a three pronged viewpoint: (1) the personnel, (2) the technology, (3) the process itself. Business process re-engineering controls change at three levels in the organisation. The sponsor levels determine the scope of the changes (Morris & Brandon 1993). The executive of the organisation sponsors the enterprise wide changes (Thorn 1989). Enterprise wide changes initiated by the executive of the organisation are usually components of the organisational strategic plans. A single executive steering committee oversees the enterprise wide projects and address issues that cross departmental boundaries. Process improvement changes are proposed by the teams involved with change, for example, departmental managers or supervisors. Process improvements initiated can improve a single process or a group of interrelated processes. Finally, the users initiate the task level changes, with some management co-ordination. Task level changes are creative responses to the need to get the job done. These are often subtle changes or modifications to existing workflows (Morris & Brandon 1993).

One or more objectives drive the re-engineering effort. The organisation drives each objective linked to the business goal. The common criteria for re-engineering objectives are that they support the organisation business plan. The objectives reduce time in completing tasks, reduce the number of staff to complete the task or establish a new service. They also improve standards and the quality of a process and or improve service. Put simply, workflow completes tasks the way the organisation expects. There are three main types of work flow contingencies and the organisation must choose the most appropriate workflow system to achieve its objective. The first of these workflows is the sequential workflows, which complete the work in a strict order. The second workflow is the pooled workflows that are unrelated but contribute to the work group objective. The third workflow is the reciprocal workflows, that produce an output that is an input for other jobs.

The design of work should have two objectives: (1) functional effectiveness, to increase productivity and to enhance the effectiveness of work; and (2) human values, to focus on the maintenance or enhancement of job satisfaction and health and safety (Thorn 1989). The two objectives closely relate to one another and to achieve one without the other is virtually impossible. The question is how to design work that will achieve these objectives.

It is impractical to consider the whole organisation can be re-engineered at one time (Fitzpatrick 1993). It is therefore necessary to increment the changes. There are nine steps to business process re-engineering:

- Identify possible efforts for business process re-engineering.
- Identify workflow categories and conduct the initial impact analysis.
- Select an effort and define the scope of the changes.
- Identify business and work processes.
- Define alternatives, simulate new work processes and workflows within the department.
- Define potential impact of each alternative.
- Select best alternative.
- Implement the selected alternative.
- Update the positioning baseline models and information (Morris & Brandon 1993).

Once there is the need to commit any plan to paper a suitable notation must be chosen. Plans can be drawings, specifications or flow diagrams, and these must all be regarded as a means of communicating information. Several notational methods and languages have been devised for timescale planning (Lock 1988).

Project management

Project management functions are, planning, organising, controlling and leading. The planning function states the activities, estimates how long it will take, and projects what it will cost. The organising function staffs the project team and brings together team members, users, and managers to achieve the project plan. The controlling function monitors progress reports and documents deliverables. It compares plans with what actually happens (Burch 1992).

Two popular project management tools are the program evaluation and review technique (PERT) and Gannt, named after Henry Gannt. A PERT chart estimates, schedules and controls numerous interdependent tasks. The PERT chart determines the minimum amount of time required to complete the project or a phase. A Gannt chart is a bar chart that illustrates phases or tasks. On the left hand side of the Gannt chart the tasks or phases are shown, whilst the number of days, weeks, months are shown across the top of the chart. The Gannt chart compares planned performance with actual per-formance, to determine whether the project schedule is on time. Gannt charts are simple to understand; however, they fail to show relationships with interrelated tasks. This is why the Gannt chart schedules a complete system project, while the PERT chart schedules interrelated tasks (Burch 1992).

Records kept by the project management inform users how the business process has changed. These records will detail the design of the change and construction of the changes. For ease of access and physical security the project library houses this documentation.

The aim of the project leader is to 'bring the project to a successful conclusion', 'successful' being to give the user what they want, working on time and to budget. Project leadership is out of the scope of this chapter, except in so far as it affects business process re-engineering.

The role of confidant is a proper one for the business process engineer and can be useful, provided the business process engineer performs it well. Effecting a relationship, where users can approach the business process engineer and discuss matters in confidence concerning, for example, mistakes made, can only benefit the project.

There are two types of delegated authority that can be given to the business process engineer (Morris and Brandon 1993). First is formal delegation with authority to

- effect small changes (small defined by cost and resources)
- deploy resources within well defined limits
- initiate studies and formulate cost benefit analysis
- halt any changes that are established as a waste of effort.

The second type of authority is informal delegation. The effect of informal delegation is to protect the project leader from unnecessary stress and an excess of information by the business process engineer reporting to the project leader on a regular basis.

The task of identifying change will inevitably come the way of the business process engineer, particularly to fulfil the role of confidant. If a change is too large or will clearly use a substantial amount of resources even before the identification of cost benefits, then the business process engineer submits a brief. This brief is to estimate the amount of time and resources to complete the analysis before commencement on the changes.

The business process engineer will at times act as an instructor, carrying out a great deal of informal education and training for users and their departments. Thorn (1989) states that staff require adequate training and gain the skills and knowledge required to perform the jobs changed by the redesign. If the organisation has not had access to computers prior to the implementation then a new education program as outlined previously, will need to be developed. The business process engineer needs to continue to perform walk-thrus and subsequent follow up discussions with user departments and or individual users.

Hardware installation

We have discussed at length the process for change in relation to performance of work. The final discussion with the user is where to install the hardware for the new system. The involvement of the Occupational Health and Safety Officer is essential to this process as they will provide the expert knowledge concerning ergonomically sound placement of the hardware. The business process engineer will have completed studies of the workflows and the collection of data in the earlier phases of implementation securing the change decisions as close to the action as possible. That knowledge will also assist in the appropriate placement of the hardware. Without the essential aspect of this process, communication, the enabling role of information technology becomes redundant.

Conclusion

In summary, when an organisation is looking at changing the work environment and work practices, the major tool used is communication. Business process re-engineering fits with the continuous quality improvement concept where commitment for change must be fully supported the executives. A system for informing everyone about any planned changes needs to be set up. Information is ideally disseminated on a regular and frequent basis. This will ensure that the organisation is up to date and really knows what is happening. It is important that the business process engineer performs regular visits to the areas where change is having the greatest impact. This will ensure the involvement of the staff in the decisions that need to be made, for these are the people who will be using the system. The provision of training to these people will ensure that they receive adequate training to gain the new skills and knowledge, to provide the ability to work in the changed work environment and to perform the job affected by change. Finally, the changes made require monitoring and evaluating to ensure development of best work practice. In so doing, learn from changes, both successful and failures. The expected outcomes from business process engineering are, first, faster delivery of patient care services, second, a higher quality of care. The third expected outcome is reduced costs and finally greater patient and employee satisfaction (McQueen 1993).

REFERENCES

Biscoe G 1986 Resistance to computers. South East Asian Regional Nursing Conference (SEARNC) Conference Proceedings, Melbourne

Burch J G 1992 System analysis, design, and implementation. Boyd Fraser, Boston

DHHCS 1991 National Health Strategy Issue Paper No. 1 The Australian health jigsaw. Department of Health, Housing and Community Services, Canberra

Ferraby L 1991 Change control: during computer systems development. Prentice Hall, Sydney

Fitzpatrick G 1993 Business process redesign-transforming care processes. In: Hovenga E J S, Whymark G (eds) HIC'93 Brisbane Conference Proceedings, HISA, Melbourne

Fulmer R M 1989 The new management, 4th edn. Macmillan, New York

Hussain D, Hussain K 1988 Managing computer resources: managing resistance to change. Irwin, Illinois

IRMC-Nursing Consultants 1992 Report on HIS site visits. NSW Health Department

James M L, Hudson C N, Gebski V J 1987 Cost benefits of planned early postnatal transfer home with nursing support. Department of Obstetrics Westmead Hospital, Westmead

Kotler P, Chandler P, Gibbs R, McColl R 1989 Marketing in Australia, 2nd edn. Prentice Hall, Sydney

Lock D 1988 Project management, 5th edn. Gower Publishing, Aldershot

McPherson J 1994 Pathology 1994 Challenges for education. Health Informatics Association NSW (HIANSW) Conference Proceedings, Pokolbin

McQueen H E 1993 The healthcare CIOs role in business process redesign. Computer in Healthcare, February

Morris D, Brandon J 1993 Re-engineering your business. McGraw Hill, New York

Purcell J 1993 Determining the impact of health information systems on practice before implementation. In: Hovenga E J S, Whymark G (eds) HIC'93 Brisbane Conference Proceedings, HISA, Melbourne

Purcell J, Feeney P 1994, Computer literacy education: introduction to computers for health care personnel: an evaluation. Health Informatics Association NSW (HIANSW) 1994 Conference Proceedings, Pokolbin

Sittig D F 1993 Work-sampling: a statistical approach to evaluation of the effect of computers on work patterns in healthcare. Methods of Information in Medicine 32:167-74

Stoner J A F, Collins R R, Yetton P W 1985 Management in Australia. Prentice Hall, Sydney

Thorn J, 1990 Managing change. The Industrial Society, London

Walker D 1993 To succeed, computers need to be irresistible, Editorial, Informatics in Healthcare Australia 2(5)

Whitten J L, Bentley L D, Barlow V M 1989 System analysis and design. Irwin, Boston

Vecchio R P, Hearn G, Southey G 1992 Organisational behaviour: life at work in Australia. Harcourt Brace Janovich, Sydney

FURTHER READING

Davenport T H 1993 Process innovation: re-engineering work through information technology. Harvard Business School Press, Boston

Dunphy D C 1981 Organisation change by choice. McGraw Hill, Sydney

Hammer M, Champy J 1993 Re-engineering the corporation: a manifestation for business revolution. Nicholas Brearly, London

Lundeberg M A 1992 Framework for recognizing pattern when reshaping business processes. Journal of Strategic Information Systems 11(3) (June)

Mukhi S, Hampton D, Barnwell 1991 Australian management. McGraw Hill, Sydney

Scott Morton M 1991 (ed) The corporation of the 1990s: information technology and organisational transformation. Oxford University Press, Melbourne

25

Information technology management

ROHAN JAYASURIYA, GRAY SOUTHON

Management of information technology in health presents a very special challenge. The IT industry itself is a dynamic, rapidly evolving field, with a continuous stream of new technologies bringing new possibilities and challenges. However IT is not merely a technological issue, as it is generally found that many of the most difficult problems are about the way the technology relates to the organisation. If technology is going to be effective in most cases, then substantial changes in the way the organisation operates is necessary (Coombs et al 1992). These changes involve many conflicting factors which can be political, managerial, industrial, cultural, and may require substantial changes in skills, and roles. Implementation is much more than a technical process, and involves skills of politicians, salesmen, project management and organisational change agents (Keen 1991). It is an area that can be highly controversial and very costly, often with considerable dissatisfaction and with significant levels of failure (Sauer 1993). In addition to these problems, health is possibly one of the most complex of environments, which makes the management of information in the health industry extremely demanding.

IT in the health environment

The health information environment itself is very complex. There are a wide range of professional specialities of varying sophistication, each with their own types of information. Much of the information is of a *high level* involving rich descriptions of complex organisms (people), with factors such as intentionality, cognition, self consciousness and behaviour (Blois & Shortliffe 1990). In addition, much information is qualitative, subjective, intuitive and transient. This information is normally handled directly by professional staff, and not amenable to technological solutions. Thus IT can contribute as only part of the information processes within a health environment. Nevertheless, the data which is computerised can be very important, and needs to be accurate, timely and secure. People's lives and privacy depend on it. Further, with the continual changing nature and requirements of information due to advances in medical technology, the need for flexibility must be high. All these factors place considerable demands on the capabilities of the systems.

Within the health industry, two major types of environments can be identified, hospital-based services and community-based services. It is in hospitals that most of the resources in staff and money is expended in the health sector. Two main types of computing in the hospitals pertain to management and clinical activities. Managerial computing originated with financial systems, and gradually expanded to include those systems required to co-ordinate and control the many supporting business functions involved in operating a hospital, including the movement of patients. Clinical systems were originally independent, specialised systems usually directly under the control of the clinicians themselves. Slowly, these systems are being brought together in various ways, with the objective of providing an integrated information system focused on the patient (Minard 1991). However, both groups of systems are often highly fragmented within themselves and most often consist of a mixture of commercial and purpose-built systems, involving different hardware and software platforms.

Expenditure on IT ranges between 7-10% of operating budget in most industries and can be much higher in transaction-intensive organisations such as insurance companies and banks (De Luca 1992). However, in the health sector, expenditure is much less. In hospital environments in the USA it is estimated to be 2.5-3.5% when telecommunications is excluded (De Luca 1992). Over the last decade investments of IT in the health sector have increased rapidly in Australia. The $800 million 10 year IT strategy in NSW Health will increase the spending in IT from less than 1% of budget to around 2% (Crawford 1992). Queensland will spend $80-100 million in seven years in their project to upgrade IT in 14 of their major hospitals (Fitzpatrick 1992). In spite of the substantial outlays in monetary terms world-wide, the development of IT in the health sector is regarded to be still relatively primitive (Joiner 1992).

The growth of computing in the health sector has typically been concentrated on hospitals. Community based information systems, despite relative growth over the years, have been neglected, resulting in rather uncoordinated, fragmented systems (Jayasuriya 1993).

Managing IT in organisations has been given more emphasis with the increasing costs of IT and the strategic importance of IT to business (Ward et al 1990, Boynton et al 1992). The most important aspect of managing IT is ensuring that the IT activities are heading in the same direction as the rest of the organisation (Glaser 1991). Schmitz (1987) considered that information must be managed as one of the most important resources of the organisation. On the lack of importance given to this he says 'many organisations give a responsibility to a data processing manager for the information that happens to reside in the computer and trust to luck that all the information in the organisation needed to make important organisational decisions will come together in a meaningful way'.

Structures for IT management

Much of the literature on IT structure in organisations has centred around the debate of centralised and decentralised IT management. The general IT literature recognises that, over time due to the decrease in economic costs and need for strategic alignment of IS to business strategy, there is a move towards decentralisation of IT function to line management (Rockart 1988). At the same time it is recognised that the roles and functions of the central IT group have also undergone major change (La Belle & Nyce 1987). Devising and negotiating an effective *IT management structure* is a crucial policy issue. Boyton et al (1992) identified four factors that affect a firm's IT management responsibility and apportioned them to be:

- the extent of the organisation's need for networking resources (i.e. exchange of information among multiple business units)
- the specific requirements to share data elements among business units and external firms
- the extent to which applying common applications across the organisation is desirable
- the requirement for specialised human resources related to IT.

If the patient is to be the focus of attention and the patient record to be the entity around which all information activities are to centre (Dick & Steen 1991), integration of information is an important strategy. Once health managers come to realise that their information requirements need to closely align with clinicians' information needs or be derived from patient management information, one might be able to vision the data network as the most powerful integrating force in operation in a modern hospital (Barone & Chickadonz 1992).

The current status of IT structures in a typical Australian hospital differs depending on a number of factors. The chief among them has been the organisational structure of the health system which varies by State. Other factors pertain to the size of the hospital and resources available. In NSW, IT services are centralised in an area/district. Typically the IT department is physically located in the major hospital, though its functions cover all IT for the area/district. In most instances these area/district organisations work within the overall State IT strategy. By contrast, in Victoria and South Australia hospitals were given guidelines for central reporting but each developed their IT independently. However, certain systems are centralised for processing such as payroll.

A recent trend is *outsourcing* which is the use of external agents to perform one or more of the IT activities (Lacity & Hirschheim 1993). Proponents argue for its increase in IS effectiveness, long-term cost savings and freedom to pursue more strategic IS issues. Opponents on the other hand highlight problems such as loss of IT expertise and the threat of the vendor taking advantage of the client. For instance, experience of the Health Department of the Northern Territory found that outsourcing was inordinately expensive and resulted in the need to rebuild the IS function in the department afterwards (Smith 1992).

Recent trends in Australia suggest that larger IT departments would be in a competitive position to provide services on a *fee for service* basis to smaller IT units. Smaller health organisations will find it cost efficient to purchase services for batch processing of financial and administrative data and to obtain 24-hour user support for their clinical systems. Developments in the communication highways throughout Australia would enable health organisations in rural areas to obtain these services. This would eventually lead towards IT departments functioning as 'provider corporations' as is occurring with some large businesses (Nosworthy 1994).

Project management

Project management refers to the co-ordination of a complex of processes associated with a major initiative. Perhaps the biggest challenge that an IT department faces is the selection (or development) and implementation of a major system.

The first requirement is to have a reasonably clear idea of the types of functions that are required to be covered (see Ch. 7). In this process it is critical to have user involvement in the decision. However simple a task might appear from the outside, it is virtually guaranteed to be more complex than expected. Users are understandably unwilling to accommodate deficiencies in the system if they weren't adequately involved in the decision making. However, involving users can be a very difficult task as well, particularly if there are a wide range of users involved. The task can be made more difficult if some of the users are too busy to put sufficient effort into understanding the system. In the final analysis, it is important for the users to have a realistic concept of how the system will help them in their work.

Once it is established what the system will do, the next question is whether to build or buy. One would normally expect that buying would have advantages over building, by being able to take advantage of the experience of other users and the capabilities of commercial developers. However, it turns out that many institutions continue to develop their own systems. This is for a combination of reasons:

- Hospitals tend to be organised in many different ways because of their history and the people involved and the legislative and administrative demands on it. They would rather have a system built around their needs, rather than accommodate structures to fit into a bought system. They also don't want to pay for superfluous functions.
- If a hospital builds its own system, then it has greater control over its development, and there is ability to modify it as required.

- Technological developments can make commercial systems obsolete, and make it more attractive to build something that uses the latest technology, and perhaps uses more efficient development techniques.
- Commercial development and marketing costs can outweigh the costs of shared development.

For example, one hospital searching for a commercial radiology system found commercial prices in the region of $400 000 and above, yet these systems did not meet important requirements for integration with other systems. A system was then purpose-built for $30 000.

Vendor selection is a critical step if the decision is taken to acquire a system. Steps in this process (De Luca 1992) are:

1 Request for Information (RFI). This is an initial screening of vendors using a short questionnaire to gather some basic data from the vendor and its products.
2 Request for Proposal (RFP). This elicits essential information from all selected vendors in a standard format to compare systems with each other.
3 Vendor demonstrations and site visits. When buying a system, it is most important that the key staff have an opportunity to see it in operation in a similar institution (not just in demonstration) and preferably to talk to people who have also purchased it, as well as the people who developed it.
4 Assessment of systems. This will consider the overall suitability of the systems including an economic analysis. Sometimes a consultant is brought in at this stage to assess the technology. The systems will be ranked and contract negotiations undertaken with the first ranked vendor.

If the decision is made to develop a system, it is important to ensure that the resources and experience are available. Building a major system requires careful management. In the 1970s a method for managing this development—the System Development Life Cycle (SDLC)—emerged as the Waterfall Model (Blum & Orthner 1989).

At each stage of the life cycle a project milestone is identified and deliverables are signed off. The cycle starts with an analysis of the needs, then the development of a functional specification. This design usually is a combination of data flow diagrams, which describe how information moves from place to place; data structures, which show how the various bits of information link together; and screen layouts, which show how data is presented on the screen, and how the various screens are linked together. These requirements must be checked with the users and signed off before proceeding. Then the design, coding and debugging is undertaken. Finally there is the installation, and maintenance, which includes updating.

In the late 1970s, structured systems development methods emerged, many of which are in use today. One of these, for instance, the Structured Systems Analysis and Design Methodology (SSADAM) has been mandated in the National Health Service in Britain (Hepworth et al 1992). They usually consist of many volumes of detailed instructions, which often need to be adapted to the task. They can, however, make the development process very cumbersome and increase development time.

One of the critical tasks of the SDLC is getting the design right before the system is built, as it is very expensive making changes at a later stage. Therefore much effort is usually put into the design stage, and careful documentation is carried out. One popular means of doing this is the Joint Application and Design (Smith et al 1992) which involves teams of users working with the developer to establish the requirements.

In the early 1980s the availability of fourth generation languages (4GLs) enabled an alternate development path to be taken. Unlike traditional SDLC, progressive iterative development or *prototyping* was more feasible. In prototyping, mock-ups of the system are developed so users can get a better feel for how the system will finally work (Sprague & McNurlin 1993).

The above methodologies are based on the assumption that system requirements are basically knowable in advance. However, as shown by Jones & Walsham (1992), there are many ways in which our ability to see into a future situation are limited. A rather different type of approach is *evolutionary* development which doesn't assume this pre-knowledge. Evolutionary development recognises that requirements are going to change, and that users have only limited knowledge initially. The system first built may be only a small part of what is finally envisaged, and once that is in use, then users can refine and expand their requirements for the next version. This can be highly successful for relatively simple systems. Evolutionary development can make it difficult to maintain technical integrity when systems are complex.

With the increasing complexity of system development it is becoming very difficult to ensure everything ties together properly, and a number of tools have been developed to help IT staff. One important tool aimed at automating the development of large applications is Computer Aided Software Engineering (CASE), which automates flow diagrams, data-base design, software engineering, and coding. The benefits of CASE are increased programmer productivity, higher quality software, easier maintenance and co-ordination of complex jobs. While these can be attractive, sometimes the training costs and other inconveniences can detract substantially from the benefits (Fenton 1993). Another development has been the use of object-oriented programming systems development methods. With both of these technologies, it is important that there is practical evidence that they achieve what one wants of them in similar circumstances to which they are being used, and that start-up and training costs are properly considered.

Management control and evaluation of information systems

The framework for management control that is widely accepted relates to a model by Anthony et al (1989). They define management control as 'all methods, procedures and devices, including management control systems, that management uses to assure compliance with organisational policies and strategies'. It is difficult to apply traditional management control concepts to control of information system activities for a number of reasons. Firstly, information systems serve three levels of management. Secondly, they include many subsystems that vary in relative importance (a good example in hospital information systems is between clinical decision support and accounting information). Finally, information systems are continually needing to work with new IT (and in the case of health, new technologies of medicine and procedures). Moreover, some of those IT activities are of an experimental or research nature.

Some of the concepts of Evaluation Research are useful in the development of a framework for discussing control measures. Formative evaluation encompasses the process of development of the information systems and their maintenance. The evaluation of a system in operation can serve a number of objectives:

- It can demonstrate whether the intended productivity improvements such as decreases in resources have been achieved.
- Show barriers and difficulties that prevent full exploitation of the system by its users and can lead to action to remove these barriers.
- Provide evidence upon which future developments and plans can be built.
- Reveal unexpected side-effects of the system; positive effects that would give direction for future development; and negative effects that need remedial actions (Eason 1988).

Much of the research in IT evaluation has grappled with the measurement of *impact* of the system. Impact evaluation in the context of information systems is the determination of how the implementation and use of an information systems application affects the organisation. A useful classification by Eason (1988) brings in the concept of levels of evaluation (and control). He identifies four levels as:

- Technical systems performance—this encompasses the technical quality of the system which is usually undertaken by quality assurance of software development.
- User evaluation of technical services—this level ascertains the functionality and usability of the system.
- User performance and satisfaction—this level assesses the impact of the system on the users and their job performance.
- Socio-technical systems performance—at this level an organisational evaluation is conducted to establish whether the system is performing efficiently and effectively. It is at this level the question of cost benefit is posed.

User satisfaction has been utilised as a construct to measure *success of IT*. An instrument to measure this construct has been applied in a hospital setting by Zviran (1992). End user satisfaction has also been used by hospital management to take decisions on acquisition of new software (Bailey 1990).

However, user perception constitutes only one viewpoint of the multiple dimensions of systems performance.

In the field of information systems, though in practice much effort is taken to justify the benefits of the system prior to its development, many organisations do not conduct evaluations of the system once the decision is taken to build it. The conduct of a post implementation review, when the conversion to a new system is complete, provides the organisation with useful information on the costs and benefits of the system. Post implementation evaluation (review) includes evaluations performed just before installation, just after installation and considerably after installation once the system has a chance to settle down (Kumar 1990). Evidence from Canada in business shows that in most cases these evaluations are conducted only after a project is completed and usually by the systems development team. Since the evaluation is to test the design and development process, it is questionable whether any basic flaws in the process or product will be discovered by such evaluations (Kumar 1990).

Assessment of IT benefits have generally focused on the measurement of efficiency though Sprague & McNurlin (1993) claim the largest payoffs from IT lie in improving effectiveness. To quantify benefits Keen (1991) suggests using operational indicators of performance that can be used over time called *anchor measures*. Curley and Henderson (1992) identified that the potential level of IT benefits differ according to level of the organisation and that IT investments extend beyond business performance. Based on this concept they developed a value assessment framework to assess IT benefit.

Evaluation of hospital information systems has tended to be limited to those done just before handing over. However, some IT managers have built in systems of quality assurance that allow them to obtain feedback from users as to their satisfaction with the IT support (Robinson 1994). In reality, though major investments in IT have occurred in the health industry in Australia, there have not been many rigorous assessments of its benefits and impact on the work of the organisations.

Early IT systems addressed quite straightforward tasks, and often made very expensive jobs cheaper. However, as the tasks became more complex and the costs increased, then the benefits became more difficult to identify. This was for a number of reasons:

- The benefits were in the capabilities that were provided. These could only be realised if people chose to make use of them. Hence, the value of a system depends very much on political and human issues that are often not properly considered in system design.
- The benefits were widely distributed and confused with many other activities. For instance, many of the benefits of IT investments in the eighties have only come about with the thinning out of middle management.
- The systems were technology driven—introduced more because people were impressed with the technology and have a simplistic belief in its benefits. Often they had not made the effort to be specific about the benefits they want achieved.

In order to improve the performance of IT, benefit realisation has been introduced as a strategy. This is directed more at the implementation process, and seeks to measure the impact of the system in terms of corporate benefit. This relies on a clear measurable output for the organisation and a high degree of stability.

However, the complexities and uncertainties of the health industry makes this very difficult to apply. The overall benefits of any system are often complex, variable, and very difficult to measure.

Lessons from IT failures: organisational system issues

Like any technology, IT has its failures, as well as its successes. In areas such as aeronautics or civil engineering, a failure is very thoroughly analysed. There is usually much learnt from such failures. Unfortunately, this is not so in the IT industry, as failures can be partial, and are often lost in a mass of organisational politics. The very definition of failure is uncertain (Sauer 1993). Nevertheless, one can identify some fairly consistent patterns in IT development among the major systems that have been developed around Australia and New Zealand.

The implementations are typically embarked upon with substantial promises of benefits, including the enhancement of clinical services, better support for staff, and better management information. Management often approves the programs with very limited understanding of the implications or the risks. Projects are undertaken by a very enthusiastic IT staff, but they find it very difficult to consult effectively with a large and very busy staff, who may have somewhat unrealistic expectations of the system. Then there are usually delays in the implementation. Throughout this period, dissatisfaction amongst users gradually develops from such causes as inadequate consultation, delayed implementation, inadequate functionality, inconvenience of use and high costs. When management may be reluctant to face the criticism from powerful interest groups, it may be difficult for them to provide unequivocal support for the system. The increasing controversy can have an effect on the IT staff, reducing their morale, and increasing their turnover. In spite of all these difficulties and often with inadequate training and preparation, the system usually does operate, but does not fulfil the original expectations. The frustrated expectations and residual problems leave a general feeling of dissatisfaction.

Following the implementation, rapid changes in technology increase the difference between what people are getting, and what they feel they ought to have, and generate pressure for the early replacement of the system. If any new system is installed, however, it faces the same pressures and may well repeat the same cycle. There is a great gulf between the enthusiasts, who focus on the system's achievements, and the sceptics, who focus on its problems.

While this scenario is not universally the case, it is relatively common, and is largely predictable (Colclough 1992). It is worthwhile considering the lessons that might be learned from these experiences:

- Recognise the limitations of initial requirements analysis, and ensure that there is flexibility for the system to grow with expectations and changing demands. Make sure expectations are realistic, and the implementation is divided into steps that are manageable.
- Take into account the complex power structures in the organisation. Ensure that the management and principle power groups understand the implications of the system and are prepared to commit themselves to coping with the political implications of it. They must recognise the complex of interests involved, and have staff of sufficient seniority to address the issues.
- Understand the nature of the corporate objectives. Corporate planning in health is relatively immature, and plans do not always relate effectively to the work that the organisation does.
- Monitor top management support, and determine any reason that support is flagging. An IT project may be seen as merely one more claim for scarce resources, rather than as a strategic asset. An IT department can easily miss out on the claim for funds, making it even more difficult to deliver promises.
- Ensure there are good relationships between IT staff and users. This is a problem that has been most prevalent with central IT staff in IT in general (Smith et al 1992), and is common in health. Any major system forces changes on the organisation that are usually difficult to understand, and tension is almost inevitable. It is important that IT staff understand the problems, and are focused on helping users cope with the system.
- Beware of the phenomenon of 'escalating commitment to a failing cause'. When decision makers do not accept failure, they will continue to commit resources without abandoning the system.

Conclusion

Management of IT in health care organisations is not merely a technological issue. If it is to be of substantial use, changes in the way health care organisations operate are necessary. This has not been the usual case, partly because of the many inherent factors in a complex organisation such as a hospital that is driven by professionals. IT management therefore requires the skills in implementing projects, managing organisational change and evaluation. Techniques and tools have emerged in recent years to help in management of IT. However, experience in Australia and overseas shows that IT has had significant failures which are very costly. Lessons from IT failures are useful in refining these methods that could address demanding organisations such as those found in the health sector.

ACKNOWLEDGEMENTS

The authors would like to thank Ian Lumb, Denis Nosworthy and Mike Robinson for commenting on earlier drafts of this chapter.

REFERENCES

Anthony R N, Dearden J, Bedford, N M 1989 Management control systems, 6th edn. Irwin, Homewood

Bailey J E 1990 Development of an instrument for management of computer user attitudes in hospitals. Methods of Information in Medicine 29:51-56

Barone C A, Chickadonz G H 1991 Organisational transformation: responding to technological innovation. In: Ball M J, Douglas J V, O'Desky R I, Albright J W (eds) Healthcare information management systems. Springer-Verlag, New York 260-269

Blois M S, Shortliffe E H 1990 The computer meets medicine: emergence of a discipline. In: Shortliffe E H, Perreault L E (eds) Medical informatics: computer applications in health care. Reading, Addison-Wesley

Blum B F, Orthner H F 1989 Implementing health care information systems. New York, Springer-Verlag

Boyton A C, Jacobs G C, Zmud R W 1992 Whose responsibility is IT management?. Sloan Management Review Summer: 32-38

Colclough I 1992 The influence of culture when implementing new systems in hospitals. Healthcover Jun-Jul: 38-40

Coombs R D, Knights et al 1992 Culture, control and competition: towards a conceptual framework for the study of information technology in organisations. Organisation Studies 13(1):51-72

Crawford P 1992 Information technology and NSW health. Healthcover (Oct/Nov 1992): 30-34

Curley K, Henderson J 1992 Assessing the value of a corporate-wide human resource information system: a case study. In: Sprague R H, McNurlin B C 1993 Information systems management in practice, 3rd edn. Prentice Hall, Englewood Cliff 319-322

De Luca J M 1992 Health care information systems. American Hospital Publishing, Philadelphia

Dick S D, Steen E B (eds) 1991 The computer-based patient record. Washington, National Academy Press

Eason K 1988 User evaluation. In: Information Technology and Organisational Change. Taylor and Francis, London 10:87-203

Fenton N 1993 How effective are software engineering methods. Journal of Systems Software 22:141-146

Fitzpatrick G 1992 Meeting health care informatics needs. a case study of Queensland Health Hospital-based Corporate Information Systems Project. Department of Computer Science Technical Report Series Number 246, University of Queensland, Brisbane

Glaser J P 1991 Managing the management of information systems. Healthcare Executive, Jan-Feb 12-15

Hepworth J B, Griffin E et al 1992 Adopting and information management approach to the design and implementation of information systems. Health Services Management Research 5(2):115-122

Jayasuriya R 1993 Computerised community health information systems: current developments in NSW. University of Wollongong Press, NSW Community Health Accreditation and Standards Program, Sydney

Joiner D 1992 Hospitals in crisis. Healthcare Informatics 9(2):62-66

Jones M, Walsham G 1992 The limits of the knowable: organisational and design knowledge in systems development. In: The impact of computer supported technologies on information systems development, Amsterdam, North-Holland, 195-213

Keen P G W 1991 Shaping the future: business design through information technology. Harvard Business School Press, Boston

Kumar K 1990 Post implementation evaluation of computer-based information systems: current practices. Communications of Association for Computing Machinery (ACM) 33(2):203-212

La Belle A, Nyce E 1987 Whither the IT organisation? Sloan Management Review 28(4):75-85

Lacity M, Hirschheim R 1993 Implementing information systems outsourcing: key issues and experience of an early adopter. Journal of General Management 19(1):17-31

Minard B 1991 Health care computer systems for the 1990s. Ann Arbor, American College of Healthcare Executives

Nosworthy D 1994 Director, Information Services, South-Western Sydney Area Health Services. Personal communication

Robinson M 1994 Manager, Computer Services, Illawarra Area Health Services. Personal communication

Rockart J 1988 The line takes the leadership: IS management in a wired society. Sloan Management Review Summer:57-64

Sauer C 1993 Why information systems fail: a case study approach. Alfred Waller, Henley-on-Thames

Schmitz H H 1987 Managing healthcare information resources. Rockville, Aspen

Smith H A, Smith M J D 1992 Computerization and management: a study of conflict and change. Information and Management 22:53-64

Smith J 1992 Health information systems for policy and planning in the Northern Territory 1987-92 Informatics in Healthcare, Australia 2(3):31-37

Sprague R H, McNurlin B C 1993 Information systems management in practice, 3rd edn. Englewoods Cliffs, Prentice Hall

Ward J, Griffiths P, Whitmore P 1990 Strategic planning for information systems. John Wiley, Chichester

Zviran M 1992 Evaluating user satisfaction in a hospital environment: an exploratory study. Health Care Management Review 17(3):51-62

26

Health informatics in general practice

LYNN M HALL

General practice forms the core of patient information management in primary care and covers a broad range of issues. The general practitioner or family physician must care for all patients who present, treating all ages, socioeconomic classes, ethnic backgrounds, and states of health. The information presenting to the doctor is often undifferentiated resulting in classification difficulties. There is usually more than one problem presenting at an encounter requiring a comprehensive approach to information gathering. The family doctor needs to maintain a longitudinal record of the patient's history with the ability to succinctly summarise the record if the patient moves to another area. There can be legal requirements to keep records for specific time periods. This may require duplication of information if a patient wishes to attend another practitioner.

Relationship to other health workers

General practitioners relate to almost all other personnel in the health area to a greater or lesser extent. Patients may attend their family doctor for general medical care, but attend primary care clinics with special interests such as womens' health clinics, family planning clinics, pain clinics, or sports medicine clinics. Communication between community nurses, paramedical staff such as physiotherapists or podiatrists, pharmacists, dentists, counsellors and alternative medicine practitioners, demonstrate the range of communication which occurs between primary health care workers.

Communication also occurs between the primary care doctor and secondary and tertiary care health workers. Communication between specialists and primary care doctors forms a major component of health information communication for the primary care doctor. This may be directly to the specialist as the treating doctor, to a secondary referral hospital such as a local mental health clinic or geriatric aftercare hospital, or to the major tertiary teaching hospitals both within and outside the local community. Much of this information is in the form of admission assessments and discharge summaries.

The secondary referral centres of diagnostic imaging and pathology transfer information with the primary care physician on a daily basis. Much energy is expended in primary care dealing with this area of health informatics.

Variability of primary care practice style

Clinics operate in a range of different administrative structures. The style of a primary care practice relates to the method by which it attracts funds. Clinics can be owned by doctors, funded directly from government expenditure, funded from hospital budgets, or owned by non medical commercial organisations.

Fee payments for patient primary care services can be either the direct responsiblility of the patient, the government, or the hospital. Patient fees may involve third parties such as governments, health insurance agencies including work related insurance claims, or primary care health claims associated with road accidents. These organisations may be responsible in part or all of the accounts on behalf of the patient.

As funding arrangements vary, so can the style of practice. Episodic care is more appropriate to accident and emergency departments provided by hospitals. Comprehensive continuous care is a feature of the traditional family practice or the hospital outpatient clinics. Community clinics, funded through local or regional governments, are able to offer a public health perspective. These clinics are likely to employ nurse practitioners and other paramedical staff such as social workers, physiotherapists and health educators. This clinic style encourages group education and is better able to assist the socially disadvantaged and people whose first language is not the native tongue.

An alternative system for general practice financial management is that of the fund holding structure being trialled in England. This places the financial responsibilty for total patient care in the hands of the primary care providers. Each of these administrative styles requires its individual accounting structures.

The principal organisational structures in primary care are practice management, clinical record keeping, clinical research and medical education.

Practice management

Practice management has four major components in the general practice setting: patient billing, appointments, practice administration and electronic tools.

Patient billing

Each style of general practice will have its own patient billing method. This has been the first area practices have taken to computerise. In a recent

Australian survey on the attitudes of general practitioners to computerised medical records(Cacek 1992), 35% of general practices were using computers in the practice. Of these 78% were using word processing functions and 63% were undertaking financial management. This is in line with the uptake of computer use in Singapore where between 30-50% of practices have computerised for routine practice management activities (Lun & Goh 1993). The UK experience differs in this regard as patient billing does not fall within the province of the family doctor but 50% of practices are using computers in an administrative capacity (Hayes 1993).

Originally the medical packages were adapted from off the shelf accounting systems, but it was soon realized the modifications required were extensive for the general practice environment or the system failed to satisfy the requirements of the practice. Modern systems software now have been purpose written for the style of practice accounting.

A good accounting system should be structured on a Clinic Master Patient File. Every member of each family should be individually listed. Each patient should be able to have multiple account types depending on their reason for presentation. An example would be a patient attending as a member of a family with a parent as the account payer, as an individual, as a patient funded under a direct account to the government, as a work injured member or as a patient requiring an insurance report. Much flexibility is required within the accounting system. Any system selected by a practice will need to consider ease of use, as this will determine the amount of time taken by office staff to train new and relieving staff. A busy practice needs to be able to give immediate accounts, receipt payments over the counter and resolve account queries. Costs of stationery need to be determined as some systems rely on expensive preprinted stationery while others enable the use of plain paper.

A computerised accounting system can form the basis of a general clinic patient register and enable the use of patient demographics (Kidd et al 1994). An age/sex register can be developed and from this age/sex register preventive care and recall programs can be developed (Hall 1992).

Appointments

The use of computerised appointments has enabled greater flexibility into the organisation of reception. Appointments can be run from the master patient index. This enables correct identification of the particular patient and the appropriate history pulled in readiness prior to the patient attending. New patients are readily identified ensuring extra allotted time if necessary. Cancelled appointments can be removed and logged and the appointment chart will remain uncluttered by altered appointments. Clarity of typing versus hand writing further reduces errors of identification.

Some appointment systems are able to time when a patient arrives and give information on waiting room times. This can assist all members of the clinic with the problem of those visits running over time and with the management of the 'drop in' patient.

For systems using computers in the consulting room for clinical records, the appointment system can be integrated and eliminate the need for the paper record and its sundry retrieving and filing tasks. This is a major time and cost saving in the general practice environment releasing the receptionist for other activities. In the integrated system, the clinician has ready access to the appointment system and is able to keep abreast of changes to the appointment list. A further benefit of a networked or multiuser system is the flexibility of any staff member to answer the telephone call when an allocated member has become preoccupied with other tasks.

Practice administration

The administrative tasks of a modern general practice have become more complex over recent years and in order to manage a practice efficiently tight control needs to be maintained on income and expenses.

Day end procedures

The day end procedures for either a manual or computerised office include a daily list of patient consultations, account status of each consultation, receipts paid to the practice that day, and the banking report for the day or period including that day. A similar series of information could be generated per doctor, and per branch practice. Similarly lists of clinical services can be produced.

Month end procedures (EOM)

The reports generated for month end should also be able to be generated over a practice defined period. This EOM process should print statements to all account holders. A facility for tracking over due debts should be instituted and form part of the EOM procedure.

Clinics may choose to include service audits in their EOM function and others use the EOM as a time to generate recall letters to patients for due clinical services. Computerisation can enable these additional EOM functions to be set automatically greatly assisting the practice in comprehensively managing both the financial and clinical responsibilities of the practice.

Service item maintenance

General practices are required to document the services performed within a consultation by means of a service item coding system. Each country has its own government determined schedule for fee paying to clinics, hospitals or individual patients. These schedules are updated regularly and the general practices must upgrade their own lists as changes occur. Computerisation of the service item data base enables clinics to audit their practice and their individual doctors for services performed, compare practitioners' practice profiles and determine fees generated per service type or per doctor or clinic.

Batching

Practices which directly bill the government for an individual consultation (fee for service) are required to prepare them in a batched format to the responsible agency for processing and payment. Computers deal with this task most efficiently, informing accounting staff when the required batch number is reached, calculating the total moneys owing and maintaining a ledger of moneys owing and moneys receipted. Each doctor will require his own batch number and the computer should be able to allocate the particular direct bill payment to the individual doctor.

Salaries

General practices are required to manage the salaries of their staff, both medical and non medical. This may be a task performed by the practice manager or in a smaller practice by one of the principals. Payroll including taxation, superannuation, holiday leave pay, work cover insurance and where required payroll tax can be performed as a manual bookkeeping task or can be managed using a payroll computer program which may be integrated with the clinic accounting system in the form of a practice ledger.

Stock control

Larger practices undertake a formal stock control to document items purchased and items utilised. This may be performed as either a manual or computer task. Larger organisations such as hospitals have sophisticated computerised stock control systems.

Electronic tools

By far the most useful tool in use in general practice today is the telephone. This piece of technology has changed the way information has moved across the health community. Recently the facsimile(fax) machine has further extended the use of this telephone system enabling the transfer of the printed word, either directly or through the computer to anywhere in the world. The introduction of the computer, initially in the form of a dedicated word processor, has further increased the scope of how information is managed in primary care. Word processing also occurs within any general practice offices particularly in the form of letters of referral, medical reports, and clinical notes. Use of the mail merge feature can generate recall letters.

Practices with multi-user networked systems can use the feature of in-house electronic mail or messaging service (e-mail). These clinics are able to leave messages electronically for clinic staff. General practitioners have a high interest in using this facility (Cacek 1992).

Clinical records

The development of a computerised medical record which can replace the paper record (see also Ch. 12) has eluded many a medical record developer. Why is it that doctors are quite ready to computerise their office but not their consulting room? A recent survey (Cacek 1992) gives us some insight into the attitudes of the doctors in Australia to computerisation. This study revealed a high degree of concern with the concept of computerising the consulting room, despite the fact 30% were performing wordprocessing tasks at home. Manual systems were considered adequate and there was little understanding of benefits to be gained from a computerised medical record system. Similarly in the United Kingdom, 90% of primary care physicians work in computerized practices but only 50% use the computer for recording progress notes (Hayes 1993).

There are three major reasons for creating medical records:

Aide-memoir. This is to refresh our memory of the past consultation. It may be adequate for another doctor to use or it may simply suffice as a memory jog for the documenting doctor. If hand written there may be little decipherable to any other clinician. This form of record is gradually becoming less used.

Patient care. Managing patient care has increased in complexity. There are now more health workers involved in an individual's care. Diagnosing has become more sophisticated, often depending on test results to determine a diagnosis. There is an ever increasing number of drugs with their various functions and side effects which need to be considered. Doctors are being encouraged to practise proactively requiring recognition that a patient should have particular preventive services, or certain routine pathology performed. This creates a heavy demand on the doctor to have the information readily available at the time of the consultation for optimum health care. The paper record struggles under this demand.

Legal documentation. The patient's medical record needs to be able to serve as a true historical document of the consultation. Historically the law has often accepted the hand written paper record as the doctor's true record. It is necessary for the electronic record to demonstrate it is a true representation of the patient's care. Electronic records need a method of demonstrating whether information has been altered after the initial input, what changes have been made, and the ability to produce the original documentation. These issues are addressed in the more sophisticated electronic record packages with date and time signatures.

Benefits of computerising the medical record

Information retrieval is the major reason for computerising the medical record. Retrieval is used for rapid real time access of clinical information, practice auditing and research. To retrieve information the data must be collected in a structured format. This will entail some degree of coding and classification.

The most frequently used coding systems used for primary care are the International Classification of Primary Care (ICPC) (Lamberts & Wood 1987), International Classification of Disease, Ninth Revision, Clinical Modifications (ICD-9-CM)(United States National Center For Health Statistic 1980), and the READ codes (Chisholm 1990) (see also Ch. 4). These coding systems are being mapped to each other so that the issue of which coding system used is not of great importance. Of more importance is the user interface.

Real time information access

To decide what information needs to be accessed in real time one needs an understanding of the information that is collected in the medical record. Patients have information related to their registration including such details as their name, address, telephone number, date of birth, sex, social security number, account status, medical insurance status, medicare number. The primary care doctor can utilise any combination of this registration information on documents, forms and prescriptions.

A patient health summary can provide the doctor with a precise during a consultation. This information could include social information, family history, allergies, past history, life risk factors and current medical ills and medications. As this is computer based, changes to data can be readily updated giving a clear picture of the patient's current health and past history.

Computer programs have been designed to manage preventive care with on screen reminders for anticipatory care and the facility to produce mail merge recall letters for those patients who have not attended the practice and would be missed by a screen prompt alone. These systems have been trialled and found to increase the uptake of influenza vaccinations and papanicolaou smears (Hall 1992).

A computer program which includes a Problem Orientated Medical Record (POMR) structure (Weed 1969), can provide a list of current problems readily updated when the patient's history is altered. Systems incorporating a computerised script writer can keep a database of current medications, and rapidly provide the history of past medications. Checking for patient allergies should reduce the inadvertent prescribing of allergic drugs, by providing an onscreen warning to the doctor. Results of tests ordered can be incorporated into an associated database. This information can be presented by test, by date or by problem in real time. Some systems can present this information in a graphical format on a time scale, for example blood glucose levels, or blood pressure levels can be plotted against time.

General practice information systems can include databases of other providers. These providers may be referring specialists, hospitals, paramedics, or companies. Reports to these sources can be documented in the system, and if created by a wordprocessor integrated into the computerised record, and be available for ready reference. Similarly database entries can be made for reports received. This may be by summary entry, by fax or scanning with indexing for access.

309

Research by practice audit

Research in primary care can be performed by practice audit and by formal research projects such as clinical trials.

Audit functions

Practice audit can be performed manually or by computerisation. Manual audits are usually based on sampling practice populations and may require the skills of a research officer. They are time consuming and consequently performed infrequently. Computerisation of the clinical record opens a new dimension to practice audit. Whole practice populations can be included with a range of inclusion and exclusion criteria. Practices can use audits for a number of purposes.

Patient care management

The principal purpose is to improve patient management. The availability of a new diagnostic test for a particular condition may require the practice to know which patients have this condition and arrange to communicate with these patients. Patients with particular risks can be identified and notified of new vaccines or medications produced.

Preventive care management

Practices are now being required to be more proactive in their approach, taking some responsibility for ensuring those patients overdue for certain preventive services are notified. From an audit program mail merge letters can be created and personalised letters of invitation can be produced.

Doctor education

An audit serves as a powerful tool for continuing medical education of doctors. Auditing rates of particular services performed such as vaccinations, blood pressure recording, pap smears or test ordering, make for interesting comparison between colleagues. The results can be provided confidentially allowing doctors to reflect on their practice behaviour.

Formal research projects

Research is a new field of primary care. Until the introduction of the computer, general practice research had been limited to the academic institutions who had a particular interest in community medicine. Computerisation has enabled the anonymous collection of whole population data. As some medical conditions in general practice occur relatively infrequently large population numbers need to be used to gain enough statistical power for useful conclusions.

With the costs of medical care ever increasing, governments are looking to primary care for information solutions and outcomes. From a community perspective general practice will need data collected into computerised records to achieve these goals. Data collection will need to be organised, requiring the use of classification and coding (see also Ch. 4 and Chs 28-30).

Medical education

Medical education includes the education of the undergraduate, the new graduate and the experienced general practitioner. It also includes the education of the patient and this has been a major role in family medicine since its inception. Undergraduate education is not addressed in this chapter.

New graduates

When the new graduate enters general practice there is much information to be learnt: community services, practice providers, trade names of drugs, preventive care management, relevant test ordering and administrative tasks to undertake. Each different community will have its own services and each practice its own style. Computerisation can help assist the new graduate by providing ready access to databases of information, screen prompts for preventive care and reference to protocols of management (Hayes 1993).

Experienced general practitioners

The more experienced doctors benefit from access to up to date knowledge basis. There are several CD-ROM programs now available based on authorative sources. Other knowledge base programs present doctors with clinical case scenarios, predictive indices of diseases, and knowledge bases incorporated into the system. These systems can be utilised in the consulting room with the aid of a CD-ROM drive incorporated into a PC or by access via modem to a site with a CD-ROM bank of resources.

Patients

The computer can effectively be incorporated into patient education. The simplest of these is the personalised patient hand out. Hand outs can be indexed to illnesses and when appropriate printed out for the patient's use. The doctor can then explain details to the patient. The information is readily accessible reducing the frustration of searching through myriads of papers. Another means of educating patients is to empower them by noting screen prompts. Preventive care prompts display to both the patient and the doctor that certain services are due for review. This may motivate both patient and doctor even when this may not be on the original agenda for the visit. For example vaccination rates for tetanus can be increased utilising this technique. Medication information is an ideal topic for computer education and pharmacists are using this widely with dispensed medications. Sophisticated programs have been created by specialists to educate patients on particular topics. Diabetes and low fat diets are topics that the computer can manage for this purpose.

Telecommunications

The use of telecommunication for health information is a new field. Doctors involved in research have used modem connections to bulletin boards and networks for research information, communication with colleagues via e-mail, and to authorative data bases. Some clinics are now transferring their direct bill accounts via modem eliminating the physical task of collating accounts. Many computer software suppliers use modem connection for maintenance to reduce costs of on site visits. In the future general practitioners will transfer their pathology and radiology requests and results via modem. They will have connections to hospitals for admission and discharge information, access to knowledge bases, and ready communication with colleagues as their research peers have today. The field of telecommunications will open up a whole new dimension to the practising family physician.

REFERENCES

Cacek J 1992 A survey of the attitudes of Australian practitioners to computerisation of medical records. Department of Community Medicine, Monash University, Melbourne

Chisholm J 1990 The Read classification. British Medical Journal 300:1092

Hall L 1992 Development of a computerised preventive care programme for use in a general practice. Department of Community Medicine, Monash University, Melbourne

Hayes G 1993 Computers in the consultation: the UK experience. Proceedings from the Seventeenth Annual Symposium on Computer Applications in Medical Care, Washington, DC

Kidd M, Carson N, Crampton R, Cesnik B, Bearman M 1994 New technology in primary care: benefits, problems and advice. In: Fry J, Yuen N (eds) Primary care and family medicine. Radcliffe Medical Press, Oxford

Lamberts H, Wood M 1987 International classification of primary care. Oxford Medical Publications, New York

Lun K C, Goh L G 1993 GP computing—the Singapore scene: present and future. Proceedings from the Royal Australian College of General Practitioners Seventh Annual Computer Conference, Australia

United States National Center for Health Statistics 1980 International Classification of Diseases, Ninth Revision. Clinical Modification, Washington

Weed L 1969 Medical records, medical education and patient care: the problem orientated record as a basic tool. Case Western Reserve Press, Cleveland

27

Casemix and information systems

EVELYN J S HOVENGA

Casemix refers to a mix of patients classified in some way. It describes a system which groups patients by predetermined factors into clinically meaningful and resource homogenous groups to describe the hospital or health service product (a measure of output). A number of patient classification (casemix) systems have been developed for various purposes. The casemix system used by Australian acute care hospitals to define their 'products' is the Australian National Diagnosis Related Groups (AN-DRGS). Similarly patients may be grouped to represent homogeneity in terms of nursing resource usage. Such classification systems are therefore 'nursing casemix systems' and are used to describe the nursing department's products which are components of the hospital products. Other departments may also use a system to classify their patient services on the basis of resource usage in order to identify other product component costs.

With a definition of the health service product it is possible to relate all inputs and processes to these products to support decision making at all levels within an organisation. This is highly desirable in a climate where ac–countability, efficiency and effectiveness are valued. Inputs consists of buildings, labour resources and supplies as well as the health status of individuals seeking health services. Processes consist of all that happens to and on behalf of the recipients of health care. Relating inputs to processes, outputs and outcomes for the purpose of performance evaluation requires effective and timely integrated information systems. Thus clinical and costing data need to be captured relative to intermediary and final products however defined.

Information systems associated with casemix may be described as grouper software, costing systems, morbidity systems, hospital information systems, departmental (feeder) systems, including nursing workload monitoring systems, pathology, organ imaging systems and executive information systems. In fact most if not all health information systems may be related to casemix in some way.

Definitions associated with casemix influence system specifications. For example an episode of care differs from the length of stay. An episode of care relates to the type of episode where each type refers to its own casemix system. For example AN-DRGs apply to acute patients only. Hospital services are now further differentiated into acute, sub-acute and non-acute type of patients. A patient may be discharged from one episode of care to another within the same hospital length of stay. In other words the term 'episode of care' is no longer used to mean the period from admission to discharge, except where the patient has only one episode of care during the period of hospitalisation. Patients may also be transferred from one hospital to another within the same episode of care.

Actual costs are influenced by the quality and quantity of all resources used to provide patient care towards achieving the desired outcome. As in industry, once costs are identifiable one can explore the most cost-efficient methods or processes to be employed to achieve the desired outcome. Through the examination of the production relationships (inputs relative to outputs) one gains an understanding of those elements which can explain cost variations between hospitals. Outputs need to be defined not only in terms of the product as expressed by casemix but also in terms of outcomes. According to Iezzoni (1987) a 'useful outcome measure would be sensitive to subtle changes in health status or well-being, thus permitting clinically meaningful evaluations of the impact of medical interventions'. The linking of quality to outcomes was explored by Shamian et al (1994). These authors state that 'an outcome is a measurable product, it is the state or condition of an individual as a consequence of health care'. This implies that outcome measures have agreed definitions and can be captured by information systems which is an essential prerequisite to the evaluation of service cost effectiveness. An understanding of the production relationships is necessary when using cost data as a basis for management decision making aimed at improving both efficiency and effectiveness of services provided.

Casemix is now well established in Australia having been placed on the national health care services agenda as part of the 1988 Medicare Agreements. The Casemix Development Program funded by the Commonwealth Government commenced in Australia in 1989. In 1991 the Commonwealth re-directed the focus of its Casemix Development Program towards implementing a national casemix infrastructure. This program was renewed under the 1993 Medicare Agreements in accordance with a five year Casemix Strategic Plan as approved by the Australian Health Ministers' Advisory Council in late 1993. The strategic plan for the casemix development program has the following priorities:

- continued development, adjustment and enhancement of AN-DRGs and the development of classification systems for all other types of hospital care

- development and refinement of Australian cost weights and service weights and improvement of hospital information systems to determine costs and set prices
- development and use of improved payment systems with the aim of ensuring the efficient delivery of high quality health care.

Clinicians are actively involved in casemix activities through the Australian Casemix Clinical Committee (ACCC).

The Casemix Development Program aims to provide the health care industry with a nationally consistent method of classifying all types of patients, their treatment and associated costs, in order to achieve better management, measurement and payment of high quality and efficient health care services. The Government has recognised the need for consistent tools to assess quality, compare costs and understand the relationships between inputs and outputs for some time. These initiatives have had major implications for health information systems used for data collection and processing to provide management decision support at multiple levels of decision making.

DRGs and AN-DRGs

AN-DRGs are modelled on the Diagnosis Related Groups (DRG) system which has been used as a basis for allocating resources via the US Medicare prospective payment system since 1983. The DRG patient classification system was developed during the 1970s by Fetter et al (Fetter 1985a) at the Yale School of Organisation and Management and the School of Public Health 'to attempt to discern and identify discrete kinds of illness for which one could expect, in a statistical sense, a relatively consistent response from any one physician or any one set of physicians with respect to the diagnostic and therapeutic services ordered to deal with that'. On the basis that physicians are primarily responsible for determining the process and hence the cost of patient care, this grouping was used in an attempt 'to establish the statistical similarity and significances of differences in resource consumptions and patterns from one kind of patient to another' (Fetter 1985a).

To classify an episode of care into a DRG the following information is needed after discharge:

- principal diagnosis
- significant secondary diagnosis
- age of patient
- gender of patient
- surgical procedures performed
- type of discharge.

This information is normally available from the discharge summary which is completed by the treating doctor after discharge. Medical record ad–ministrators code the conditions treated and the procedures performed using the International Classification of Diseases—9th Revision Clinical Modification (ICD9-CM) system which was discussed previously in Chapter 4. These codes plus the other information are then used by grouper software to classify the in-patient episode. Advantages of grouping are that there are considerably fewer case types (products) than ICD9-CM. The DRG system has been widely tested and the data needed for classification purposes are now available from every medical record in every Australian hospital. This is largely the result of improvements in infrastructure, mainly funded and facilitated through the casemix development program.

The first version of DRGs contained 327 groups, and these were later expanded to 383 groups based on the International Classification of Diseases, Eighth Revision (ICDA-8). ICD9-CM was published in 1978 and produced a greater refinement in diagnostic coding and a wider spectrum of diseases and disorders (Hornbrook 1982). Subsequently an entirely new set of DRG definitions were developed resulting in 467 groups using the ICD9-CM coding which has around 12 000 diagnosis codes and 4 000 procedure codes. A fundamental change was to organise the major diagnostic categories by organ system (rather than aetiology) since this follows the organisation of medical specialties. This became the First Revision and was used for prospective payment in the US in 1983. This version was also used for many of the original Australian DRG studies.

In 1986 the Second Revision was adopted by US Medicare and this version was used widely in Australia. Later in 1986 the Third Revision was implemented in the US and Victoria. The Fourth Revision, consisting of 475 DRGs, came in use late 1987. In October 1988 the Fifth Revision, consisting of 477 DRGs was introduced. In addition to these versions New York State has extensively modified version 4 for use in its own payment system, the National Association of Children's Hospitals and Related Institutions (NACHRI) in the USA developed an extension of the DRG system and Yale University developed a Refined DRG (RDRGs) system (Palmer & Reid 1989). In 1991 the New York State version 8 was issued. It has 614 DRGs (Verco 1991). By 1990 there was no common version in use in Australia. However by 1992 the ACCC had developed Australian National DRGs (AN-DRGs) in conjunction with 3M who also developed the related software to aid the grouping of cases into AN-DRGs.

Versions of the DRG classification as used by the US federal government agency, the Health Care Financing Administration (HCFA) responsible for the operation of US Medicare and other health care programs, are referred to as HCFA DRGs such as HCFA-3 introduced in 1983, HCFA-4 etc. The tenth version applied in 1993.

Each year amendments are made to the ICD9-CM code lists. The later additional diagnosis codes relate mostly to HIV infection and there have been many new codes for surgical procedures (Palmer and Reid 1989). A new version, the International Statistical Classification of Diseases and Related Health Problems, 10th Revision (ICD10), is now available and plans are under way to introduce its use in Australia and to use this as the basis for the AN-

DRG version 4. Procedures are to be coded using the Commonwealth Medicare Benefits Schedule (CMBS). These many changes have implications for information systems, especially when there is a need or desire to make comparisons over time. It means that some form of mapping between the different versions must be possible. Furthermore the number of digits used for the codes determines the size of data fields. Thus an addition of one digit is likely to have major cost implications for information systems.

Australian DRG development

A proposal by the Commonwealth Department of Community Services and Health to the Australian Health Ministers Advisory Council (AHMAC) in early 1990 led to the endorsement of the establishment of a national standard casemix classification system. Another related Commonwealth initiative was the National Health Strategy Review. An important component of this review was to assess the use of casemix for funding purposes.

An interim clinician steering group, now the ACCC, was established to coordinate the development of a standard inpatient classification method for use in Australia. The ACCC was of the view that 'a more clinically precise classification and one reflecting Australian Health Care would be more effective for use in funding and in clinical management' (Verco 1991). Other casemix working groups were responsible for formulating all project requirements, including education, cost weights, finance design, documentation standards and conventions, and information technology. Changes needed to be consistent to ensure that Commonwealth policy objectives were met.

Major difficulties identified affecting the empirical data analysis were the absence of a 'single authoritative sample of Australian patient discharge data that uniformly represents the practices of Australian health care providers'; 'resource measures throughout Australia do not consistently include the cost of services rendered'; plus 'standards and conventions for documenting DRG data elements differ across the States' (McGuire 1992). Notwithstanding these difficulties the AN-DRGs version 1 released in 1992 were said to be 'a synthesis of state-of-the-art US DRGs with clinical modifications that better characterise the organisation of acute care in Australia' (McGuire 1992). AN-DRGs version 2 became available during 1993 and were used for the second National Costing Study. Version 3 is expected to be in use for 1994/95. Later versions are expected to be based on ICD10. AN-DRGs have a higher level of grouping consisting of 23 Major Diagnostic Categories (MDCs).

A variant of the AN-DRG was developed to define neonates by age to suit all neonatal in-patient episodes defined either by age under 29 days or by the presence of a neonatal diagnosis or both. There are 30 neonate AN-DRGs. Paediatric sub-groups are also defined as the Paediatric modified DRGs (PM-DRGs). The split is at age 10 in AN-DRGs, and usually at 18 in other variants of the DRG system. As the use of casemix systems is expanding the need for new classification systems is emerging. It has become apparent that the same principles may be applied to other, non-hospital health services. As a consequence casemix systems have and continue to be developed for the extended care sector, ambulatory care, and a variety of community health services.

New Australian casemix classification systems

The Australian Ambulatory Classification (AAC) system was developed during a national study in 1992 as a result of the National Ambulatory Casemix Project (NACP). It was developed for use in all Australian hospitals, excepting specialised paediatric hospitals, and has been proposed as the national standard. Paediatric hospitals use the Australian Paediatric Ambulatory Classification system (APAC) which was developed concurrently with the AAC system. Western Australia has developed the Urgency Related Groups (URGs) classification system to categorise all services in hospital emergency departments, including those services provided to patients who are admitted directly from the emergency department.

The National Non-acute Inpatient Classification project led to the development of the Non-Acute Inpatient (NAIP) classification system in 1992. This system suits inpatients whose condition necessitates institutional but not necessarily acute hospital inpatient care. It is also used for patients who require only maintenance nursing, and those who are awaiting placement to care in another setting. It is used when an episode of care cannot appropriately be classified by AN-DRG. It defines 19 classes.

Overseas developed casemix systems

Activities of daily living index is a measure of overall dependence based on tasks such as toileting, eating, dressing, bathing and ambulation. This is used by the Resource Utilisation Groups (RUGs) and may be referred to as the RUG ADL index. RUG-3, which has 43 final classes, was introduced into US nursing homes in 1992 as a basis for funding. Another casemix classification system for nursing homes developed in California is the California Long Term Care Classification (CLTC) system. Episodes of rehabilitation in the USA are categorised into Function Related Groups (FRGs) or the San Diego Rehabilitation Acuity Instrument may be used. Also used is the Functional Independence Measure (FIM) to measure patients' functional abilities and carer burden.

Adjacent Diagnosis Related Groups (ADRG) are clusters of similar diagnoses or procedures, which may be split using age or clinical complications (CCs) to form final classes in the DRG classification system. The All-Patient Diagnosis Related Groups (AP-DRGs) is a variant of the DRG classification developed originally for use in New York State to support a DRG-based payment system. It was originally known as New York DRGs.

The United Kingdom has developed its own DRG variant called Health care Resource Groups (HRGs) to reflect the view that not all cases are diagnosis related. Also the UK uses ICD-9, not ICD-9-CM to code diagnosis. Procedures are classified using a UK classification system, OPCS. The Information Management Group and the Centre for Coding and Classification have initiated a national project to create a comprehensive multiprofessional thesaurus of clinical terms associated with the further development of the Read codes. These new clinical codes were originally developed for primary health care and are now expanded for use throughout the UK health system. Grouping to HRGs will be possible directly from the Read codes eliminating the need to associate Read codes with ICD-9 and OPCS codes. Canada has developed Case Management Groups (CMGs) to describe medical conditions treated.

Ambulatory Care Groups (ACGs) were developed in the US to categorise episodes of ambulatory care provided in a period of time, typically a year. Ambulatory Patient Groups (APGs) is another system also designed in the US to classify ambulatory episodes of care both in and outside hospitals. Other similar systems are the Ambulatory Service Weighting System (ASWS) and the Ambulatory Visit Groups (AVGs). A higher level of grouping of patients with similar diagnoses is the Major Ambulatory Diagnostic Categories (MADCs). Patient care episodes in emergency departments may be classified into Emergency Department Groups (EDGs) developed in the US. Several ambulatory casemix classifications, including APGs use the Current Procedural Terminology version 4 (CPT-4) classification of medical services which is used mainly for billing purposes in the US. CPT is roughly equivalent to our Commonwealth Medicare Benefits Schedule (MBS).

Also developed in the USA is a casemix classification system, the Psychiatric Patient Classes (PPCs) for psychiatric acute inpatient episodes as a refinement of psychiatric classes in the DRG system. There are two levels of classification: 12 psychiatric diagnostic groupings (PDGs), which are then further split into the 74 psychiatric patient classes. There are many other older patient classification (casemix) systems developed for a variety of purposes such as the Computerised Severity of Illness Index (CSI), Disease Staging, the Acute Physiology and Chronic Health Evaluation (APACHE II), the Medical Illness Severity Grouping System (MEDISGRPS) and Patient Management Categories (PMCs)

Using casemix for funding purposes

The use of casemix for decision making frequently centres around costing and financing aspects of the health system. Details of the financing of health services tend to change over time and differ between countries, and between Australian States and Territories. There are also differences between the private and public sectors. One needs a good understanding of the issues, principles and details associated with both casemix data requirements and funding formulae adopted in order to use specify system requirements and to use casemix data optimally for decision making purposes.

One should not confuse a patient billing model, as is used in the US known as the prospective payment system (PPS), with a budget allocation funding model. The former is most suitable to reimburse costs on an individual patient basis such as for the care of individual private patients in either the private or public sector. It uses the fee for service principle as it incorporates a price per DRG, an outlier definition, a payment rate and an outlier payment pool as well as adjustments for those cases which do not fit the DRG classification. A patient billing model is generally speaking not suitable for Australian public hospital funding, although elements of the model are relevant for some purposes; for example, for the transfer of funds between the States for cross boundary flows of public hospital patients or for compensable and repatriation patients in public and private hospitals. A budget allocation model on the other hand uses casemix as an input into the allocation of aggregate funds from a State or Territory health authority to individual public hospitals or area health services.

According to Palmer (1993) formulae using casemix as a basis for funding public hospitals are heavily influenced by existing relationships between the funders and the providers of hospital services and by the policy objectives of the government or other funding agencies. This model is used to distribute a fixed pool of funds between all hospitals administered by the funding authority. That is there is a ceiling referred to as 'capping'. A number of modifications may be made to this model depending upon the policy objectives. For example Victoria used a separate funding pool to adjust individual hospital budgets based on the number of cases serviced (throughput) as an incentive for hospitals to reduce public hospital waiting lists. In other words rather than using one pool, several pools may be created. Each funding pool is then exclusively used for the purpose for which it was created; for example, teaching or rural hospital or defined geographical area funding pools. The latter is population based.

The Victorian government was the first to introduce output based funding as from July 1993. This government now considers itself to be paying for services provided to hospital patients instead of providing funds to service hospitals. Hospitals receive a fixed annual grant plus a payment based on the hospital's casemix as defined by AN-DRG. Additional grant allocations are made for extra costs associated with teaching staff and for aspects of hospital care for which current AN-DRGs do not apply. New accountability processes were introduced through Health Service Agreements between the Victorian government and hospitals (H&CS 1993).

South Australia introduced casemix based funding in an ongoing operational environment a year later using its own formula as explained by Filby and Gaston (1994). The Queensland Government aims to do so in July 1995 (Read 1994). In Tasmania casemix information is incorporated within its Resource Allocation Model (TRAM) mainly used for costing inter-regional patient flows. Western Australia has adopted the purchaser-provider model of funding and uses casemix data for operational purposes and for purchasing health care services (Anderson 1994).

New South Wales uses casemix as a component of its resource allocation formula used to fund all health services. This was designed to reallocate resources on a population and needs basis. An additional allocation based on a comparison of AN-DRG cost weights and total occasions of service is made to teaching hospitals to cover additional expenses incurred for teaching. According to Newman (1993) NSW Health has formally endorsed the use of casemix based funding models within Area Health Services, districts and hospitals.

Before any casemix system can be used as a basis for funding one needs to place a value on each category. These may be expressed in relative (weights) or absolute (price) terms. Either way it is desirable to have some idea of actual costs incurred per category. There are essentially two different approaches which may be used to cost the products of health services. The first is referred to as clinical or product costing. It uses a bottom up approach by capturing data about all cases and the many services provided during an episode of care. The second option is to use what is referred to as cost modelling. In Australia the Yale Cost Model is used for this purpose. It is a top down approach where all costs associated with the organisation's service provision are distributed to the products, however defined, using this model which expresses the relationships between costs, activities and casemix products. These distinctions are not clear cut as some cost modelling does occur in the first approach depending on the available detail of cost information. However the use of product costing by some organisations provides more accurate data for use in the Yale Cost Model enabling others to more confidently use this method.

It is essential that cost centre and accrual accounting is in place to use either method. Cost centres facilitate the tracking and allocation of costs by product. It should be noted that some hospitals also undertake teaching and research, the products of which require their own definition. Some services are provided which do not directly contribute to the organisation's main product. For example a hospital kiosk or the local meals on wheels service are services provided for other organisations or individuals. Such activities do provide additional hospital income and as such are part of the financial system.

Product costing

Accounting costs are expenses classified by a standard chart of account. Costs are then allocated directly or distributed according to a uniform method of apportionment and transformed into unit costs by dividing the total costs by consistently defined and generally accepted units of service or work units. The sum of these units may be referred to as the departmental workload. The costs incurred in providing clinical services are directly related to the workload generated by patients, the staff provided to service these needs, and to materials used.

For example nursing labour resource usage is measured in terms of staff category (skill mix), the associated hourly cost and time. Staff hours required to produce a defined product represent the labour resource input cost. The cost per staff hour varies relative to staff category, shift and day of the week worked. The latter two variables are dependent on penalty and shift allowances. Thus both staff mix and rostering practices influence nursing costs. Other clinical services have similar variables influencing costs.

The time taken by a worker to carry out an operation or to provide a service is influenced by the nature of the work to be performed, the skill and knowledge of the staff member, the circumstances within which the work is performed, the methods employed, and the perceived time available. Actual costs will reflect all of these factors, including inefficiencies. To arrive at a cost per product, there is a need to first identify all resources used per unit of work relative to each product. Secondly the associated costs are identified. Thus to cost departmental services, accounting systems need to be merged and related to information pertaining to:

- all labour resources used by that department
- actual services provided per patient type (intermediary products or work units).

These costs are then related to the output measure in use e.g. AN-DRG. In this manner defined input costs relative to defined outputs are traced. According to Picone et al (1993) valid and reliable measures of nursing services must be established before the cost of nursing services can be determined. These comments apply equally to other departments. The importance of the validity of the source data used for the costing of such departmental services is directly related to the proportion contributed to the total product cost. This will vary for each category. Because nursing costs comprise a large proportion of the total costs for most AN-DRGs, the tracking and accuracy of nursing costs are very important.

Various methods may be employed to establish departmental and product costs. Different allocation methods of the same data result in different final costs per product. Another cost accounting issue to be aware of is the fact that many health care agencies continue to predominantly use a cash accounting system. However with the introduction of casemix based funding they are now switching to accrual based accounting. Cash accounting systems tend to exclude costs associated with the depreciation of capital costs as no cash transactions are associated with these costs. However such items purchased from the recurrent funding allocation are included.

Palmer (1991) noted that by 1991 it was only feasible to apply costing methods to inpatients. The reporting of non-inpatient activities required considerable improvement before these other products could be costed. This is slowly occurring.

The Australian National Costing Study, first conducted during 1992 and now regularly updated, identified the following component costs for each AN-DRG: ward nursing, medical, pathology, imaging, theatre, drugs, critical care, allied health, medical and surgical supplies, overhead allocation, patient catering and other (KPMG 1993). Individual organisations may decide to break this down further into individual responsibility centres or departments. Such breakdowns or unbundling of total costs is also dependent upon the funding formula in use. For example, if the organisation is funded separately for intensive care or medical services or non acute patients or outliers, then there is a need to identify costs associated with the components of every output measure in use. This has implications for casemix information system development.

Tracking departmental costs by output measure(s) serves a number of different purposes:

- to support departmental managers in their decision making
- to establish a price for departmental services provided
- to support corporate management in their decision making
- to establish a cost or price per product
- to develop service weights for use by the Yale Cost Model.

Costs per product could also be used as the dependent variable to improve homogeneity of any casemix system in use in respect of resource usage. In any event the data set used for such purposes must be easily available, well standardised for consistency and be reliable.

The development of departmental service weights has ususally begun in the form of a research project. The first in Australia was conducted by Stoelwinder et al (1986) in conjunction with a clinical costing project. The development of National Service Weights for organ imaging, pathology, operating rooms and critical care was undertaken during 1994. National Nursing Service Weights were originally developed during 1992/93 and are undergoing continued refinement. Note that service weights refer to relative departmental costs per AN-DRG and cost weights refer to relative costs per product.

Palmer (1991) discusses the importance of the 'marginal cost' concept. The estimated marginal cost of each AN-DRG may be used by some funding formulae. It is a concept developed by economists and represents the cost of one more unit of output. That is, the increase in the total costs associated with the treatment of an additional patient. The average cost which includes fixed and variable costs is normally greater than the marginal cost. Marginal costs are not synonymous with variable costs.

The quantification of any departmental workload requires the measurement or estimation of labour resource usage from which a model is developed. The model then continues to be used as a proxy for that workload. Departmental workload monitoring (feeder) systems are a prerequisite to product cost accounting. Nursing is the single biggest department contributing to the total product cost.

Costs versus charges (price)

The determination of hospital charges, needed when using a patient billing model as a basis for funding hospitals, is not necessarily based on an analysis of actual costs. Pricing policies may be arbitrarily determined or be based on a number of alternatives (for example full cost, cost plus). Most of the US literature which refers to costs per DRG use the terms 'costs' and 'charges' interchangeably. Consequently it has been difficult at times to identify whether the costs referred to are actual costs or charges. This is further complicated by the fact that in some instances charges do in fact reflect actual costs incurred per patient, or alternatively they reflect an average cost per patient type, however defined.

There is therefore little consistency in charge structures between hospitals in the US. Intra- and inter-facility cost comparisons are distorted when charges are used to reflect costs (Young et al 1986). In addition there are a number of reasons why the total charges for individual cases in any DRG will vary between hospitals. These include hospital pricing policies, demand and supply conditions in each local area, level of graduate medical education in the hospital, differences in practice patterns, variations in the quality of care, hospital care and availability of specialised facilities (Pettengill & Vertrees 1982). Differences in charges between hospitals therefore do not necessarily reflect differences in economic efficiency. In Australia this applies to private health care facilities. Similar comments could be made about differences in costs between Australian public hospitals.

Finkler (1982) adds another caveat when comparing costs between hospitals in his discussion regarding the use of charges data as a proxy for costs. He demonstrated that ultimately the cost assigned to the patient may be wrong due to allocation methods meant to secure maximum reimbursement rather than to accurately reflect resource consumption on a department by department basis. He differentiates between the identification of how a hospital spends its dollars (economic cost) and how much a hospital must collect to break even (accounting cost). He states that the use of an accounting cost as a proxy for economic cost is 'of questionable value due to the potential differences between economic and accounting cost for a specific patient'.

The issue of price setting for Australian public hospitals is that of deciding which cost to use in the funding formula—the national average cost or the State average cost or the hospital group average cost etc. It is also important to know exactly what this cost covers. In other words, what is in the bundle? Are medical costs or capital costs included? Thus a basis for pricing each product must determined. Should prices used for resource allocation be determined exclusively on the basis of costs? Given that the health budget is finite there may be a need to cap total expenditures which may be achieved in a number of different ways. Decisions regarding these questions are reflected in the funding formula adopted which in turn determines information system data requirements including reporting specifications.

With casemix based funding of Australian public hospitals there may be an associated desire to maximise income and minimise costs by manipulating casemix. This possibility raises ethical issues which one will need to be aware of.

Clinical (product) costing systems

The first clinical costing developmental work in Australia was performed in conjunction with McDonnell Douglas Information Systems. The original development site has since switched to the Transition clinical costing system. This fully integrated computer software system was developed in Boston, USA to support hospital cost accounting, case mix and product line management, simulation and budgeting (Transition Systems Inc. 1989) and is now widely used in Australia. It views hospital activity as a three-stage production process referred to as intermediate products, such as procedures and services provided in the patient-care process; end products or individual patient cases typically defined by AN-DRG; and product lines which are strategic groupings of the services a hospital provides. Product lines may be defined by clinical service or case type or any other characteristic which defines the 'strategic business units' of a hospital used for marketing, budgeting or strategic planning purposes.

These three stages reflect the differences in control and management. The first stage is controlled by departmental managers, the second stage by medical practitioners and the third stage by executives and administrators. Departmental costs are identified as intermediate products under the control of departmental managers. At the departmental level fixed and variable costs are identified and the intermediate products are defined for subsequent costing and for the development of standard unit costs, using any costing methodology. Also indirect costs are allocated as defined by the user. Cost and volume interfaces are automatically created, productivity and management reports may be generated and trends can be analysed. Furthermore it is possible to generate comprehensive cost variance analysis reports, conduct flexible budget variance analysis and departmental cost simulation. Many other management reports are available relative to product lines and end products.

The system employs two kinds of cost accounting systems: process cost accounting at the intermediate product level, because these units are perceived to be repetitively produced within each department using well-defined cost standards, and actual volumes of production. Job order cost accounting is used at the end product or patient case level as each patient case is different representing a unique bundle of intermediate products. For this purpose the exact numbers and types of intermediate products are usually captured.

Feeder data for any user-defined period of time, such as patient dependency data reflecting nursing costs, are loaded into the Department Cost Manager (DCM) module of the Transition system to form the information base. Thus the user decides how to identify and build intermediate products such as nursing services. Cost information is provided by the hospital's general ledger system and/or payroll data via an interface, created by the end user, that maps cost data to the DCM. The DCM is designed to be a standard cost accounting system where budgeted volumes and costs are used to generate standard unit costs. Actual volumes and costs are captured by the system which is then able to produce comprehensive variance analysis reports. Actual unit costs by intermediate product, such as a nursing cost per patient day, may be arrived at by spreading actual costs to these products based upon actual volumes and the relative value units used to develop the standard costs. Other similar systems, such as Panacea, Trendstar, and others are in use.

Clinical costing systems provide detailed management information. This consists of the best possible estimate of actual costs incurred relative to defined products such as AN-DRGs. Some cost modelling is required. A criticism and issue for consideration is whether the cost of obtaining this type of detailed information is justified relative to the benefits of greater precision. It is relatively expensive to implement and maintain a clinical costing system. It takes some time from implementation before meaningful information becomes available. Furthermore clinical costing relies on the use of feeder systems such as nursing workload monitoring systems and other departmentally based systems in order to provide detailed information which is usefull for all levels of decision making. These feeder systems use Relative Value Units (RVUs) as a basis of distributing total departmental costs on a per patient basis. RVUs are determined by the intermediary product description in use. For example nursing work units are defined by the nursing workload monitoring or patient dependency system in use. These RVUs should not be confused with those used as the basis for developing service weights by AN-DRG even though the same data are used for both purposes.

Relative value units

Actual costs need to reflect how departmental resources available at the time are actually distributed between patients. That is, costing methods need to account for situations where the staff available is less than the workload measurement systems suggests is needed and vice versa. Nursing workload monitoring systems are crucial to providing the data from which all nursing costs are obtained. The validity of these systems is dependent upon the work measurement technique used to develop the system and the way in which this is applied to generate a staffing formula. Such systems automate the process of converting patient characteristics and care requirements into staff hours and relative values, in terms of nursing resource usage, between patients.

Relative value units (RVUs) are measures of relative resource usage or relative costliness of defined units. When used to cost nursing services then a unit may be defined as a patient/nurse dependency category. Such relative values were incorporated into Australia's first clinical costing system developed by Stoelwinder et al (1986). They reflect the relative values of departmental work units. On the other hand a RVU was defined by Picone et al (1993) as a scale of items of service and measure of relative costliness of each item. A nursing RVU was defined as nursing minutes per episode of care. Here the RVUs referred to the aggregate nursing intensity per patient discharged defined by AN-DRG which was related to a similar unit. More specifically they achieved a model of relative nursing intensity by regressing nursing time on length of stay to produce a beta weight (Picone et al 1993). Note the difference between the two: the former is used as a basis for cost modelling used by clinical costing systems, a bottom up approach, and the latter is ultimately used for cost modelling using a top down approach.

Feeder systems do have other uses. For example patient dependency systems are concerned with using patient characteristics and care requirements as a means of predicting nursing resource needs. As such they are management information systems used mainly by nurse managers, although they may be used for a variety of other purposes, including strategic management, planning, for costing nursing services, development of nursing service weights, and to assist in the management of length of stay by case.

Service weights

Service weights are the end products of a process which begins with work measurement or the estimation of relative departmental work unit values. For example in nursing, work measurement is used to develop a nursing workload monitoring system from which relative values are derived which in turn are used to develop nursing service weights. A service weight is a measure of the mean cost of the specified service for any patient type relative to the mean cost for all patient types. When service weights are derived from data collected within one hospital, then they reflect a weighting applicable to that hospital only. Standard weights for national use may be developed by pooling such data from a randomly selected group of hospitals. The National Costing Study (KPMG 1993; KPMG 1994) used service weights first from the US and later Australian developed service weights, for their cost modelling approach. Individual hospitals may have a desire to compare their own resource usage, expressed in terms of time, costs or service weights, against national standards to evaluate performance.

Yale cost model (YCM)

Cost modelling does not require the detailed data collection described above; instead the relationships between costs, production processes and hospital products are modelled. Clinical costing is desirable to gain a better understanding of the various cost relationships per DRG. This does not imply that every hospital needs a clinical costing system.

According to Palmer (1991):

the YCM (Yale Cost Model) is the only feasible method of generating estimates of cost by DRG in circumstances where information about the costs or charges associated with individual patients is not routinely collected. This is (was) the case for all public hospitals and most private hospitals in Australia.

The YCM evolved from the cost per case data set, referred to by Fetter (1985a) as one of two data sets assembled, which consisted of amounts charged to the patient per service category. The data did not represent costs of care but service charges. Fetter (1985b) defines the cost allocation process used by the Yale team as 'an absorbing Markov process to find the accounts as a matrix in which the rows are the definitions of the accounts and the columns are the values of the accounts', the matrix is then inverted. The answer thus obtained is not in terms of the actual allocations but in terms of the matrix of coefficients which identifies the destination of every dollar. This is different from what is called a 'stepdown process' which results in different answers depending upon the ordering of the stepdown used. According to Fetter et al (1977) 'The usual step-down method will not suffice in this application since it is too costly computationally when one preserves the identity of the source accounts in the final allocations'.

The YCM as described by Chandler (1988) represents a specific application of linear algebra to cost accounting in a hospital setting. This requires the definition of cost vectors and mapping matrices. Costs are mapped in a four step process from a hospital general ledger into AN-DRGs. First costs are allocated to cost centres, then overhead costs are allocated to the various clinical departments using a separate formula for each overhead cost. The third step consists of adjustments so that only costs for inpatient treatment episodes are included (some cost centres service both in and out patients). Finally costs from the clinical departments are mapped into AN-DRGs using charges (or costs) as the allocation statistic. Nursing and some other departmental costs are allocated on the basis of service weights by AN-DRG for each clinical department. Reports can be prepared to give labour, materials, total, direct and allocated costs per AN-DRG, costs per bed-day per AN-DRG and costs per allocation statistic per AN-DRG. Other facilities for displaying the various allocation matrices in the mapping process are also available.

Palmer et al (1991) describe the YCM as consisting of several computer programs designed first to allocate costs from each overhead cost centre to all patient care cost centres, second to allocate the total costs from the patient care cost centres to each DRG. The latter is described as 'conceptually the most complex of the modelling processes'. Palmer et al (1991) described the first use of this model in Australia. This cost modelling approach has since been used by KPMG Peat Marwick who were the successful tenderers for a Commonwealth government contract to undertake a National Costing Study to produce national cost weights by AN-DRG. This project began in February 1992. Cost weights for the AN-DRG Version 1 were released in August 1993. An extension of this project enabled the production of cost weights using AN-DRG Version 2. Chapter 4 of their report details the assumptions used in the cost modelling process.

Data inputs required by the YCM were summarised and listed by Palmer (1991) as follows:

• Expenditure by cost centre, classified by type of expenditure, for example, salaries and 'other', and by type of cost centre, for example, 'overhead', 'patient care'.

- Proportion of total resources used in each patient care cost centre which are associated with inpatient activities - the inpatient fraction of each of these cost centres.
- A statistic for each overhead cost centre such as total costs, staff numbers, floor space, bed numbers, bed days and admissions, which can be measured for all relevant cost centres and used to allocate expenditure by overhead cost centres to all patient care cost centres.
- Number of patients discharged and the number of patient-days, by patient care cost centre, for each DRG.
- Measures of relative resource use (service weights) by DTG for specified patient care and ancillary services.)

The validity of service weights, is very important for those hospitals which rely on using this cost modelling approach to cost their services by AN-DRG. The original YCM software has been modified to make it easier to use and is referred to as COSMOS. This micro-computer based software, complete with a user's guide for the model has been available to Australian hospitals since mid 1991.

Critical (clinical) paths

The management of length of stay by case has become an important component of managing within a casemix based funded environment where it is desirable to achieve a close to the average length of stay for each AN-DRG for every case. In project planning terms a critical path is the shortest possible length of time within which a project may be achieved. Critical or clinical paths in health care refer to multidisciplinary outcome based care plans. It requires the development of care plans on a case by case basis. They could be seen as an extension of the nursing care plan. Any care plan may be developed for each patient by the patient's care manager or a standard plan may be developed for each diagnosis using any product description such as the ICD-9-CM codes, or AN-DRGs. In any event such plans must be developed in consultation with all care givers. The use of clinical paths is expected to increase productivity, improve quality and control costs. Obsolete or unnecessary practices may be identified during the development process. Many hospitals have begun to develop clinical paths for high volume or high cost AN-DRGs to assist management to achieve this. Managing each case relative to the clinical path is referred to as case management.

Components of the path include a timeline identifying all required or anticipated interventions, outcome indicators against which progress may be monitored relevant to each discipline associated with the care, expected health status at the time of discharge, and individualised special needs. Once such plans are in place, one is able to monitor progress relative to the corresponding plan. This in turn permits the implementation of exception reporting. In other words any variation from the plan is noted and analysed so that corrective action may be taken as soon as possible. This is one way by which to manage individual length of stay and patient throughput as a whole.

It is an important tool for using casemix data for decision making. In particular it is useful for improving organisational efficiency and outcome effectiveness. It is a useful aid to discharge planning and to identify areas for continuous quality improvements. The system also permits input from the patient and significant others providing a customer focus. It is a mechanism for achieving financial objectives without compromising the standards of care. The system will only work effectively if there is a supportive infrastructure which facilitates prompt problem solving when variations are noted. Such variations may be relevant to an individual patient only or they may reveal organisational wide problems.

Clinical path care plans are developed so as to achieve high quality care, effective communication between all disciplines, collaboration and optimum resource utilisation. The use of standardised care plans and terminologies will facilitate computerisation of clinical data and as a result improved capacity for clinical research at less cost than is the case with a paper based system. Case management on the other hand is about coordinating all activities identified as required in the clinical path by a case manager. Nevertheless individual patients can be case managed in the absence of such a path by an experienced health professional. Nurses are ideally placed for such a role both in hospital and community settings, although in some instances it would be more appropriate to appoint an allied health professional. Case management is particularly cost effective for complex cases requiring many different types of services. Managed care, case management and clinical paths are being implemented in a number of Australian hospitals. There are some variations regarding the terminology and the use of the concepts outlined.

Information systems are now being developed to support this. These management activities are heavily dependent upon accurate and timely information. Historical data are used to first develop each clinical path and secondly to modify these as required. Continual patient assessments with feedback regarding outcomes lead to adjustments in services provided. There is an extensive body of literature on this topic.

Discharge planning

The process of discharge planning is closely linked with case management. O'Hare and Terry (1988) define discharge planning as 'assessing needs and obtaining or coordinating appropriate resources for patients and clients as they move through the health care system'. The aim is to provide care continuity and to ensure that patients move through the system in the shortest possible time without adverse effects or the need for re admission. For many hospital cases this requires follow up care by community based services. Such care needs to be anticipated and organised in advance. Casemix based funding provides an incentive for effective discharge planning.

Problems following discharge can occur where a patient or the family are unable to support daily living needs or do not understand directions for follow-up care or are unlikely to comply with advice given. Also the home environment may not be suitable for satisfactory self care. The home location relative to the treating centre may prevent care on an outpatient basis. Discharge planning must occur in consultation with the patient, the home based care givers where relevant, community based services and the health professionals providing inpatient care. An interdisciplinary approach is highly desirable. Discharge planning needs to commence on admission ᵁᵃnd in some cases prior to admission. Length of stay can be reduced only in conjunction with effective discharge planning.

Performance indicators

Indicators are signs, flags or signals, some of which may indicate desirable events where others indicate negative events. There are two types of quality performance indicators. The first is a rate based indicator which designates a level of occurrence; the second is a sentinel event. Rate based indicators are measured against predetermined acceptable thresholds, whereas sentinel events are so serious that no rate of occurrence is considered acceptable. Thresholds must be achievable. The Australian Council on Hospital Standards (ACHS) defines a clinical indicator as 'a measure of the clinical management and outcome of care' (Lawson & Collopy 1993). The ACHS assists medical colleges with clinical indicator development and health care facilities with its implementation. The use of clinical indicators, which began with hospital wide indicators such as infection rates, unplanned re-admissions and others, is now an integral part of the accreditation process.

Performance indicators are used to identify areas which would benefit from further investigation so as to improve performance and quality. Indicators are chosen as much for their data availability and collection feasibility, as for their relevance or established link with that which is desired to be measured. Where the quality of a service cannot be measured directly, it may be measured indirectly through the use of any number of indicators. Such indicators are pointers from which one may infer that the desired quality and outcomes were achieved. Alternatively they are used to indicate areas for further investigation. Workload and service utilisation statistics together with cost and outcome data may be used as indicators of quality.

There are a number of possible cost efficiency performance indicators for acute hospitals. Examples are average AN-DRG weight, average inpatient unit cost, average length of stay, relative length of stay indicator, occupancy rate percentage of registered beds, and total admissions. None of these are very precise measures, but when compared over time or with other hospitals they should indicate relative cost efficiency. Such indicators do not assist in explaining cost variations; rather they indicate where further investigation is warranted. These data need to be associated with outcome data, including patient satisfaction data, to get a sense of the quality and effectiveness of services provided.

The ACHS has established a database, the Inaugural National Clinical Indicator Data Evaluation System (INCIDE). As from 1993 this is being used to store all accreditation survey data to monitor the use and usefulness of hospital wide clinical indicators. It will also be used to observe trends in patient care on a national level and permit facility specific comparative performance evaluation. The intention is to link trend results to AN-DRG and other casemix funding.

Quality

Quality is defined in the Australian Department of Administrative Services and the Australian Office for Better Buying quality assurance policy (DAS 1992) as: .

> Fitness for purpose, or conformance to requirements—the totality of features and characteristics of a good or service that bear on its ability to satisfy the user's stated or implied needs at the time of purchase and during its useable life. Quality is not a synonym for excellence; a quality product is the one best suited to the purpose intended rather than the best that money can buy. An appropriate level of quality may be determined by balancing factors such as performance, reliability, cost, consequences of failure, etc.

The quality of a country's health service is generally speaking assessed by the mortality rates and incidents of morbidity. These types of statistics are reported world-wide as death rates, major causes of death, life expectancy, live births, maternal and infant mortality rates and others. Such measures are indicators of ill health and provide the big picture. This information may lead to the identification of areas warranting closer scrutiny.

Another way of looking at quality is to examine what constitutes health. After all, health services aim to promote, maintain and restore health. The Australian Institute for Health and Welfare defines health as social, economic, environmental, spiritual or existential well being. It also includes life satisfaction and other characteristics valued by humans. The World Health Organisation defines health as 'a state of complete physical, mental and social well being and not merely the absence of disease or infirmity' (WHO 1946). Thus a quality health service produces and maintains healthy people. Consequently measures of health may be used as indicators of quality.

At an institutional level quality may be measured in terms of the physical and organisational structures which contribute to or provide an appropriate environment for the delivery of quality health services. Another perspective on the measurement of quality is through the examination of processess, procedures and outcomes. Consumers are concerned with getting the most appropriate service provided competently by a qualified person at an optimum time and place, within an acceptable time frame, which achieves what it is intended to do and which meets consumer expectations at every encounter. Thus quality is the degree to which the above expectations are met.

In a casemix environment we are concerned with more detailed information than has traditionally been available to begin to explain some of the variations which may be identified by the previously mentioned crude measures. Casemix as an output measure lends itself to scrutinising all planned and systematic actions as well as the management of the production processes associated with each case or case type. Quality assurance requires evidence that the services provided will or have been provided consistently in accordance with customer requirements. Thus if we assume that customers of the health service industry expect to achieve or optimise general health, then evidence of health status needs to be provided.

Health status

Health status may be defined in many different ways. The concept of health varies between people. There are a number of unresolved issues associated with quality measurement in health. The most significant ones are issues of definition. The concept of health is subject to many different interpretations. Perspective or the position from which we view health influences the definitions used. There are healthy but disabled people for example. Individuals will place different values on health. Concert pianists are likely to value their ability to hear and their dexterity more than others. Loss of function creates greater problems for some people than for others. The value individuals place on health stems from whether our state of health allows us to lead a fulfilling and satisfying life. For some this leads to more risk taking behaviour than for others. Thus individuals contribute to their own state of health. The value of any health status is also age related. What is effective functioning for some individuals is not for others; it depends on one's perception and values.

So another significant issue regarding quality measurement is the fact that there are many variables which influence health. There is no obvious direct cause and effect relationship in many instances. According to Mooney (1986) health services have all the characteristics of uncertainty, irrationality, unpredictability, large monopoly elements, paternalism and important externalities. It is the combination of these factors which makes health care unique as a commodity.

Defining what is to be measured

Quality measurement in a casemix environment is concerned with the identification of inputs, processess and outcomes and the relationships between these. Input measures consist of raw materials and other resources made available. In the health care industry the raw materials are the people who seek health services. Admission policies are developed within this context and state the conditions within which a person may be admitted to receive specified health care services. A person's health status on admission becomes the benchmark against which outcomes may be measured.

A major factor influencing admission policies is the acceptance of risk. Risk assessment is about an analysis of the probability that a person considered for admission to a particular service will benefit from that service. For example existing health, severity of illness, personal support systems, socioeconomic and lifestyle status will influence the probability of complications, adverse outcomes and extended length of stay.

Other inputs are buildings, equipment, materials and labour resources necessary for the delivery of health services. The quality of these and the environment in which these are used will influence the cost and quality of the services provided as well as health outcomes. So these factors need to be defined and measurable.

Casemix is used to define output measures. This system may be used for quantitative purposes. On the other hand outcome measures have a qualitative dimension. A useful outcome measure would be sensitive to subtle changes in health status or well being, permitting clinically meaningful evaluations of the impact of medical interventions (Iezzoni 1987). Thus outcome measures could double as measures of health status on admission. According to Nash and Markson (1991):

> Outcomes management, at its best, will systematically approach the topic of health care quality and costs through mechanisms that enable us to engage in ongoing analysis of the uncertainty that exists in the art of delivering high-quality medical care. We may not be able to predict with certainty the outcomes of care, but we should be in a better position to identify and prevent highly variant behaviour and to make more informed decisions.

Two types of outcome measures are required, disease specific measures to permit comparisons to be made between treatment options for individual cases or AN-DRGs, and generic outcome measures. The latter need to incorporate a means of evaluating the cost or benefit to the patient or client or society. Benefits may be defined in terms of functional improvement, pain relief, improved general well being, improved psychological outlook, improved quality of life, life years saved or increased life expectancy, improved employment opportunities or prospects, reduction in dependency on others or a reduction in the number of morbid days or ill health episodes. Some of these measures refer to life utility and functional health status which are outcomes of particular importance to individuals or their family members.

In order to use any of these measures in the future we will need to ensure that the data available permits such usage. This requires careful structuring of clinical data and knowledge, using a standard language throughout the health care system, and enabling these data to be processed electronically. The meaning of standard data elements must be clear and universal.

Conclusion

The introduction of casemix (output) based funding has had major implications for health information system development. Most systems need to be linked to casemix in some way to maximise their usefulness. Indeed health information systems need to be fully integrated so as to enable timely, accurate and comprehensive information to be provided to support all levels of decision making, from the operational (clinical), to middle, executive and corporate management. In particular clinical and financial data need to be merged to enable effective management. Information systems need to be able to support decisions leading to the productive efficiency of the intermediate outputs and also support decisions which result in the effective utilisation of these services for the treatment and care of individual patients. Thus the measurement of organisational performance requires data collection which records both the utilisation of goods and services and expenditures incurred in their production.

Now that casemix defines health care products, all inputs, processess and outcomes need to be related to these products. This means that all systems now need to be patient or client focused although there continues to be a need for a departmental focus to support management decision making at that level. Clinical information systems must have a user interface that supports the needs of all clinical disciplines. Effective use of casemix based information systems permits the understanding and control of health service expenditures and requires a provisional casemix category assignment on admission to permit analysis of variance throughout the production process (episode of care or length of stay) enabling continuous quality improvement.

REFERENCES

Anderson S 1994 Western Australia adopts purchaser-provider model, a report of Anderson's presentation at the Sixth National Casemix Conference, Hobart. Australian Casemix Bulletin 6(5)

Australian Institute of Health and Welfare 1994 Australia's Health 1994. Australian Institute of Health and Welfare, AGPS, Canberra

Chandler I R 1988 The Yale cost model. Proceedings of the Second International Conference on the Management and Financing of Hospital Services, Sydney

Department of Administrative Services (DAS) 1992 Commonwealth of Australia, May 1992, Quality Assurance Policy. AGPS, Canberra

Fetter R B, Shin Y, Freeman J L, Averill R F, Thompson J D 1980 Case mix definition by diagnosis related group. Medical Care Supplement Feb. vol. 18 no. 2

Fetter R B, Mills R E, Riedel D C, Thompson J D 1977 The application of diagnostic specific cost profiles to cost and reimbursement control in hospitals. Journal of Medical Systems 1(2):137-149

Fetter R B 1985a DRGs: fact and fiction. Australian Health Review 8(2):105-115

Fetter R B 1985b Cost models and DRGs: an international comparison. Australian Health Review 8(2):16-125

Filby D, Gaston C 1994 A casemix based payment system in South Australia. In: Proceedings of the Sixth National Casemix Conference, Hobart, Commonwealth Department of Human Services and Health, Canberra

Finkler S A 1982 The distinction between cost and charges. Annals of Internal Medicine 96(1):102-109

Health and Community Services 1993 The elements of the new formula. In: Casemix funding for public hospitals, Victoria's policy. Health and Community Services, Melbourne

Hornbrook M C 1982a Hospital casemix: its definition, measurement and use: Part I, The conceptual framework. Medical Care Review 39(1):1-43

Hornbrook M C 1982b Hospital casemix: its definition measurement and use: Part II, Review of alternative measures. Medical Care Review 39(2)73-123

Iezzoni L I 1987 Case classification and quality of care: issues to consider before making the investment. Quality Review Bulletin April 135-139

KPMG Peat Marwick 1993 National Costing Study 1993 Report to the Commonwealth Department of Health, Housing, Local Government and Community Services. KPMG Peat Marwick, Adelaide

KPMG Peat Marwick 1994 Report to the Commonwealth Department of Human Services and Health, National Costing Study Production of cost weights for AN-DRGs version 2, Adelaide

Lawson M J, Collopy P C 1993 Australian Council on Healthcare Standards Care Evaluation Program. In: Hovenga E J S, Whymark G K., (eds) HIC'93 Proceedings, Melbourne

McGuire T 1992 Australian acute patient classification project—evaluation and refinement final report. In: Proceedings of the Fourth National Casemix Conference Augus, Gold Coast. CDHH&CS

Mooney G H 1986 Economics, medicine and health care. Harvester Wheatsheaf, New York

Nash D B, Markson L E 1991 Managing outcomes: the perspective of the players. Frontiers of Health Services Management 8(2):3-65

Newman J 1993 Teaching and research. Paper presented at the DHHLG&CS workshop on casemix funding formula options, December, Canberra

O'Hare P A, Terry M A 1988 Discharge planning strategies for assuring continuity of care. Aspen Publishers, Rockville

Owens H J 1990 DRGs and hospital financing in the Australian health system. Proceedings of the Australian Nursing Federation and the Department of Community Services and Health Nursing and Casemix Conference, Sydney

Palmer G, Reid B 1989 DRG system developments. Australian Casemix Bulletin 1(1):3

Palmer G 1991 The costing of a hospital's products: some theoretical and empirical perspectives. Paper presented to the Annual Conference of the Australian Health Economists Group, September

Palmer G, Aisbett C, Fetter R, Winchester L, Reid B, Rigby E 1991 Casemix costs and casemix accounting in seven major Sydney teaching hospitals. Centre for Hospital Management and Information Systems Research and School of Health Services Management, University of New South Wales, Sydney

Palmer G 1993 Casemix funding models for use in Australian public hospitals. Paper presented at the DHHLG&CS workshop on casemix funding formula options, December, Canberra

Pettengill J, Vertrees J 1982 Reliability and validity in case mix measurement. Health Care Financing Review 4(2):101-128

Picone D, Ferguson L, Hathaway V et al 1993 NSW nursing costing study. Sydney Metropolitan Teaching Hospitals Nursing Consortium. September

Read P 1994 Casemix in Queensland for 'management purposes': a report of Read's presentation at the Sixth National Casemix Conference, Hobart. Australian Casemix Bulletin 6(5)

Shamian J, Petryshen P, O'Brien Pallas 1994 Outcomes monitoring: adjusting for risk factors and severity of illness when determining outcomes. Nursing Informatics '94 invitational post conference. Austin, Texas

Stoelwinder J U, Stephenson L G, Wallace P G, Abernethy M A, Putt C M 1986 Clinical costing at the Queen Victoria Medical Centre. Australian Health Review 9(4):372-386

Transition Systems 1989 Transition I: a functional overview. Boston, Product Information

Verco C 1991 Development of the Australian inpatient casemix classification standard. Australian Casemix Clinical Committee, Adelaide

Young W W, Carson M S, Lander S A 1986 Patient management care and the costs of nursing services. In: Shaffer (ed) Patients and purse strings. National League for Nursing, New York

World Health Organisation (WHO) 1946 Constitution of the WHO. Reprinted in: Basic documents, 37th edn. Geneva

FURTHER READING

Bender J, McGuire T 1994 AN-DRG based hospital financing: benefits and risks. Healthcover 4(2)

Calore K A, Iezzoni L 1987 Disease staging and PMCs: Can they improve DRGs. Medical Care 25(8):724-737

Cope I 1992 Performance indicators: their place in health care evaluation. Australian Health Review 15(1)

Department of Human Services and Health (DHSH) 1994 Better health outcomes for Australians. AGPS, Canberra

Eagar K, Hindle D 1994 The Australian casemix dictionary. The National Casemix Education Series. DHS&H, Canberra

Field M J, Lohr K N (eds) 1992 Guidelines for clinical practice: from development to use. National Academy Press, Institute of Medicine, Washington DC

Gonnella J S, Hornbrook M C, Louis D Z 1984 Staging of disease: a case-mix measurement. Journal of the American Medical Association 251(5):637-644

Gray P A, Abernethey M A, Stoelwinder J 1988 Models for costing patient care services, part 2: Costing organ imaging services. Australian Health Review 11(2):98-105

Henderson N, Tate R 1991 Hospital finance, understanding the basics. The Victorian Hospitals' Association, Melbourne

Herkimer A G 1989 Understanding health care accounting. Aspen, Maryland

Hindle D 1994 Product costing: the costing of health care services. The National Casemix Education Series, Department of Human Services and Health, Canberra

Hofman P A 1993 Critical path method: an important tool for co-ordinating care. Journal on Quality Improvement 19(7)

Horn S D, Horn R A 1986 The computerised severity index: a new tool for case-mix management. Journal Medical Systems 10(1):73-78

Hovenga E J S 1994 Casemix, hospital nursing resource usage and costs. PhD Thesis UNSW, Sydney

Knaus W A, Zimmerman J E, Wagner D P, et al 1981 APACHE—acute physiology and chronic health evaluation: a physiologically based classification system. Critical Care Medicine 9:591-597

Knaus W A, Draper E A, Wagner D P, Zimmerman J E 1985 APACHE II: a severity of disease classification system. Critical Care Medicine 13(10):818-829

Levy V M 1992 Financial management of hospitals, 4th edn. Law Book, North Ryde

Magnus A, Abernethy M, Stoelwinder J 1988 Models for costing patient care services Part 3: Costing operating theatre procedures. Australian Health Review 11(4):311-318

Palmer G 1986 The economics and financing of hospitals in Australia. In: Butler J R G, Doessel D P (eds) Proceedings of the Eight Australian Conference of Health Economists—Australian Studies in Health Administration No. 59 Economics and Health, School of Health Administration, University of New South Wales, Sydney 1-24

Palmer G 1993 The development of service weights for the national costing study. Paper presented at the Annual Casemix Conference, Canberra

Pilla J 1994 Development of AN-DRGs: meeting the concerns of clinicians. The Medical Journal of Australia 161(Suppl 5)September

Reeve T 1993 Coherent and consistent quality assurance and utilisation review activities in public and private hospitals in Australia. Report to the Commonwealth Department of Health, Housing, Local Government and Community Services

Stoelwinder J U, Stephenson L G, Hughes A D, Putt C M 1984 Improving the funding of Australia's public hospitals: using DRG's to monitor for efficiency and control. Australian Health Review 7(2):32-39

5

Health research and informatics

28

Research in health care

CHRISTOPHER SILAGY

Research is often described as 'organised curiosity' that is coupled with systematic problem solving. The main purpose of research is to increase our level of knowledge and understanding of a subject. Research has always been an important and integral aspect of the health care system. It spans a wide spectrum of interests and endeavour, ranging from the molecular and genetic basis of disease through to broader community issues involving the structure and effectiveness of the health care system. For example, in the area of breast cancer researchers are involved in sorting out the intricacies of genetic profiles which may predispose women to the development of the disease; clinicians in a variety of disciplines are engaged in trials to try to find effective therapies; behavioural research scientists are concerned with examining the psychosocial implications of the disease; and health service researchers are examining the benefits of providing community-based mammography screening services. At all of these levels, research has helped to improve our understanding of both health and disease, and has frequently formed the basis for developing effective therapeutic interventions which can be offered to individuals or communities.

This chapter is concerned with describing the different types of research that are most frequently used in health care, particularly in clinical settings. Later chapters will deal with specific aspects of the research process where information technology has a particularly important role to play.

Classification of research

Health care research can be broadly defined into two categories: laboratory based and clinical.

Laboratory based research is usually concerned with trying to find explanations for *how* and *why* the human body is structured or functions in a particular way. Although a lot of laboratory based research involves complex genetic, molecular, or physiological procedures, information technology is being used increasingly as part of such research. Sophisticated computer software is now available to assist in areas as diverse as gene mapping, prediction of pharmacokinetic effects with various drugs, and dissecting anatomical structures and pathways. Laboratory based research provides an important foundation for many developments in health care; however, it will not be described here in further detail.

Clinical research, which is the main focus of this chapter, can also be divided depending on the *type of data* or the *study design*.

Type of data

Researchers often distinguish between use of *quantitative* data and *qualitative* data. Quantitative data involves collection of data which is measurable and which can lend itself to analysis using various statistical methods. Most clinical and epidemiological research draws heavily on quantitative methods. Measurements of parameters can be compared between people with, or without, a particular disease as well as between people who receive, or do not receive, a particular therapy. Statistics are an integral part of quantitative research. However, this does not mean that every researcher must be an expert statistician. Various computer software packages are available to assist researchers manage large amounts of data and deal with complex mathematical calculations. As a result, the important issue for researchers who rely on quantitative methods is to have an understanding of the basic concepts of data management and statistics, a working knowledge of the various software programs available, and the ability to seek out expert advice as required.

Qualitative research is concerned more with meanings and processes than simply measurements. It allows an analysis of a broad range of topics (including symptoms, processes, decisions, and outcomes) using in-depth enquiry which elaborates on data in a descriptive rather than quantitative manner. Qualitative research seeks to understand human behaviour from the subject's own frame of reference. Frequently, this type of research has been confused with subjective enquiry. This is incorrect; qualitative research has its own unique methods of data collection and rigour. These include direct (or indirect) observation, interviews, focus groups, questionnaires, videotape or audiotape recordings and narratives. Analysis of qualitative data often involves trying to identify themes or recurring patterns in how people think or behave. Although this can be a very tedious task, specific computer software has recently been developed to assist.

Study design

It is usual to distinguish between *observational* and *experimental* designs (Table 28.1) In observational studies, nature is allowed to take its course and changes or differences in one characteristic are related to changes in another.

Table 28.1 Classifying clinical research study design

Observational	Experimental
Descriptive	Random allocation
• Cross-sectional survey	• Randomised controlled trial
• Case series	Non-random allocation
Analytical	• Quasi-randomised trial
• Cohort study	
• Case-control study	

Observational studies are usually further sub-divided into *descriptive* or *analytical.* One of the simplest forms of descriptive research is a case series, which provides an account of one or more patients with a particular condition, syndrome, or pattern of symptoms. Often a combination of quantitative and qualitative data are collected in the process. The case series is the equivalent to applying a spotlight or using a microscope.

Probably the most widely recognised type of descriptive research is a cross-sectional study. This type of research usually examines a particular subset (or sample) chosen from the community at a single point in time. It enables data to be obtained about the proportion of the sample with a particular characteristic(s). Cross-sectional studies often use survey methodology to collect the data. If such studies follow a group of people forward in time and are repeated at various intervals, they can be useful in monitoring whether changes in a characteristic are occurring over time. For example, what proportion of people who have just had a myocardial infarction will die in the next five years? The major limitation of descriptive research is that it does not enable associations or causal links to be established between various characteristics and outcomes.

Analytical studies can be subdivided into non-experimental or experimental. Case-control and cohort studies are examples of non-experimental analytical studies. In an analytical study the investigator is concerned with attempting to explain the relationship between a variable and a particular outcome. One way in which this can be done is a cohort study, which involves identifying a group of people and following them forward (prospectively) over time. By measuring whether people within the group who are exposed to the variable (say, cigarette smoking) are more likely to develop an outcome (such as lung cancer) it is possible to make inferences about the likely association between cigarette smoking and lung cancer.

In a case-control study, the investigator begins by identifying people with the outcome of interest (i.e. 'cases') and then identifies another group of people who are similar in most ways except that they do not have the outcome of interest (i.e. 'controls'). After suitable cases and controls have been selected, exposure to the variable of interest is measured and compared in the two groups. The relationship between brain tumours and exposure to high tension power lines is an example. Firstly, a group of patients with brain tumour are identified. Secondly, a group of people with similar backgrounds, but no brain tumour, are selected as controls. Then the past and/or current exposure to

343

high power tension lines is compared in the two groups. The major difficulty with a case-control study is selection of the control group. Frequently, the group from which controls are chosen is not representative of the study base from which the cases arose.

Experimental studies are one of the strongest weapons available to a researcher who wishes to test a hypothesis. The main reason for choosing an experimental design is to minimise the chance of bias interfering with the effect of an intervention on a particular outcome. In an experimental design, individuals are allocated to either an *intervention* or *control* group and the effect of this on the outcome of interest can then be measured. A common example is evaluation of a new drug, where 50 patients may be allocated either to receive the new test drug or a standard drug.

Randomised controlled trials are often described as the *gold standard* of experimental design because they effectively eliminate the major sources of bias that are present with the various research designs described previously. Unfortunately, it is not always possible to use this design and various modifications are necessary, which are referred to as quasi-experimental studies.

Uses of research in health care

Research is potentially of limited value if it is ultimately not applied to produce desired changes in the health care system. No matter how much is known about the molecular basis of a particular disease and the effectiveness of a particular therapeutic agent, if the therapy is not offered or used appropriately then individuals may miss out on receiving health care of an appropriate quality.

The need to ensure that research is translated into action has become a major effort in its own right in a number of health care systems in recent years. Set in a context of contracting resources, health care providers are being increasingly encouraged to ensure that resources are used most effectively. This type of thinking is part of a paradigm shift in attitude emerging within the health care system. The role of evidence based practice is being valued more highly than unsystematic reports of clinical experience in influencing decision making. High quality clinical research needs to underpin clinical practice and policy decisions.

Clinical audit, which involves documenting what currently happens in clinical practice, comparing that against a pre-determined standard, and then instituting appropriate modifications to clinical practice has become a routine part of many health care settings. For clinical audit to be effective and efficient, there is a need to have satisfactory information systems available in order to facilitate the collection and monitoring of relevant data.

Outcomes research is concerned with determining the effect of a particular intervention or service on some measurable outcome. For example, the effect of a new treatment for stomach ulcers could be measured against a range of laboratory based outcomes (such as the level of acid secretion), investigational outcome (such as ulcer healing as detected by endoscopy), or clinical outcomes (such as symptom improvement). Incorporating measures of quality of life and economic indices as part of the outcome assessment is important if the overall effects of an intervention are to be fully assessed.

Stages in research

Conducting a research project involves a number of discrete stages. Each needs to be considered in detail, and generally, the greater the effort that is put into the design phase, the more likely the project is to be successful. Listed below is an outline of the six main stages in undertaking a research project. In addition to these steps it is important to set a realistic timetable and budget for the project and to give due consideration to any ethical issues that may be relevant.

- Asking a research question
- Selecting appropriate methods
- Data collection
- Data management
- Data analysis
- Presentation and dissemination of results.

Role of information technology in research

With the growing complexity of health care research, there is an increasing role for information technology to be utilised at various stages of most research projects. The potential uses of information technology in this context are summarised as follows:

1 Research design
   - bibliographic management/literature searching
   - determining sample sizes
   - randomisation
2 Data collection
   - use of existing computer databases (e.g. for medical records)
   - design of data collection forms
   - multi-centre data collection systems
   - data coding systems
   - safety checks on data accuracy
3 Data analysis
   - software packages (both for quantitative and qualitative analyses)
4 Presentation and dissemination of results
   - report preparation (including use of graphics)
   - dissemination via on-line systems

In some areas, information technology has almost revolutionised the ability of the researcher to access and summarise data. For example, the availability of bibliographic databases provides researchers with the tools to catalogue references from a variety of sources, to link these with large international on-line databases, and to search and organise these databases in an almost endless number of combinations. Tasks that previously required extensive statistical calculation, such as sample size estimates, or tedious manual manipulation, such as randomisation of subjects in a study, can now be undertaken in a few minutes with the aid of purpose written software. Furthermore, the variety of data management and statistical analysis software that is now available means that even a novice researcher can manage large data sets simply and effectively.

Some of the special purpose software packages that are available for health care research cover multiple stages of a project, such as from the design of a questionnaire, through to data entry, analysis and then writing up the final report and preparing graphics for slides. Despite the benefits that technology has brought to the mechanics of research, it is important to remember that the most crucial aspect of a research project, asking a good question, is still very much dependent on the critical faculties of the researcher.

One of the growing trends in health care research is towards large scale multi-centred studies which involve co-ordination of data collection from a number of sites. With the advent of small portable computers and the ease of networking, it is now possible to link many sites to a central data management site.

With the increased use of computerised patient record and data man-agement systems in a variety of health care settings, it is now possible to access large databases which contain a variety of patient information. If patient identifying details are removed from these databases, it is possible to use the non-identifiable patient data for research purposes. The quality of data extracted from these large computer-based record systems is frequently superior to that contained in written medical records. One such system which is based in the UK, known as VAMP, has been used to study adverse effects of various drugs, and sentinel practice monitoring of infectious diseases. The advantage of these large practice based systems is that results of research can be fed back into the system to use for clinical audit.

One of the least exploited uses of information technology in a research context has been the dissemination of research findings. However, as the pressure grows on health care providers and policy makers to make greater use of available evidence in their decision-making processes, it will be necessary to have ready access to research findings. On-line systems, such as INTERNET, and disk based methods can be used to disseminate research findings. Several electronic based research journals have recently been developed, which allow their subscribers to access on-line research outputs as they become available. There is obviously an enormous potential for research disseminated in this way also to be regularly up-dated.

Future applications of information technology in health care research

As the knowledge and technical skill with information technology systems continues to develop, the possibility for introducing innovative developments in health care research will continue to expand. The potential for developing computer aided decision support systems that use large research databases as their source of 'expert knowledge' is huge. Such systems can only help to facilitate the linking of research and health care decision making. Technical advances in storing data on Smart Cards has potential application as a method of storing information about participants in research studies. Similarly, with increased networking and linkage between a variety of different points within the health care system, it may be possible to open up new avenues of research that were previously logistically impossible.

FURTHER READING

Armstrong D et al 1990 Research methods for general practitioners. Oxford Medical Publications, Oxford
Gardner M J, Altman D G 1989 Statistics with confidence. British Medical Association, London
Geyman J (ed) 1978 Research in family practice. Appleton-Century-Crofts, New York
Howie J G R 1989 Research in general practice, 2nd edn. Chapman and Hall, London
Sackett D R, Haynes B, Tugwell P 1984 Clinical epidemiology: a basic science for clinical medicine. Little Brown, Boston
Silverman W A 1985 Human experimentation: a guided step into the unknown. Oxford University Press, New York
Swinscow T D V 1983 Statistics at square one. British Medical Association, London

29

Information technology in research

RITA AXFORD, GARY GRUNWALD, ROB HYNDMAN

Health care information exists in both paper based and computer based recorded forms. Health care information appears in formally published literature in journal articles, books, and conference papers. Other kinds of documents that help researchers access the literature include indices to and abstracts of these published documents.

Health care information also consists of important, but more difficult to access, informal literature. This includes unpublished, noncopyrighted reports, databases from other studies and surveys, and patient care protocols or facts relating to practice, education, research or management in health care.

Bibliographic and library information retrieval systems are important research tools and also exist in both paper (book) and computer form. Computer based retrieval systems may be available on-line or stored on CD-ROM or magnetic tape. They are extremely powerful tools because of their ability to be updated rapidly and accessed widely. Computer networks allow many users to access the same tools and information from a variety of geographic locations at virtually the same time. These networks may be local in nature (local area networks or LANs) or may be extensive, even world wide and include use of the Internet (see also Ch. 10).

Electronic bibliographic retrieval systems enable researchers to identify documents and the location of these publications. Some systems contain more than just the citation and allow the user to access an abstract or even the entire text of a document via their computer terminal or printer. These tools vary according to the scope and content of their databases. The most common ones contain citations to published journal articles, books and monographs. Others contain references to newspaper articles, technical reports, unpublished theses, audiovisual materials, computer software packages and other media forms.

Bibliographic databases vary in their focus. For example, citations indexed in a given database may cover a specific topic, such as gerontology, bioethics, or toxicology. The collection may be limited to a specific type of literature (e.g. journal or newspaper articles only), a specific time period (publications since 1980), or certain languages (such as English only or English, German and Russian). Similarly, databases vary in terms of their organisation. One may be able to search according to an author's name, a key word or topic of interest, titles of articles or books, citations (or references to a given writer), or other such categories.

When searching a database for a topic of interest, knowledge about the specific vocabulary used in the database is essential. Databases require the user to describe their topic using only words specified in a thesaurus of terms. For example, information relating to cancer may be located only through use of the designated term 'oncology' or 'neoplasm' depending upon the terms in the thesaurus for the database.

Searching the database is best undertaken using a methodical search strategy. This might include the following steps: (1) decide the topic; (2) check the thesaurus for the term or heading; (3) if found, check for related topics and conduct the search; (4) if not found, cross check for related terms and depending upon success at this step, either proceed, rephrase the heading, or reconsider the topic. This search strategy can be used for both paper and computerised databases. Although paper databases can also be searched in non-methodical ways by browsing through the pages, computer based searches are powerful tools because they are methodical. Users enter commands which appropriately broaden or restrict the search to identify the most relevant literature for their purpose. For example, the words 'and' and 'or' are common commands for many bibliographic databases. A command which asked the database to search for 'neoplasms or adolescents' would identify all publications in the database which relate to neoplasms and all which relate to adolescents. A command which stated 'neoplasms and adolescents' would locate only those references which referred to both terms, i.e. adolescents with neoplasms. In this case, a much more specific list of resources would be generated.

Many electronic bibliographic databases are designed to be searched by the researchers themselves. Others require the skills and experience of specialist librarians. Many times it is some combination of both that results in the best access to the research literature. One can improve ones searching skills by trial and practice. Similarly, one should not be afraid to ask for help.

Health-related electronic bibliographic databases

The following electronic bibliographic retrieval systems have been selected either because of their wide use or their unique capabilities. This is neither a comprehensive list, nor a recommendation to use only these. An introduction to some common and some unique databases will hopefully spark further inquiry.

MEDLARS (Medical Literature Analysis and Retrieval System) is one of the largest databases in the world. It is a computerised system of databases and databanks offered by the National Library of Medicine (NLM) in the United States. The NLM enters into bilateral agreements with public institutions throughout the world to serve as International MEDLARS Centres. These Centres assist health professionals to access these databases. The National Library of Australia in Canberra, ACT, is the International MEDLARS Centre for Australia. MEDLARS is a set of over 20 databases and was begun as MEDLINE in 1966 as a means of preparing the *Index Medicus*. It contains over 7 million references to the journal literature from over 3800 biomedical journals from 1966 to the present and is updated weekly. The system is searched using a unique vocabulary called MeSH (Medical Subject Headings). This consists of a hierarchical tree structure with broad categories and a large number of headings and subheadings (some 17 000). The database search provides a citation that lists author, title, publisher, key words and in approximately 65-70% of the cases also provides an abstract.

GRATEFUL MED is a software package that allows one to access MEDLARS directly from one's personal computer at any time of the day or night at very low cost. It is complemented by an electronic ordering system so that subscribers can obtain the full text of many articles. This system is called LOANSOME DOC.

CINAHL refers to the Cumulative Index to Nursing and Allied Health Literature and is another bibliographic retrieval system that provides on-line searching. This database is housed in paper form and electronically on-line, on magnetic tape, and on CD-ROM. It contains references to over 580 serial publications on nursing and allied health dating back to 1982. It also provides access to health care books, nursing dissertations, selected conference proceedings, standards of professional practice, the serial publications of the American Nurses' Association, the National League for Nursing, the Division of Nursing of the US Department of Health and Human Services and nursing associations from all 50 states in the USA. CINAHL is updated bimonthly. It can be accessed through the Internet and is also available commercially through two vendors, Silver Platter and Paperchase. As from June 1994 CINAHL includes the bibliographic citations for the references from articles in selected journals.

HealthROM is the Australian reference source on public and environmental health in electronic form for PC (DOS and Windows based) and Macintosh computers. It contains information on public health policy, HIV/AIDS, drug and alcohol use, food and nutrition, casemix, therapeutic drugs, family health, clinical and nursing practise, Aboriginal health, health economics, and sports medicine. It is produced by the Department of Human Services and Health in collaboration with the Australian Institute of Health & Welfare, the National Health and Medical Research Council (NH&MRC), the National Library of Australia, and the Alcohol and Other Drugs Council of Australia. HealthROM contains bibliographic citations plus the full text of over 100 Australian health publications plus the following journals: *Australian Prescriber*, *Communicable Diseases Intelligence*, *Australian Casemix Bulletin*, and *Health Expenditure Bulletin*.

ERIC stands for Educational Resources Information Center and is a paper-based and electronic bibliographic retrieval system developed by the US

Department of Education. It consists of two databases. One covers periodicals indexed in the *Current Index to Journals in Education* and the other, *Resources in Education*, includes other printed documents on education including complete coverage of all educational literature, including that relating to a number of health care professions. It is available through the Internet and vendors such as DIALOG and BRS.

SOCIAL SCISEARCH (Social Sciences Citation Index) is an electronic bibliographic retrieval system prepared by the Institute for Scientific Information. It consists of a database with citations to over 3700 journals in the social, behavioural, and related sciences (which include health care disciplines). In addition to the usual author, title, and source listings, SOCIAL SCISEARCH produces a list of references cited in the indexed journals. This database is also accessed via commercial vendors such as DIALOG and BRS.

The Virginia Henderson International Nursing Library is a recently developed 'electronic library' accessible through the Internet. This unique computerised collection of databases and knowledge resources incorporates the Directory of Nurse Researchers and includes biographical data about registered nurse researchers, projects funded by Sigma Theta Tau International, and the *Online Journal of Knowledge Synthesis for Nursing*.

Research data

Thorough access to the relevant literature is fundamental to identifying good research questions that build upon previous knowledge. With the widespread introduction of electronic databases into libraries, researchers now have worldwide access to the literature.

Collecting and interpreting data for new research undertakings is the second major area of the complex process of research that this chapter explores. It should be noted that many data collection tools and instruments can be located through electronic databases. Research data may be collected expressly for a given study, or they may be extracted from data housed as client data or as care protocols within currently existing clinical information systems. There are many important issues relating to IT and the conduct of research that are beyond the scope of this chapter. These include issues about organisation of data, data standards, data sets, language and taxonomies, integrity and quality of data, confidentiality and the ethical use of health data for research (see Chs 8 and 25).

The purpose of this chapter is more technical. This discussion will therefore focus on how research data are handled in order for them to assist researchers in answering their questions. This is not to detract from the importance of the other issues in health informatics referred to above.

Software for handling research data

There is a range of computer software packages designed to help researchers store, manage, analyse and interpret data. For quantitative studies, a statistics package can play an important part in determining the value and effectiveness of the study. Although they are a more recent development, computer programs for handling qualitative data likewise are proving to be valuable research tools.

Data entry

Bioinstrumentation may allow for quantitative data to be collected and entered directly onto a computer, such as with cardiac monitors and blood chemistry analysis. Quantitative data are also often collected in the form of questionnaires, surveys or in experimental log books. In these cases, getting the data from paper into a computer is a necessary step before much use of the data can be made. A popular approach is to use a spreadsheet package (see Ch. 6) for data entry. However, data may then have to be transferred to a statistics package for analysis. If this approach is followed, it is important that the statistics package is able to input data stored in the format of the spreadsheet. It is very frustrating to have data stored in one format but not accessible by other programs.

Alternatively, some statistics packages have their own spreadsheet-like interface which can be used for data entry. While this avoids the problem of transferring data between programs, it has its own problems. The spreadsheet interfaces offered by many statistics packages have limited facilities compared with full spreadsheet packages. For example, one sometimes needs to record the same value (e.g. dose of drug) many times, but some packages require the value to be entered repeatedly rather than allowing automatic repetition.

The best data entry facilities allow error checking as data are entered. For example, entering an age of four years for a married man should trigger a warning message. Most packages do not have these useful checks, however.

Qualitative research consists of data gathering strategies that generate narrative as opposed to numerical data. Qualitative data can take the form of verbatim transcripts of interviews, field notes, and reflective journal entries. Most of these activities can be greatly facilitated by data entry using electronic word processing capabilities.

Data management

Qualitative research methodologies often require concurrent data collection, entry, coding and analysis. Coding of qualitative data consists of examining the text line by line, and in some instances word by word, to abstract meanings or categories that describe situations, processes, or concepts. As more data are collected, or current data are re-examined, new categories may be identified and prior categories reconceptualised, eliminated, or subsumed within new categories. Analysis for theory development involves an additional data management activity, examining the relationships between categories. Management techniques for qualitative data are complex as they must permit categories to be examined in reference to the original text, by prior coding schemes, and by comparing and contrasting selected data clusters.

353

When managing quantitative data it is equally important to be able to access the data from a variety of vantage points. Having entered the data, it is usually necessary to make some modifications before producing graphs, tables and statistical analyses. For example, it may be useful to look at subsets of the data — only results for females or only results after a certain time. A statistics package should make such data management tasks easy.

Another common requirement is to allow more informative labelling than the stored data contains. For example, instead of treatment levels 1 and 2, one may wish to recode 1 as 'experimental drug' and 2 as 'placebo'.

Data summary

Quantitative data can be summarised in various ways. Numerical summaries usually consist of averages, medians, standard deviations and other statistics. Any statistical package should be able to produce a range of summary statistics easily for each variable of interest. Some packages will churn out dozens of largely meaningless statistics, which is not very helpful. The best packages will give a few key statistics by default and others if specifically requested.

Most statistics packages will compute cross-tabulations of categorical data. For example, one may have data from 500 people indicating their sex and blood-type. A cross-tabulation of the data would show how many people of each sex fell into each blood-type. An extension of this idea is to compute the average weight of people in each sex by blood-type combination. Many statistics packages will generate cross-tabulations with more than two categorical variables but these are harder to display. Not only should a good statistics package be able to compute such tables, but it should display the results in a format that is easy to read and understand.

Graphical summaries

An alternative method of summarising data is by the use of graphs. A statistics package should be able to produce histograms of numerical variables, scatterplots showing one numerical variable plotted against another, and so on. As with numerical summaries, it is easy to generate many graphs of limited value. A good statistics package should be able to provide highly informative graphics by default.

When exploring data and trying to uncover interesting structure, it is more important to be able to produce informative graphs quickly than very high quality graphics slowly. Some packages concentrate almost entirely on producing high quality graphics and so are obviously better suited to presenting rather than investigating or exploring data.

Data analysis and modelling

Data analysis and modelling are the areas most people think of as 'real statistics'. Producing a statistical model for a set of data is an important part of drawing conclusions from the data. Using a statistical model, one can calculate the probability that data could have arisen given a certain hypothesis. This means more objective inferences can be drawn than are possible from graphical or numerical summaries.

There is a huge range of statistical tests and models that have been used and are available in statistics packages. All statistics packages should be able to do simple tests such as t-tests (testing whether the mean of one group of data is significantly different from the mean of a second group of data). Likewise, statistical packages should be able to fit simple models such as straight line regression models (modelling one variable as a linear function of another variable).

Most packages can also do a wide range of standard but more complicated tests and models. Some packages aim to cover almost all of the methods that are widely used in applied statistics. One or two packages are designed to enable the user to develop and implement new methods.

Presentation—text, graphs, and tables

At the end of a study, it is usually necessary to present the results by giving a talk or by writing a report or research paper. Word processing is an extremely useful tool for developing text, but graphs and tables may be needed to summarise some aspects of the study more succinctly. Often these graphs are the best of those found when exploring the data in the earlier stages of the study, but tidied up by using informative headings and axis labels. Legends are often added and, if available, colour may be used.

In the past, the quality of graphics in statistics packages has varied enormously. These days, most packages make some attempt at producing graphs suitable for publication. Nevertheless, there are still packages which produce graphs which are hard to read because of clotted lettering and shading by diagonal lines.

If a statistics package does not produce sufficiently high quality graphics, it may be necessary to produce the final graphs in another specialised graphics package. In this case, it is important that the data are stored not only in a format suitable for the statistics package, but are also easily accessible by the graphics package.

If a report is to be written, it is usually desirable to be able to enter the graphs directly into the word processed document rather than sticking them in with glue later on. Therefore, it is useful if graphs can be saved in a format that the word processor can input and print.

Tables of summary statistics are often also required for presentation. Many statistics packages do not present tables in a form suitable for presentation. Often they have to be heavily edited in a word processor or simply re-typed.

Examples of statistics packages

There is a huge range of programs that can make some claim to being statistics packages. In order to illustrate the wide range of packages available, brief descriptions of several types of computer packages that do some degree of statistical analysis are presented in this section. An indication of their usefulness to professional statisticians has been made in order to benchmark the use of these tools. Examples of each type are given, but inclusion (or exclusion) is not meant to be a recommendation (or otherwise) of the package, though packages mentioned are among the standards of that type.

Spreadsheets

Many spreadsheet packages include some statistical and/or graphical functions. The range of functions available is usually quite limited, but it is increasing with newer versions so that the line between interactive statistics packages and spreadsheets is becoming less defined. Often spreadsheets do not provide the tools needed for exploratory analysis or checking model assumptions, but rather function as statistical calculators. A working statistician would not get far with these packages, but someone interested in a whole range of spreadsheet operations, presentation graphs and tables, and a bit of statistical analysis, all easily interfacing with other packages, could find them quite useful. Examples: Excel, Lotus 1-2-3.

Interactive statistics packages

These packages have a simple structure, with data stored and entered in spreadsheet format. They are easy to learn and use and are good for many kinds of standard data analyses and graphs. They contain many standard statistical methods as built-in functions. Professional statisticians doing general consulting could perhaps do somewhat more than half of their work with one of these packages. Some packages allow some customisation and programming, but users familiar with computer programming may find these interactive packages somewhat tedious in this regard. Because of simplicity, general applicability, and fairly low cost, these packages are very popular in a variety of settings, including teaching. Examples: JMP, Minitab, Stat–graphics, Systat.

Large statistics packages

These large scale packages were originally written for mainframe computers, though now some PCs run them. They do a very wide variety of analyses and do them fast. They can handle very large data sets (millions of cases), which would cause havoc with most other packages. They allow some level of programming and customised analysis, and have good graphics, particularly for presentation purposes. They tend to be less interactive and flexible than some of the other packages discussed here, and can be tedious for those used to working with more interactive packages or languages. Examples: BMDP, SAS, SPSS.

Statistical programming languages

These are interactive programming languages designed especially for statistical applications. They allow extreme flexibility in data handling and application of statistical methods to data. They contain many built-in standard statistical functions, including very modern methods, and also have a language that allows virtually any kind of calculation to be done. Users can write specialty programs to perform the desired analyses, using the built-in functions as building blocks. These languages are most useful to experienced statisticians who are developing new statistical methods, applying existing methods in new or non-standard ways, or customising existing methods to new situations. All of this flexibility and power has its advantages, but these languages are not for the novice. They require good computer skills and a high level of statistical knowledge. Even the simplest analyses require a large initial investment in learning the basics of the language. Example: S-Plus.

Specialty quantitative data analysis packages

Sometimes packages are written to do a certain type of analysis, rather than a full range of statistical analyses. These packages often include analyses not available in other packages. These are not generally substitutes for statistics packages but can be indispensable to those who need the particular analyses. Some of these analyses are now available in the large statistics packages or in S-Plus. Here are a few examples.

EGRET (Epidemiological GRaphics, Estimation and Testing) performs analyses common in epidemiology and other medical research areas. For instance, logistic and Poisson regression and variations of them, exact contingency table analysis, and survival analysis are available.

GLIM (Generalized Linear Interactive Modelling) is an interactive package for fitting Generalized Linear Models. These models are very commonly used in social sciences and medical research, and require a fairly high level of statistical knowledge.

TIME SERIES: There are various packages such as ITSM, Forecast Pro and TSP specifically designed for the analysis of time series data.

Qualitative data analysis packages

Qualitative research is not a single methodology, but includes a range of methodologies grounded in the humanities and social sciences such as sociology and anthropology. The range of methods includes ethnography, content analysis, and grounded theory construction. Qualitative data management and analysis software packages are a recent development and those available are designed to suit the specific methodology employed. The Ethnograph was developed in the late 1980s and is particularly suited to ethnographic methods as the name implies. NUDIST (Non-numerical Unstructured Data Indexing, Searching and Theorizing) is a qualitative data analysis system developed in the early 1990s. It was developed to support a range of methods for the analysis of unstructured data, with emphasis on the building and testing of grounded theory. HyperQual2 is an Apple Macintosh program which incorporates the features of a common Macintosh program called HyperCard. It is designed to store, manipulate and present data in the form of written reports. It frees the mind of the researcher as much as possible from the mechanics of qualitative data analysis so that the analyst can concentrate on the conceptual aspect of data analysis (Padilla 1993).

Choosing a statistics package

Since there is such a bewildering number of different packages to choose from for statistics and data analysis, many researchers have difficulty in selecting an appropriate package for their needs. The questions below may be useful to keep in mind when selecting a statistics package.

A good resource for finding out about various packages is the Statistical Software Guide, which is planned to be an annual feature in the journal *Computational Statistics and Data Analysis*. In the 1992-93 guide (Koch & Haag 1993), 80 packages were summarised with brief descriptions obtained from vendors. Note, however, that several major packages were not included in this list.

Does the package do what you want?

Many people purchase software before carefully evaluating exactly what their needs are. It is important to consider the data analysis facilities one will require and then purchase a package which provides at least those facilities. If the research requires the fit of a sophisticated logistic regression model, it is unlikely that a spreadsheet will suit this requirement. On the other hand, if one is using a statistics package only for producing graphs, it is unnecessary to spend large sums of money and time learning a high-powered statistics package such as SAS or S-Plus. Likewise for qualitative research, if counting the frequencies of certain words and word groupings is what is required, word processing may fulfill this function. If theorising is planned, more sophisticated qualitative research software should be sought.

What platforms is the package available on?

If one is a dedicated Macintosh user, it is unlikely a PC-based package will suit. Even if one has access to a variety of computing environments, it may be necessary to transfer graphics or data from the statistics package to a word processor or some other package. It is easier and more efficient if all commonly used software tools are available on the same computer platform.

Do you require customised statistical analyses?

If there are a number of packages which do what is needed on the computer available, the choice between packages often comes down to one's own requirements about user friendliness and flexibility. Some packages are very easy to use but are relatively inflexible—they provide standard statistical analyses quickly but do not allow the user to modify the methods used or implement new methods easily. Other packages are extremely powerful and flexible but are more time consuming to learn and to use. Ease of use and flexibility are not necessarily incompatible characteristics, but to some extent, greater flexibility in the possible analyses available tends to make a package more difficult to use.

Do you require interactive or repetitive data analysis?

Some packages are best suited to interactive, exploratory data analysis, while others are designed for more repetitive tasks. If the analysis involves the same operation applied to many different data sets, then a menu-driven package designed for interactive use may be tedious. A more appropriate package would enable a short program to be written to carry out these analyses. Some packages attempt to allow for both styles of data analysis by providing a choice between a menu-driven interface and a command-driven interface with some simple programming functions.

Do you have very large data sets?

Many statistical packages will be unable to cope adequately with very large data sets. With more than 100 000 observations, most small or medium size statistical packages will struggle. Be wary of advertised claims that a package can cope with very large data sets. These claims are sometimes based on the assumption that they will be run on an extremely powerful computer. This is often not the case. To analyse large data sets adequately it is usually necessary to use a large scale statistical package such as SAS, SPSS or BMDP on a high powered computer.

Is there any local support?

Having someone nearby to help is invaluable. Such a person may be a fellow user in the same organisation, a member of a local users' group, or a contributer to an Internet news group. Similarly, good documentation is essential. Most programs are now accompanied by understandable user manuals and classes are run for many of the quantitative and qualitative packages available on the market.

General comments on using computer data analysis software packages

The wide availability of inexpensive, easy to use packages makes sophisticated analyses available to nearly everyone. The following comments relate to how best to use packages as well as some common sense suggestions that reflect many years experience consulting on research projects and analysing a variety of kinds of data.

The research methodology one uses will play a large part in identifying groups of data analysis packages best suited to ones needs. Within these groups, often, familiarity is what makes for the 'best' software package. While choice is more restricted among packages which support specific qualitative research methodologies, most major statistics packages do most standard things. Rather than constantly pursuing the 'best' packages and switching whenever a new one appears to offer some new advantages, a better strategy is to select a good package (or possibly a combination of two complementary packages) and become familiar with it. One will then be able to use the package more efficiently and will feel more confident with the analyses.

A picture is worth a thousand words. In quantitative data analysis, good graphs are essential in finding interesting patterns, checking assumptions, and understanding how analyses relate to the variables and raw data. For presentation in papers or talks, a few good graphs can summarise the results of a study clearly and concisely. As discussed above, most packages have features for making these graphs. Expect to spend time at this. It is often challenging to think of a good way to present results in graphical form, and many attempts will end up in the rubbish. Once a good graph is decided on it is often just as challenging to get the package to make the graph exactly as desired and to place it automatically in a document.

The advantages of having access to good, easy to use packages are clear; one can now perform a great many statistical analyses, and do them very quickly. But with this power come potential disadvantages; one can now make a great many mistakes, and make them very quickly. It is wise to learn the packages one uses and the analyses one chooses well enough to be able to cross-check results of more difficult or unfamiliar analyses with simple data summaries or graphs. It's best to make sure all results make sense when considered from various angles.

A common misconception is that all statistical packages give the same answers. Unfortunately, mistakes have been made, even in some very well known and widely used packages. It is a good idea to check output from the package against published results or output from an equivalent analysis in a competing package.

Some errors result from numerical inaccuracy, particularly when very large or very small numbers are involved (Sawitzki 1994). This is a particular problem with most spreadsheets. Other errors result from statistical misunderstandings (programmers are usually not statisticians) or from programming bugs.

Don't hesitate to ask for help from an appropriate consultant. Computer packages can answer many questions but are no substitute for expertise and experience. Just as most statisticians are not expert health care practitioners, neither are most health care researchers experts in statistics. Qualitative data analysis is likewise vulnerable to inappropriate analyses. Successful researchers plan and budget for the cost of a good statistical or qualitative research consultant and value this commodity.

Finally, think. No computer package can substitute for careful thinking about the limitations of various research designs, the meaning of variables, possible problems with the data, expected or hoped for patterns, and other such issues. The best data analysis comes not from keystrokes and printouts, but from spending time thinking.

REFERENCES

Koch A, Haag U 1993 Statistical software guide '92/93. Computational Statistics and Data Analysis 5:241-266

Padilla R V 1993 Qualitative analysis with HyperQual2. Chandler, Arizona

Sawitzki G 1994 Report on the numerical reliability of data analysis systems. Computational Statistics and Data Analysis 5:289-301

FURTHER READING

Baker C A 1988 Computer applications in qualitative research. Computers in Nursing 6(5):211-214

Bryant J, Ryder R 1993 Grateful Med (Version 6.0) Training Workbook. Outreach Kentucky Project, Medical Centre Library, University of Kentucky, Lexington, Kentucky

CINAHL Information Systems 1993 Glendale, California

HealthROM information brochure, Department of Human Services and Health

Hudgings C 1992 The Virginia Henderson International Nursing Library: Improving access to nursing research databases. In: Arnold J M, Pearson G A (eds) Computer applications in nursing education and practice. National League for Nursing Publication no. 14-2406

National Institutes of Health, National Library of Medicine 1993 Factsheet. Bethesda, Maryland

Norman E M 1989 Applications: how to use word processing software to conduct content analysis. Computers in Nursing 7(3):127-128

Richards T, Richards L 1991 The NUDIST Qualitative data analysis system. Qualitative Sociology 14(4):307-324

Saba V K, Oatway D M, Rieder K A 1989 How to use nursing information sources. Nursing Outlook. July/August 37(4):189-195

Tesch R 1990 Qualitative research: analysis types and software tools. The Falmer Press, New York

30

Research, public health and policy development

DAVID RANSON

The avenues for research in medicine are almost unlimited. There is little doubt that information technology has made a major impact in the research carried out in many of the medical discipline areas. The field of public health and the related area of health policy formation has benefited very greatly from the rapid developments that have been made in the area of health informatics. Indeed medical epidemiology as a specialist area probably could not have developed the way it has in recent years were it not for the rapid advancements made in the field of medical informatics at a technical and organisational level. It must be remembered, however, that advances in technology and information theory do not of themselves lead to changes to medical research or practice. It is the acceptance by medical professionals of such new technology and the integration of new information handling practices into medical research and practice that has resulted in the advances we have seen in the fields of public health, medical epidemiology and health policy development (Paul-Shaheen 1989).

It could not be said that developments in information technology have been the underlying stimulus for the development of new directions in health policy. Whilst the field of public health and health policy formation is highly reliant upon information technology much of the drive to advance these areas has come from the changing economic structure of health care. The economic pressures now placed on health care resources allocation and national and international health care budgets have been considerable. The upward spiral of health care costs seems inevitable. This appears to have prompted an almost frantic drive towards rationalisation of health resources which in turn has stimulated many of the advances in information systems related to health care (Davis 1993).

The insatiable demand for health care information on the part of policy makers now faced with the economic reality of rising health care costs and effective reductions in health care budgets has artificially stimulated the field of health informatics. In layman's terms this scenario might be described as the field of health informatics having had a sudden rush of blood to the head. The explosion of ideas, network information systems, hardware and software platforms that resulted was both productive and destructive. Productive in that new information systems were appearing almost every week but destructive in that attempts to develop health informatic standards came too late. In many cases by the time the standards were published the health information field had moved ahead and developed in a way that made the new standards obsolete. Hopefully we are beginning to achieve a level of integration between the emerging standards and the technology itself. Indeed as the field of health informatics begins to spread into non medical areas and to integrate with other governmental, social and community based information systems the need for standards to facilitate data interchange has reached a high priority. Indeed health informatics providers at a technical information services level are now working with standards groups in a way that has not been seen before.

Medical health care providers have in the past been largely immune to the issues of cost efficiency at commercial level. Health care standards were set by professional medical bodies with little or no interest in the economic consequences of the health care policies. In the last ten years this attitude amongst health care professionals has almost completely died out. It is now clear to all that resources are limited and that economic factors will have an increasing role in shaping global and individual health care practices. Like it or not, health care providers are having to accept the fact that health policy is being determined by individuals from the fields of business and economics whose attitudes to health care outcomes, resource allocation and medical effectiveness may be very different to that traditionally found in health care professionals (Feinglass & Warren-Salmon 1990). The health power equilibrium has changed. If health care workers are to continue to play a part in health policy development they need to be empowered with the information and the skills in data analysis in order for their voices to be heard amongst national and international policy makers. The development of health informatics as a specialty for health care professionals is at last providing them with a new role as stake holders in health care planning.

Communication and data processing

When considering some of the technologies involved in health informatics it is important to recognise the distinction between information networks (communication) and the technologies involved in data processing. Health informatics in its broadest sense involves a very wide range of information technology including data processing, communication, networking and telecommunication. Indeed today telemedicine is one of the new emerging fields of health informatics and one which has the capacity to significantly alter the delivery of health care, particularly in rural areas and communities that are geographically isolated. A recent study (Schneider et al 1992) predicted that in the US 28 billion dollars could be saved in health care costs through the efficient use of telecommunications in the movement of patient man-agement information. This study also identified that health care administrative costs could be reduced by 6.8 billion dollars through the use of modern electronic communications and data processing technology.

Recognition of the importance of electronic communications and the value of networking has resulted in a number of initiatives around the world. In Australia the development of the Health Communications Network is a sign of the significance that is placed on networking by health care policy makers. Medical information networks today comprise systems with advanced developments of central hubs and main data trunk lines. Many of the major medical and health care institutions are already connected electronically and developments in the links between these central sites will in the next few years lead to advances in the complexity and quality of the electronic data that can be communicated. Four major problems remain to be solved however before telemedicine and the widespread use of health care information networks becomes practical reality.

The first of these is the education and training needs of health care professionals. A large commitment to training is required by health care institutions before these modern technologies become truly effective in the work place.

The second major problem to be overcome is that whilst the major institutions are well networked electronically the vast bulk of primary health care providers and indeed their clients are as remote from health care information and communication systems as they were ten years ago. This 'last mile of wire' is almost certainly the most important mile as far as electronic communication and networking in health care is concerned (Blau 1993). The third major problem to be overcome relates to communication standards and electronic data interchange standards in health informatics. As commented before, it is essential that technology and standards develop in concert and until such a balance is achieved the absence of implemented international standards will remain a significant impediment to the establishment of world-wide health care related communications.

The final problem in health communications that has the capacity to significantly impair the development of research and health care policy is the community and social attitudes to telemedicine and health care networking. In particular issues in relation to medical ethics and the law with respect to privacy and confidentiality must be addressed. It must be said that medical ethicists and the legal professional have been slow to come to grips with modern information technology and the implication that it has for their discipline. Again it is essential that these areas are integrated with the development of health communications networks for such systems to be accepted by the community at large. For the field of health informatics to make any major impact on public health and policy development these issues relating to networking and electronic communication must be resolved.

For whom the bell tolls

The ability of policy makers to formulate health policy is intricately bound to the health care information service which provides them with the data they need. It has to be remembered, however, that the source of such health data ultimately comes from the grass roots level of health care. As we have already noted this is the very area which is least developed and prepared with regard to information systems. Despite this, health care workers in the field recognise the importance of information for health care planning. Whilst the task of data collection is onerous, there is now an increased understanding of the need for information in order that health services might be improved.

Where health interacts with non-health related agencies recognition of the importance of interchange of core information is less well recognised. This network disconnection can be seen particularly in the area of mortality data and death investigation. In many cases the individuals with access to this information do not come primarily from the health care field but instead from the legal and administrative organs of government. For health care planning to be truly effective health policy makers must be informed and provided with data from both the health care community and the associated legal and administrative services that impact upon health.

The legal profession and the medical profession have at their roots a work practice that is related to the individual handling of cases so that work is carried out on a case by case basis dealing with each case as an isolated event. For many years, however, the medical profession in particular has reaped the benefits, in terms of research into the understanding of disease and health care planning, of the analysis of groups of cases that show similar features. Not only do such group analyses lead to increased understanding of disease processes, therapeutics and health care but they increase the efficiency in which medical professionals can undertake their work. Such analysis of groups or collections of like cases is rare within legal systems including death investigation systems such as coroners or medical examiner systems. Yet if we are to learn from those defects in society that result in death and injury we need to be continually reminded of the risks and dangers in the community. Similarly those who have the responsibility and power to make our society safer including health care policy makers need to be reminded and continually charged with that duty and alerted to the information that is available from the organisational areas outside health care.

The development of health care policy and health care plans for prevention of disease and injury remains at the forefront of public health. Many of the initiatives and directions taken to improve health and safety fall within the framework of community education. There are many clinicians, pathologists, epidemiologists and indeed lawyers who see this educational and preventative role as one of the most important goals of any health care information system. The reality, however, is that at the grass roots level those charged with the social investigation of death and injury are not integrated with the health care information system. If each injury and death is to play a part in moulding and shaping public health policy leading to a healthier and safer community the information revealed by such tragedies has to be communicated and analysed by policy makers. The absence of such data communication makes us all vulnerable. As Donne said 'Ask not for whom the bell tolls, it tolls for thee'.

Disaster and diffuse disaster

In examining the ways in which health informatics resources can contribute to public health and policy development it is useful to consider the notion of diffuse disaster. In a mass disaster the entire society including its medical, political and administrative officials is alerted. This in turn stimulates sympathy, concern and practical action in the form of response activities designed to deal with the injured, the loss of life and destruction of community and property. Inevitably in the case of mass disasters there is a post disaster investigation process that examines the cause and the response to the disaster. In addition detailed investigations are directed to determine processes and mechanisms to prevent the hazardous situation occurring again. Essentially it is the manner in which the extent of the disaster is communicated to the public and the response agencies that determines the nature of the eventual investigation and preventative processes.

The diffuse disaster is very different. Deaths, injury and disease are with us every day. They form part of our unconscious acceptance of life in our community. Not all of us will experience deaths or severe injury, not all of us are informed of death or serious injury, not all of us are aware of the suffering deaths or injuries cause but nonetheless such morbidity and mortality is present throughout our community. It is the wide temporal and geographical distribution of these events that prevents them being perceived by the community as a disaster. Yet if one was to view the incidence and prevalence of such morbidity and mortality with the temporal and geographical factors removed they would indeed form a true mass disaster. For example, if one-tenth of the murders in Australia were to occur at a single place at a single point in time from the actions of a single person there would be a national outcry yet murders and other forms of violence and non accidental injuries occur throughout our community all year round. As a result of this failure to identify the collective nature of such diffuse disasters, their investigation is impeded and their significance is lost on the community. As a result the drive from the community for action in relation to the prevention of such deaths or injuries never occurs.

The above issue is easy to comprehend when one examines death, non-accidental and accidental injury. However, the concept of the diffuse disaster can also be found in the area in natural disease. The concept of the diffuse epidemic is well recognised and much medical research today involves the identification of similar or like cases of disease. Such pattern based disease analysis forms one of the cornerstones of medical epidemiology. However, our ability to identify patterns and trends in disease in the community is strictly limited by the quality and quantity of the data that are obtained and analysed.

367

A disease process may be so rare that only a single case occurs in the world each year. Yet if we have one hundred years' worth of data a pattern and trend might be identifiable. The information gained on the diseases aetiology and pathogenesis might have implications for a number of co-related disease processes whose origin continues to remain obscure.

Examples

Infectious disease

Possibly the best example of the way in which health information has influenced research, public health and health policy development can be seen in relation to communicable diseases. Indeed the very foundations of medical epidemiology come from research that led to an understanding of the infectious nature and pathogenesis of communicable diseases. The outstanding success of organisations such as the Center for Diseases Control in Atlanta and the various Departments of Epidemiology, Community Medicine and Social and Preventative Medicine worldwide have established the place of medical epidemiology and statistics in medical science. Information gathering and data processing has certainly been one of the major tools employed in these disciplines. In recent years the rapid expansion in health informatics together with network and communications services has led to a transformation in communicable disease surveillance including the identification of infectious hazards. In 1984 an information system was established in France to provide for national surveillance of communicable diseases (Garnerin & Valleron 1992). This information system allowed both data entry and information retrieval as well as interpersonal communications. The backbone of the system was a relational database and a telephone dial-up network to a Videotext server provided the access to the system. This network was established by the National Department of Health and the National Institute of Health and Medical Research in France and was based on the belief that

> improving the quality, adequacy and rapidity of response of public health systems depends mainly on the ability to refine the processes implemented to collect, analyse and distribute needed information and reinforce interpersonal communication between different partners.

It should not be thought that the use of information and communication networks solves all problems with regard to the notification of infectious diseases. Studies from the Center for Diseases Control in Atlanta have demonstrated (Birkhead et al 1991) that delays occur even when data is reported via the National Electronic Telecommunications Systems Surveillance in the US. These delays were recognised to occur across a very wide geographical area and reinforces the difficulty for health care planning when there is little standardisation between the organisations that provide the basic data. It is clear that the difficulties in timeliness of data on national electronic networks does not relate to the complexity of the technology employed nor to the network structure. Instead the major difficulties are experienced at the grass roots level with the data providers. Education of staff and standardisation of human organisational procedures involved in the provision of primary data sources is an essential step to take in ensuring the success of these national networks.

Quality assurance

Current economic models of health care delivery are looking more and more towards output measurement for identifying successful health programs and efficient health care services. Quality assurance and control are two essential elements in ensuring that health care provision is both effective as well as efficient. Whilst quality assurance systems can be found at all levels within the health care system they are most clearly identifiable within a hospital and laboratory environment.

Hospital information systems have in the past tended to concentrate upon the areas of financial management and patient administration. In recent years, however, there has been increased recognition that hospital based information systems have a role to play in health care quality assurance (Selbmann & Pietch-Breitfeld 1990). An important factor in these quality assurance systems is that if data are collected from the global health environment of a hospital it is possible to identify not only quality levels of individual items of health service but also information relating to total patient outcome. This while highly desirable in an economic and health policy sense carries with it a number of potential dangers if such global data taken alone is used to influence individual patient based health care practice.

An example of this issue can be seen in the situation that arose in the Ford Pinto case. Here a situation arose in relation to vehicle manufacture. The company identified that a minor increase in the cost of the vehicle would have led to increased safety for the occupants. While this would add a very small amount to the cost of each car it amounted to a substantial overall sum for the manufacturer. An individual purchaser of a car may have been prepared to pay the small increased cost of the modification had they known of the risks of not having the modification to the vehicle. The manufacturer would not have seen this small purchase cost factor as they saw the cost in terms of the millions of dollars of additional manufacturing costs. In the final event, however, the manufacturer when looking at global costs decided not to proceed with the modification. Subsequently successful legal action was taken against the manufacturer by injured parties demonstrating the danger of taking this global cost saving approach.

Quality assurance issues in medical informatics also overlaps with the field of infectious diseases particularly in the area of infection control and antibiotic therapy (Scott Evans & Pestontnik 1994). Health informatics systems have much to offer in the area of monitoring of adverse drug reactions within hospital audit systems, patient outcome measures and planning of new or reviewed health care systems.

369

Assessing the quality of health care is now a mandatory task in almost all major health systems. The financial limitations placed on the growth of the health care industry in modern times make the need for information, that can be used for health care planning, all the more intense.

Death investigation

Death investigation takes place at many levels. Death investigation processes can be seen at their simplest level in the case where a medical practitioner assesses the death of their patient and signs a death certificate. In a hospital setting this same process can occur but with the added facet of a hospital autopsy and/or a clinicopathological audit process. Where formal investigations are performed it is the coroner's or medical examiner's systems that bear the brunt of detailed death investigation.

The legal process of such investigation processes, albeit carried out by medical practitioners, has in the past resulted in cases being investigated on a case by case basis with little concern given to the patterns of injury that might be identified by a systematic analytical approach to death investigation. The analysis of collections of like cases is rare within coroners' systems and yet if we are to learn from those defects in society that result in death we need to be continually reminded of the risks and dangers around us. On a random case by case basis this is extremely difficult for a coroner's system to identify potentially significant fatal hazards in our society and yet at the same time coroners and their supporting investigatory medical agencies are in a position of having access to a wide body of information relating to such groups of death. It is of particular interest that the coroners' and medical examiners' systems have within them the means to make public the issues and factors that have contributed to the death. While several countries today are attempting to collate and analyse national data from death investigation systems there is no coherent system available anywhere in the world.

Coronial systems were originally created to gain wealth for the Crown. Despite this their potential use as agents for the identification of preventable hazards in society has been long recognised. In 1907 William Brend wrote that:

> the value of the (Coroners) statistics is diminished by the absence of coordination...hence we have the anomaly that while a full enquiry is conducted into deaths from violent and unnatural causes, practically no subsequent use is made of the information for public health purposes.

In 1915 the same author wrote: 'if prevention of death is not now regarded as the main purpose to be served by inquest, the inquiry becomes of relatively little value' (Brend 1915).

In Australia today the role of the Coroner in the prevention of deaths is well recognised and medical informatics including data analysis, networking and communication systems is playing an increasing part in bringing together death and injury data for the benefit of the community.

The National Injury Surveillance Unit is actively pursuing information system networking to allow investigatory agencies to analyse group death and injury data. National databases are becoming established with regard to particular health problems and Australia has the world's only national sudden infant death database which is available to researchers in the fields of medical epidemiology and basic medical science.

In 1991 the Australian Royal Commission into Aboriginal Deaths in Custody (1991) stated that:

> moreover, in human terms, thoroughly conducted coronial enquiries hold the potential to identify systemic failures in custodial practices and procedures which may, if acted on, prevent future deaths in similar circumstances. In the final analysis adequate post-death investigations have the potential to save lives.

The construction of a national coroners' database is now underway in Australia. Recent case studies in Victoria have demonstrated the success of such an approach. In the three year period between 1987 and 1990, 20 fork lift related deaths occurred in Victoria. These deaths represented a significant increase over the 22 such deaths that had occurred in the previous ten years. Group analysis of these cases by the coronial systems led to identification of a number of risk factors resulting in these fatalities. Fork lift operation and design factors associated with fatal hazards were identified and a number of recommendations were made. The implementation of these recommendations have resulted in a significant reduction in such fatalities (Coroners Case 1990).

Analysis of deaths related to Methadone overdosage in 1989 in Victoria revealed a sudden and unexpected increase in fatalities amongst intravenous drug addicts who had just commenced a Methadone maintenance program. As a result of the identification of these, recommendations were made regarding the assessment of drug dependent persons admitted to the program. Medical education and training regarding drug addiction treatment programs was increased and deaths from Methadone toxicity were substantially reduced (Drummer et al 1992).

The difficulties of data collection and analysis in the area of death investigation are considerable. Countries with national death investigation systems are at a considerable advantage in having a uniform and consistent data source. The reality, however, is that legal death investigation systems are most commonly based on local jurisdictions which operate independently from each other. In the US there are over 2000 separate death investigation jurisdictions, each operating essentially independently of the other. Such a situation makes the task of integrating information systems almost in–surmountable. The Center for Diseases Control in Atlanta has been working with the national association of medical examiners to resolve this problem. Today their stated goals are:

- to obtain more timely, accurate and complete information on sudden unexpected deaths
- to better understand the causes of those deaths

- to reduce the mortality from those causes that are amenable to public health intervention (AJFMP 1989).

Death investigation is of course only a part of the picture. Injury analysis is receiving the same attention from public health practitioners and medical epidemiologists. The National Injury Surveillance Systems are beginning to address these issues. The cost of injury to our society has been grossly undervalued in previous years and injury control and prevention is only now becoming part of national health policy.

Organisation theory and health care

The organisation of health care systems has undergone a paradigm shift in recent years. Fiscal restraint, increasing commercialisation of health care, community pressures and re-evaluation of health goals has led to a much changed environment. In many ways, changes in health care provision have followed the changes that have occurred in the world of business and commerce.

> The war of business has shifted onto a new battleground. In the 1960s marketing was the watchword to achieving competitive advantage. In the 1970s manufacturing became the hot topic and in the 1980s quality. Now competition has arrived at the fourth battlefield customer service (Davidow & Ittal 1990).

The shift towards client services and client satisfaction as a marker for the success of health care systems represents a fundamental change in the way health care is delivered. The classic centralised systems of state based health care where policy decisions percolate down to the periphery of the health care system, are being replaced by regionalised systems where much health policy is made at a local level in response to the stated needs of communities. This devolution of policy and control represents an enormous challenge for health informatics systems in the next decade. Indeed it could be argued that for such a diffusion of health policy and power to be successful, health information systems will have to play a major part in providing the glue that holds these regional health care systems together. Current analysis of modern information technology itself recognises the way in which informatics systems are becoming a crucial component of modern organisational structures.

There are major strategic developments in IT itself which are now maturing to the point of practical commercial application. Of key importance are:

- office systems and applications for the workplace
- communication technologies which provide open networks and value added network services
- information management techniques including imaging, hypertext and object orientated paradigms which enable the electronic capture and use of unstructured records and soft information, and also a richer interpretation of knowledge

- growing maturity in the management of IT with the recognition that this function should be managed in the same way as for other parts of the business. This includes the need to manage IT expenditures as investments with the assets generated being managed as are other assets, including the concept of return on investment and life cycle maintenance (Lovell & Olson 1991).

Many of the old views of information technology including those originally applied in the area of health informatics are being eroded. Today we do not see health informatics simply in terms of databases to be used for research, hospital administration, patient record systems or appointment systems. The availability of new technologies for the electronic communication of images and the analysis of textual and relational information have radically changed the way in which health informatics can take part in the formulation of health policy and contribute to medical research and public health.

REFERENCES

AJFMP 1989 American Journal of Forensic Medicine and Pathology 10(1):88
Birkhead G, Chorba T L, Root S et al 1991 Timeliness of national reporting of communicable diseases: the experience of a national electronic telecommunications system for surveillance. American Journal of Public Health 81(10):1313-1315
Blau A 1993 Bringing the promise home: policy options and strategies to promote medical information networking. Journal of Medical Systems 17(6)
Brend W A 1907 Bills of mortality 5. Trans. Med-Legal Society
Brend W.A 1915 Enquiry into the statistics of deaths from violence and unnatural causes in the United Kingdom. A thesis approved for the degree of Doctorate of Medicine in State Medicine at the University of London, Charles Griffin
Coroners Case No. 2272/89, heard May 1990
Davidow W H, Ittal B 1990 Total customer service: the ultimate weapon. Harper Perennial, New York
Davis K 1993 Health care reform in the United States. The contribution of health services research to the debate. Annals of the New York Academy of Science, December 31, 703:287-90
Drummer O H, Opeskin K, Syrjanen M et al 1992 American Journal of Forensic Medicine and Pathology 13(4):346-50
Feinglass J, Warren-Salmon J 1990 Corporatisation of medicine: the use of medical management information systems to increase the clinical productivity of physicians. International Journal of Health Services 20(2):233-252
Garnerin P, Valleron A 1992 The French communicable diseases computer network: a technical view. Comput. Biol. Med. 22(3):89-200
Lovell M, Olson M 1991 IT Planning for the nineties: designing new organizations. Computer Control Quarterly 2:10-15
Paul-Shaheen P A 1989 Overlooked connections: policy development and implementation in state local relations. International Journal of Health Services, 19(3)
Royal Commission into Aboriginal Deaths in Custody—National Report. Vol. 1, Para. 4.7.4, April 1991
Schneider M K, Mann N, Schiller A 1992 Can telecommunications help solve America's health care problems? Arthur D. Little, Boston

Scott Evans R, Pestontnik S L 1994 Applications of medical informatics in antibiotic therapy. In: Poupard J A et al (eds) Antimicrobial susceptibility testing. Plenum Press, New York

Selbmann H, Pietsch-Breitfeld P 1990 Hospital information systems and quality assurance. Quality assurance in health care 2(3-4):335-344